POSTTHERAPEUTIC NEURODIAGNOSTIC IMAGING

POSTTHERAPEUTIC NEURODIAGNOSTIC IMAGING

Editor

J. Randy Jinkins, M.D.
Director of Neuroradiology
University of Texas Health Science Center at San Antonio
San Antonio, Texas

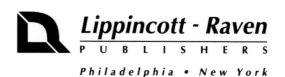

Lippincott - Raven
P U B L I S H E R S

Philadelphia • New York

To Carol

Acquisitions Editor: Jim Ryan
Developmental Editor: Brian Brown
Manufacturing Manager: Dennis Teston
Production Manager: Larry Bernstein
Production Editor: Nicholas Radhuber
Cover Designer: Diana Andrews
Indexer: Jayne Percy
Compositor: Tapsco Inc.
Printer: Courier-Westford

Printed in the United States of America

9 8 7 6 5 4 3 2 1

Library of Congress Cataloging-in-Publication Data

Posttherapeutic neurodiagnostic imaging/edited by J. Randy Jinkins.
    p. cm.
    Includes bibliographical references and index.
    ISBN 0-397-58406-7
    1. Central nervous system—Imaging. 2. Head—Imaging. 3. Neck—Imaging. 4. Central nervous system—Diseases—Treatment—Complications—Diagnosis. I. Jinkins, J. Randy.
    [DNLM: 1. Central Nervous System Diseases—diagnosis. 2. Diagnostic Imaging—methods. 3. Central Nervous System Diseases—therapy. WL 141 P858 1996]
RC349.D52P67 1996
616.8′04754—dc20
DNLM/DLC
for Library of Congress   96-42057
                                                    CIP

Contents

Contributors

Darryl J. Ainbinder, M.D. *Chief of Ophthalmic Oncology, Ophthalmic Pathology, Staff Surgeons Oculoplastics, Department of Ophthamology, Madigan Army Medical Center, Fort Lewis, Washington 98431-5000*

Carlos Bazan III, M.D. *Associate Professor of Radiology, Department of Radiology, University of Texas Health Science Center at San Antonio, 7703 Floyd Curl Drive, San Antonio, Texas 78284-7800*

Carl V. Bundschuh, M.D. *Associate Professor of Radiology, Department of Diagnostic Radiology, Norfolk General Hospital, 600 Gresham Drive, Norfolk, Virginia 23507*

Mauricio Castillo, M.D. *Associate Professor and Chief of Neuroradiology, Department of Radiology, University of North Carolina, School of Medicine, Campus Box 7510, Chapel Hill, North Carolina 27599-7510*

Barrett G. Haik, M.D. *Chair and Hamilton Professor, 956 Court, Suite D228, Department of Ophthalmology, University of Tennessee, Memphis, Tennessee 38163*

Stig Holtås, M.D. *Professor, Department of Radiology, University Hospital, S-221 85 Lund, Sweden*

Ava Huchun, M.D. *Department of Ophthalmology, Walter Reed Army Medical Center, Washington, D.C. 20306*

J. Randy Jinkins, M.D. *Director of Neuroradiology, Department of Radiology, University of Texas Health Science Center at San Antonio, 7703 F. Curl Drive, San Antonio, Texas 78284-7800*

Denis Laurent Kaech, M.D. *Doctor of Medicine, Leitender Arzt, Neurochirurgische Abteilung, Kantonsspital, Loestrasse 170, CH-7000 Chur, Switzerland*

Claudia da Costa Leite, M.D. *Medical Doctor, Neurology Fellow, Department of Radiology, University of Texas Health Sciences Center at San Antonio, 7703 F. Curl Drive, San Antonio, Texas 78284-7800*

Mahmood F. Mafee, M.D. *Professor of Radiology; Director MRI Center; Chief, Radiology, Eye and Ear Infirmary, Department of Radiology, The University of Illinois Hospital, MRI Center, M/C, 830 S. Wood Street, Chicago, Illinois 60612*

LTC Robert A. Mazzoli, M.D. *Clinical Assistant Professor of Surgery, Uniformed Services University of the Health Sciences, Bethesda, Maryland; Director, Department of Ophthalmology, Madigan Army Medical Center, Tacoma, Washington 98431*

Blake M. McClarty, M.D. *Associate Professor of Radiology, Department of Radiology, St. Boniface Hospital—University of Manitoba, 409 Tache Avenue, Winnipeg, Manitoba R2H 2A6, Canada*

Kevin W. McEnery, M.D. *Assistant Professor of Radiology, Mallinckrodt Institute of Radiology, Washington University, St. Louis, Missouri 63110*

Gregory J. McGinn, M.D.   *Lecturer, Department of Radiology, St. Boniface Hospital, University of Manitoba, Winnipeg, Manitoba R2H 2A6, Canada*

Guido Meier, M.D.   *Orthopaedic Surgeon, Orthopaedic Section of the Surgical Clinic, Ratisches Kantons-und Regionalspital, Loestrasse 170, CH-7000 Chur, Switzerland*

Suresh K. Mukherji, M.D.   *Assistant Professor of Radiology and Surgery; Chief, Head and Neck Radiology; Adjunct Professor, Diagnostic Sciences, School of Dentistry, Department of Radiology, University of North Carolina School of Medicine, 3324 Old Infirmary, Chapel Hill, North Carolina 27599-7510*

Harsh Rastogi, M.D.   *Clinical Fellow of Neuroradiology, Department of Radiology, University of Texas Health Sciences Center at San Antonio, 7703 F. Curl Drive, San Antonio, Texas 78284-7800*

Kent B. Remley, M.D.   *Assistant Professor of Radiology and Otolaryngology, Department of Radiology, University of Minnesota Hospital and Clinic, Box 292, 420 Delaware Street S.E., Minneapolis, Minnesota 55455*

Farid F. Shafaie, M.D.   *Neuroradiology Fellow, Mallinckrodt Institute of Radiology, Washington University School of Medicine, 510 South Kingshighway Boulevard., St. Louis, Missouri 63110*

Richard M. Slone, M.D.   *Assistant Professor of Radiology, Mallinckrodt Institute of Radiology, Washington University School of Medicine, Barnes-Jewish Hospital, 510 South Kingshighway Boulevard., St. Louis, Missouri 63110*

Michelle Smith, M.D.   *Instructor, Section of Neuroradiology, Department of Radiology, University of North Carolina School of Medicine, Chapel Hill, North Carolina 27516*

Jill Thompson, M.D.   *Clinical Instructor, Section of Neuroradiology, Department of Radiology, University of North Carolina School of Medicine, Chapel Hill, North Carolina 27599*

Pamela Van Tassel, M.D.   *Associate Professor, Department of Radiology, Section of Neurology, Medical University of South Carolina, 171 Ashley Avenue, Charleston, South Carolina 29425*

Preface

One of the most challenging areas of diagnosis is to be found in acquiring and interpreting medical images in the patient who has undergone one or more forms of therapy. This may have involved conservative treatment, surgery, radiation therapy, chemotherapy, or other forms of medical treatment. The imaging findings may be either of an expected or unexpected nature. In some instances, the treated tissues may be left with benign scarring; in other cases, there may be a recurrence of disease or spread of the disease beyond the original site. In still other situations, the observation may represent a true complication of the therapy. All of these possibilities complicate medical image analysis.

In order to critically evaluate the posttherapeutic patient, it is imperative to understand several factors in reasonably specific detail. These include (a) the primary diagnosis, (b) the treatment(s) undergone by the patient, (c) the elapsed time since the various therapies, and (d) the current clinical syndrome. The answers to these questions will in large part determine which imaging modality or modalities are chosen for the work-up, how the images are acquired, and whether or not an enhancing agent is used.

The chapters in this textbook move step by step through the various subdivisions of the central nervous system and related tissues and the regions of the head and neck in order to illustrate the features of expected and abnormal posttherapeutic neurodiagnostic imaging. These discussions provide the background, practical information, and graphic examples necessary to enable the imaging physician to better approach the clinicoradiologic work-up and analysis of the posttherapeutic patient.

J. Randy Jinkins, M.D.

Acknowledgments

A great deal of thanks and respect goes out to those who made the production of this textbook possible. These individuals include Cheryl Portenier Howard and Renee Rodriguez, the secretarial staff at the University of Texas Health Science Center at San Antonio; and Brian Brown, Jim Ryan, and Nick Radhuber at Lippincott-Raven Publishers. I salute your talent and professionalism.

PART I

The Cranium

Posttherapeutic Neurodiagnostic Imaging,
edited by J.R. Jinkins,
Lippincott-Raven Publishers, New York © 1997.

CHAPTER **IA**

The Posttherapeutic Cranium

Harsh Rastogi, Carlos Bazan III, Claudia da Costa Leite, and J. Randy Jinkins

The recognition of both expected and abnormal alteration of the brain as a consequence of surgery, radiotherapy, chemotherapy, or other types of medical management has improved since the introduction of computed tomography (CT) and magnetic resonance imaging (MR). These noninvasive imaging modalities have revolutionized the art of the practice of modern medicine.

Complications occurring in the immediate postoperative period are a significant cause of morbidity and mortality (1). Hemorrhage and parenchymal swelling are two of the most common problems encountered in the immediate postoperative period. Infection and infarction may also complicate some surgical procedures (1,2). Prompt diagnosis is extremely important. Computed tomography remains the modality of choice for initial evaluation of the cranium in the acute postoperative period (3,4). Modern CT scanners provide high-resolution images of the brain in a very short period of time. Critically ill patients on life-support devices and the presence of aneurysm clips are not contraindications to CT examination. Contrast enhancement in the immediate postoperative period is usually not indicated; however, it may be useful in some cases in order to differentiate among infection, infarction, and residual tumor.

The role of MR in the immediate postoperative period is currently being evaluated (5). Despite its high resolution and multiplanar imaging capabilities, MR has not become the imaging modality of choice in the evaluation of critically ill patients. Prolonged examination time, problems associated with the use of life-support devices and patient monitors in a strong magnetic field, and potential danger of displacement of cerebral aneurysm clips with catastrophic hemorrhage remain major limitations. However, MR coupled with paramagnetic contrast agents (e.g., gadolinium, Gd) is the study of choice in the late postoperative period to evaluate for residual or early tu-

mor recurrence, meningeal or subependymal tumor seeding, parenchymal or meningeal infection, and postradiation changes (1,2,5–7).

Angiography plays a limited role in the immediate postoperative period, although it may be helpful in the detection and identification of residual vascular lesions or regrowth of highly vascularized tumors of the cranium. It is the study of choice for the evaluation of treated aneurysms, arteriovenous malformations, and dural arteriovenous fistulas.

The role of single-photon-emission computed tomography (SPECT) and positron-emission tomography (PET) in the evaluation of the brain during the early postoperative period has not yet been established. However, in the chronic phase, PET with ^{18}F-fluorodeoxyglucose (FDG) has been shown to be useful in some cases in differentiating radionecrosis from regrowth of metabolically active high-grade glioma (8).

The remainder of this chapter is devoted to analyzing the role of imaging in specific pathologic states of the posttherapeutic cranium.

SCALP AND SKULL VAULT

During the first few postoperative days, a number of subtle but important findings may be encountered involving the superficial operative site. These include scalp hematoma, extraaxial collections (e.g., CSF, blood, air), pseudomeningocele, and abnormalities of the meningogaleal complex overlying the craniotomy site. Both CT and MR examinations are quite helpful in correctly diagnosing infection, hematoma, and other collections early in the postoperative period and in enabling clinicians to make more accurate decisions regarding reexploration, initiation of antibiotic therapy, or simple clinical observation of the patient's condition.

Scalp swelling encountered over the operative site in the early postoperative period is often a nonspecific finding. This is commonly a sign of edema or a collection of CSF mixed with blood or air in the soft tissue of the scalp

H. Rastogi, C. Bazan III, C. da Costa Leite, and J. R. Jinkins: Department of Radiology, The University of Texas Health Science Center, San Antonio, Texas 78284.

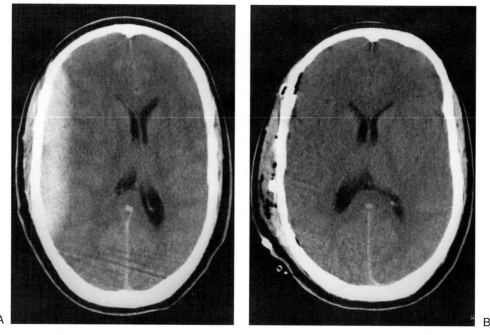

FIG. IA-1. Postoperative subgaleal swelling hematoma in a 27-year-old man involved in a motor vehicle accident. **A:** Unenhanced axial CT shows a right-sided epidural hematoma with midline shift to the left and compression of the right lateral ventricle. There is only a small amount of overlying scalp swelling. **B:** Unenhanced axial CT following evacuation of the epidural hematoma shows thickened scalp tissues with edema, blood, and air overlying the craniotomy.

(Fig. IA-1). This swelling slowly resolves over a period of weeks. Persistence or increase in the size of the swelling is ominous and should suggest wound or bone flap infection, frank empyema formation, expanding hematoma, or CSF fistula.

Immediately following uncomplicated craniotomies, several distinct layers may be identified on T_1-weighted MR images. Most superficially, a band of intermediate signal intensity represents the skin, followed by a layer of hyperintense subcutaneous fat; the temporalis muscle, edema, and blood appear as a zone of moderate intensity. The bone flap appears as a tram track with areas of discontinuity at the site of burr holes and along craniotomy lines. Immediately subjacent to the bone flap, a high-signal layer may be seen representing CSF-containing blood products. The dura may be seen as a thin band of low signal intensity just internal to this last layer. Metallic MR artifacts from surgical sutures are often encountered at the margins of the craniotomy site.

Some authors have noted important differences in the enhancement pattern at the postoperative site demonstrated on CT versus MR images (9); a thin, regularly enhancing dura mater or meningogaleal complex has been observed on MR after Gd contrast administration within 24 hr of the operation. The CT did not show such enhancement until the end of the first week. This normal postoperative enhancement can persist for several years on MR, but on CT it disappears by the end of 6 months (Fig. IA-2). The most likely explanation for this discrepancy

is the differential contrast resolution sensitivity of CT and MR.

Infection of the operative site in the early postoperative period is a potentially serious complication. The diagnosis may be difficult based on imaging because expected postoperative imaging changes can mimic infection. Postoperative infection often begins at the surgical suture line and may spread to the bone and meninges to cause bone flap infection, meningitis, or CSF fistula (10–12). The earliest radiographic signs of postoperative infection are encountered as alterations in the baseline appearance of the meningogaleal complex that may change from a well-defined dark dural line to a thick, ill-defined, nodular, and densely enhancing membrane on CT and MR. These findings correlate histologically with edema, inflammation, and granulation tissue seen along the meningogaleal complex.

Fluid collections seen in the scalp region are often sterile. They usually represent pockets of CSF mixed with blood or its breakdown products. However, progressively enlarging subgaleal lesions may be the result of infection or an abnormal communication with an epidural or subarachnoid collection through a defect in the bony cranium. When the fluid collection is infected, the source of infection may on occasion be traced to the bone flap. After craniotomy, the bone flap is more or less devascularized and therefore devitalized. For this reason, it may promote bacterial growth and suppuration (Fig. IA-3). On CT, infected calvarial bone appears as lytic areas with or without bone fragmentation associated with subgaleal and/or

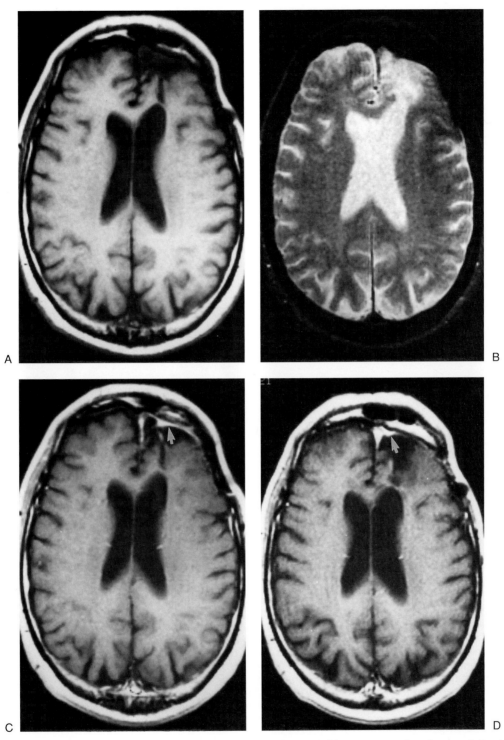

FIG. IA-2. Benign postoperative dural thickening in a 54-year-old man presenting 5 years following resection debulking of a grade III astrocytoma. **A:** Unenhanced axial T₁-weighted (600/20) conventional spin-echo (CSE) MR obtained 1 month after surgical debulking shows left frontal lobe area of low signal intensity without associated mass effect. **B:** Axial T₂-weighted (2000/80) CSE MR shows an ill-defined hyperintensity in the left frontal area. **C:** Enhanced axial T₁-weighted (600/20) CSE MR acquired at the same time as **A** and **B** shows postoperative peripheral enhancement of the dura over the left frontal surgical site (*arrow*). **D:** Enhanced axial T₁-weighted (550/20) CSE MR obtained 5 years after those of **A–C** reveals subtotal resolution of the dural enhancement in the left frontal area adjacent to the anterior aspect of the superior sagittal venous sinus, with minimal residual (*arrow*). There is no evidence of recurrent enhancing astrocytoma.

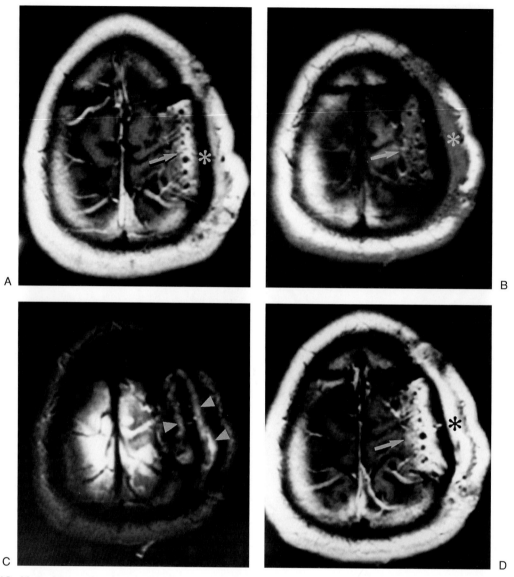

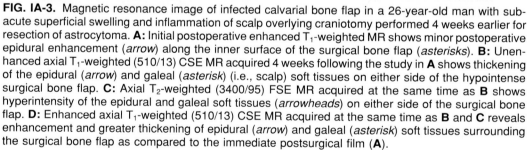

FIG. IA-3. Magnetic resonance image of infected calvarial bone flap in a 26-year-old man with subacute superficial swelling and inflammation of scalp overlying craniotomy performed 4 weeks earlier for resection of astrocytoma. **A:** Initial postoperative enhanced T_1-weighted MR shows minor postoperative epidural enhancement (*arrow*) along the inner surface of the surgical bone flap (*asterisks*). **B:** Unenhanced axial T_1-weighted (510/13) CSE MR acquired 4 weeks following the study in **A** shows thickening of the epidural (*arrow*) and galeal (*asterisk*) (i.e., scalp) soft tissues on either side of the hypointense surgical bone flap. **C:** Axial T_2-weighted (3400/95) FSE MR acquired at the same time as **B** shows hyperintensity of the epidural and galeal soft tissues (*arrowheads*) on either side of the surgical bone flap. **D:** Enhanced axial T_1-weighted (510/13) CSE MR acquired at the same time as **B** and **C** reveals enhancement and greater thickening of epidural (*arrow*) and galeal (*asterisk*) soft tissues surrounding the surgical bone flap as compared to the immediate postsurgical film (**A**).

epidural collections of pus or granulation tissue (Fig. IA-4). The standard treatment is removal of the infected bone flap and abscess drainage. However, an otherwise normal but devitalized bone flap over many years may become irregular in its density and lose its well-defined cortex and diploic space, giving it a mottled appearance. Similar sterile bony changes may be evident after radiation therapy. The clinical picture of an absence of signs of suppurative inflammation should distinguish these latter two conditions from infection.

Finally, after craniectomy in which the bone flap has been removed, a muscle flap may be interposed between the skin and the underlying brain in order to afford long-term protection to the cerebrum (Fig. IA-5) (13,14). This should not be confused with inflammation or neoplastic alteration. Postoperative pseudomeningoceles are occasionally encountered after suboccipital craniectomies when the dura is left open or is sutured to the craniectomy margin. Pseudomeningoceles can progressively dissect into the soft tissue planes to form blind pockets, which may release their contents into the subarachnoid space from time to time, presenting clinically as episodes of aseptic meningitis. This condition is known as the "post-craniectomy dumping syndrome" (10).

CRANIAL EXTRAAXIAL SPACES

Intracranial extraaxial collections are usually seen at the site of surgery early in the postoperative period. This serosanguinous fluid collection may persist as an epidural/subdural effusion beneath the bone flap. Simple effusion is crescentic in shape and appears similar to CSF on both CT and MR. Most resolve spontaneously and do not require treatment (2).

Infected extraaxial collections are known as empyemas. They are a sequel to wound infection, osteomyelitis, or meningitis complicating surgery. Cerebritis, cerebral abscess, and cortical vein and venous sinus thrombosis may subsequently ensue. Commonly, the inflammatory collection becomes encapsulated in the subdural space. It is of low density on CT, iso- to hyperintense compared to CSF on T_1-weighted MR sequences, and iso- to hypointense to CSF on T_2-weighted acquisitions. The encapsulating neomembrane and septae are quite vascular; they enhance intensely after contrast administration (15). If the empyema is not drained, the capsule may calcify in the chronic stages.

Even a relatively simple neurosurgical procedure such as shunt placement may be complicated by a life-threatening extraaxial hematoma (16,17). Rapid decompression of obstructive hydrocephalus during posterior fossa surgery, ventricular drainage, or a shunt operation may induce the formation of a subdural or extradural hematoma (17). These hematomas are either consequences of sudden cortical collapse with tearing of superficial cortical veins or rupture of bridging epidural veins into the potential epidural space between the dura and the inner table of the skull.

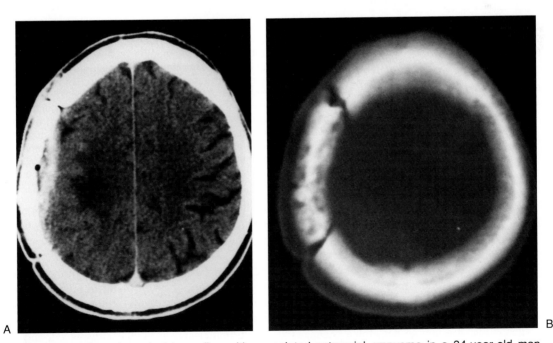

FIG. IA-4. Infected surgical bone flap with associated extraaxial empyema in a 34-year-old man presenting following resection of a right parietal astrocytoma, now complaining of fever and focal pain over the surgical region. **A:** Enhanced axial CT shows a convex enhancing extraaxial collection associated with air bubbles contiguous to the bone flap on the right side. **B:** Axial CT filmed with bone window settings at a level above that of **A** shows lytic lesions in the right-side surgical bone flap.

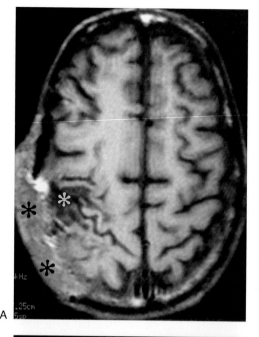

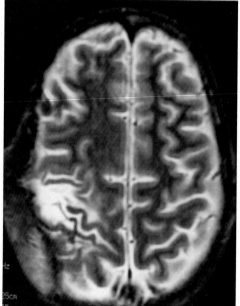

FIG. IA-5. Superficial cranial latissimus dorsi muscle flap implant following craniectomy for bone flap infection in a 34-year-old man. The patient had a cerebral astrocytoma resected 2 months earlier. **A:** Unenhanced axial T_1-weighted (550/13) CSE MR shows the latissimus dorsi muscle implant (*black asterisks*) overlying the craniectomy site. The surgical resection site (*white asterisk*) is also noted. **B:** Axial T_2-weighted (3500/95) FSE MR again shows the surgical resection site and the implanted latissimus dorsi. **C:** Enhanced axial T_1-weighted (517/13) CSE MR shows enhancement of the implanted muscle flap (*asterisk*) and the underlying dura. There is also a small area of enhancement in the surgical site (*arrow:* recurrent astrocytoma) and diffuse enhancement of the left hemispheric cerebral cortex (postradiation necrosis).

The diagnosis of simple hemorrhage into the extraaxial space is in part based on the shape of the hematoma. In the unoperated patient, extradural hematomas are usually lentiform, whereas subdural hematomas are crescentic in shape (18). However, in the postoperative patient, this distinction based on configuration may not be reliable (Fig. IA-6). On CT, attenuation of the hematoma is a reflection of hematocrit, water, and protein content. In addition, the attenuation of a simple hematoma changes as it evolves. Acute hematomas are uniformly hyperdense, subacutely they become isodense, and chronically the lesion is hypodense as compared to the adjacent brain parenchyma. Small hematomas adjacent to the calvaria or

at the skull base may be easily overlooked on CT; a change in the window width and level may be required to separate small hematomas from the adjacent dense bone.

In a severely anemic patient, an acute hematoma may be isodense to brain. Bilaterally symmetric isodense hematomas can be very difficult to recognize. In these patients, the adjacent ''cortex'' appears unusually thick, the sulci and gyri are effaced, the gyral processes of cerebral white matter appear medially displaced, and mass effect on the lateral ventricles is usually observed. On bolus contrast-enhanced CT, the superficial cerebral vessels are seen to be displaced away from the inner table of the skull. Later, chronic hematomas may become encapsulated; the

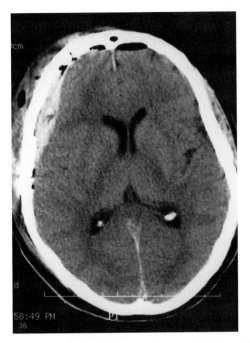

FIG. IA-6. Postoperative extraaxial hematoma in a 61-year-old man presenting following clipping of cerebral aneurysm. Unenhanced axial CT shows a right-sided extraaxial acute postoperative hematoma beneath the craniotomy site. Air is present within the calvarium as well as within the swollen scalp overlying the craniotomy site.

neovascularized wall around the encapsulated hematoma will enhance intensely after contrast administration (18). If untreated, 0.3% to 0.7% of chronic subdural hematomas develop calcification or ossification (Fig. IA-7) (19).

On MR, extraaxial hematomas generally evolve in a pattern similar to intracerebral hemorrhage (discussed later). Hyperacute extraaxial hematomas are isointense to gray matter on T_1- and hyperintense on T_2-weighted sequences (oxyhemoglobin). A thin, hypointense line of dura separating the blood clot from the adjacent brain may sometimes be seen. Acute hematomas may be iso- to hypointense on T_1-weighted and hypointense on T_2-weighted acquisitions (deoxyhemoglobin). Subacute extraaxial hematomas are hyperintense on both T_1- and T_2-weighted MR sequences (extracellular methemoglobin). Chronic subdural hematomas are hypointense to gray matter on T_1-weighted studies and hyperintense on T_2-weighted sequences, representing final blood breakdown products (proteinaceous fluid). The neovascular capsule of the hematoma or fibrous subdural mass will enhance intensely after i.v. Gd administration. Rehemorrhage may complicate these hematomas; this will appear as a mixed-signal-intensity mass with multiple membranes, with or without a fluid–fluid level (20–27).

Spontaneous delayed intracranial extraaxial hemorrhage is a known complication of craniectomies when Silastic dural substitutes are utilized (18). Dural substitutes are used to close large surgical defects that are cre-

ated during some procedures. A neomembrane arising from the dura slowly encases the dural substitute. Fragile vessels associated with this new dural membrane may be a source of hemorrhage. Hemorrhage has been observed at the operative site up to 12 years after surgical implantation (18). This extraaxial hematoma may mimic recurrent neoplasia, but it can be differentiated on MR by the characteristic signal intensities of blood and its breakdown products (19).

CRANIAL MENINGES

Local dural or generalized meningeal enhancement observed on MR images in the postoperative period is often benign and should not necessarily be considered a sign of infection or meningeal spread of CNS neoplasm (28). This nonneoplastic meningeal enhancement most likely represents a sterile inflammatory response caused by surgical trauma or spillage of blood into the subarachnoid space at the time of surgery. It is speculated that this aseptic chemical meningitis may lead to meningeal fibrosis and dense pial–arachnoid adhesions (28). The CT is relatively insensitive to the detection of meningeal enhancement over the convexities because of the imperceptible difference in density of enhancing meninges and the high attenuation of the adjacent bone. On i.v. Gd-enhanced MR, however, the enhancing meninges stand out against the signal void of the cortical bone. More extensive meningeal enhancement after surgery may result from infectious meningitis, leptomeningeal metastasis, or local tumor invasion (28–32). In more than 50% of cases of bacterial meningitis, contrast-enhanced CT may appear normal (33). However, i.v. Gd-enhanced MR is felt to be much more sensitive for the detection of meningitis.

Spillage of the contents of a craniopharyngioma or epidermoid or dermoid tumor into the subarachnoid space during surgery can produce chemical meningitis, which appears as intense leptomeningeal enhancement on enhanced CT or MR in the early postoperative period (34). Nodular meningeal enhancement may appear months to years after resection of choroid plexus tumors, primitive neuroectodermal tumors, and glial tumors. These tumors have a predilection for meningeal dissemination (Fig. IA-8) (35–40). Although repeated CSF examination may be abnormal, actual malignant cells are less frequently detected (30). The proof of CSF seeding of tumor may only be attained on open surgical biopsy of the dura or at autopsy.

An unusual pathologic cause of leptomeningeal MR signal alteration in the late postoperative period is superficial siderosis (31,32). It is typically a sequel of repeated episodes of subarachnoid hemorrhage from brain tumors, aneurysm, or arteriovenous malformation (AVM) rupture but also can be a complication of surgical procedures

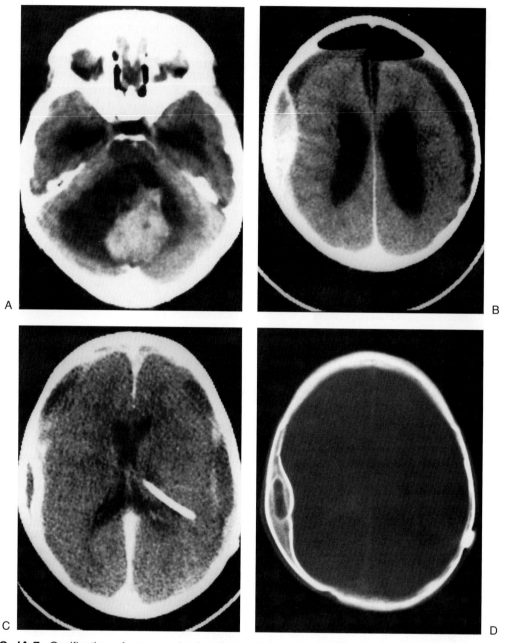

FIG. IA-7. Ossification of an extradural collection in an 8-year-old girl presenting with history of prior medulloblastoma and resection. **A:** Preoperative enhanced axial CT shows an enhancing fourth ventricle mass (medulloblastoma) associated with marked ventricular dilation. **B:** Enhanced axial CT obtained immediately following surgical resection shows a hyperdense extradural hematoma along the right convexity. Bilateral subdural collections and hydrocephalus are also present. **C:** Enhanced axial CT obtained 5 months after that in **B** shows persistence of the right extradural collection as well as bilateral subdural collections. A ventricular shunt catheter is in place. **D:** Axial CT acquired on bone window settings 5 years after **C** shows that the extradural collection has ossified and fused with the inner table of the calvarium.

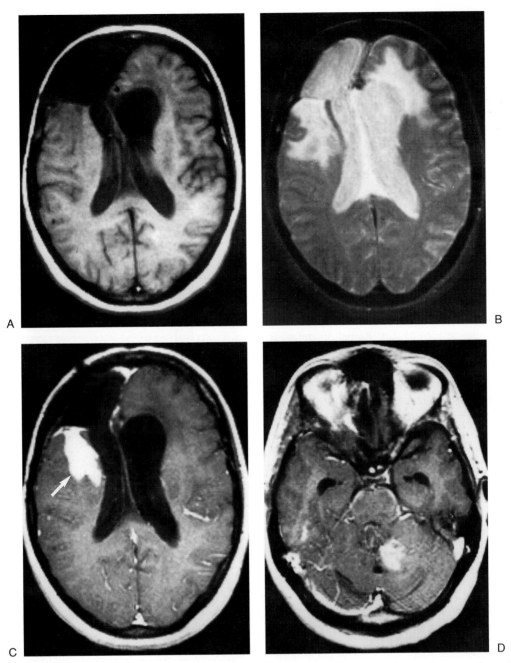

FIG. IA-8. Recurrent oligodendroglioma with CSF seeding in a 42-year-old woman presenting with progressive signs and symptoms following multiple resections of an oligodendroglioma followed by radiation and chemotherapy. **A:** Unenhanced axial T_1-weighted (500/20) CSE MR shows the site of surgical resection in the right frontal lobe and *ex vacuo* deformity of the lateral ventricles. **B:** Axial T_2-weighted (2400/80) CSE MR shows hyperintensity adjacent to the resection site as well as in the left frontal white matter. **C:** Enhanced axial T_1-weighted (500/20) CSE MR shows enhancement of a mass (*arrow*) adjacent to the right frontal lobe resection, indicating recurrence. **D:** Enhanced axial T_1-weighted (500/20) CSE MR through the posterior fossa shows an enhancing nodule bordering on the fourth ventricle area compatible with subarachnoid seeding of tumors.

such as hemispherectomy. Siderosis is characterized by deposition of hemosiderin in the leptomeninges covering the brain, spinal cord, and cranial nerves. Siderosis typically stands out as a low signal of hemosiderin outlining the brain surfaces (especially the brainstem and the cerebellum) against the bright signal of CSF on T_2-weighted conventional spin-echo MR images. Gradient T_2-weighted recalled echo imaging can demonstrate superficial siderosis better than can conventional spin-echo acquisitions.

CEREBRAL VESSELS

Patients who undergo radiation therapy to the head and neck are at a small risk of experiencing serious or fatal stroke long after cure or resolution of their clinical condition for which the radiation treatment was administered (41). Postirradiation vascular insufficiency syndrome usually manifests itself clinically during the late phase following radiation therapy (6,41,42). Radiation injury to the cranial and neck vessels can lead to accelerated atherosclerosis, "foam" cell arteritis, and vascular occlusion (6,41,43–46). Small arteries and capillaries are more affected by endothelial damage than are medium-sized vessels. Arteriography may show stenosis or occlusion involving not only the intracranial arteries and their proximal branches but also the cephalic arteries in the neck; a moyamoya collateral pattern may accompany the proximal intracranial arterial occlusion, or the picture may simulate a diffuse arteritis (46). Both CT and MR demonstrate associated parenchymal infarcts. Spontaneous rupture of these vessels with hemorrhage has also been described (47–49). In combination with methotrexate, radiation therapy may result in mineralizing microangiopathy in children being treated for leukemia and other malignant CNS tumors (Fig. IA-9) (6,50).

Recently, intracranial AVMs have been successfully treated by radiosurgery (51–55); CT, MR, and angiography have reliably documented the evolution. After a latent period of 6 to 24 months after radiosurgery, the majority of small and medium-sized high-flow AVMs demonstrate nonfilling of the nidus on angiograms. Larger AVMs may take years to evolve to complete obliteration (51). The MR was found to be superior to CT and cerebral angiogram in documenting a regression in size of the nidus (51). The MR also detected hemorrhages and thromboses within the AVM after ablation that were not demonstrated on CT (51). At the time at which angiography showed complete resolution of the AVM, CT demonstrated minor enhancement at the site of the nidus, presumed to be caused by leakage of contrast into the interstitium, while flow voids on MR were replaced by intermediate signal of the thrombus. However, CT was better in defining late calcifications within thrombosed AVMs that were missed by MR. The white matter change associated with radiation

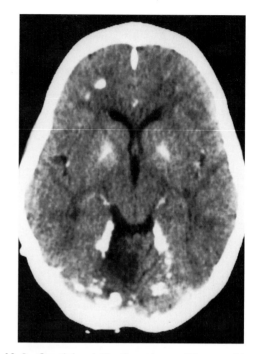

FIG. IA-9. Cranial calcifications in an 18-year-old woman presenting with prior resection of a posterior fossa medulloblastoma in childhood followed by radiotherapy and chemotherapy (methotrexate). Enhanced axial CT shows multiple marked hyperdense lesions (calcifications) in the basal ganglia, frontal lobes, interhemispheric fissure, tentorium, and cerebellar hemisphere. (Case courtesy of P.C. Davis, M.D., Atlanta, GA.)

injury (i.e., radiation leukodystrophy) is seen as a halo of low attenuation on CT that on MR has a prolonged T_1 and T_2 relaxation times (see Sequelae: Diffuse Radiation-Induced Leukoencephalopathy).

The reevaluation of aneurysms following surgical clipping is best carried out by selective conventional angiography for several reasons. Successful aneurysm clipping (Fig. IA-10), slipped aneurysm clips (Fig. IA-11), and residual aneurysm lumens are clearly analyzed only by conventional angiographic techniques (56). In addition, aside from spatial resolution considerations, the metallic artifact on CT precludes adequate evaluation of the region of the aneurysm; similarly, magnetic susceptability artifact obscures regional MR detail, to say nothing of the risk of rupture of the aneurysm by torque being placed on the ferromagnetic cerebral aneurysm clips (Fig. IA-12) (57–63).

BRAIN PARENCHYMA

Edema

Pathologic postoperative edema often presents clinically as intracranial hypertension. The development of cerebral edema in the postoperative period result from a

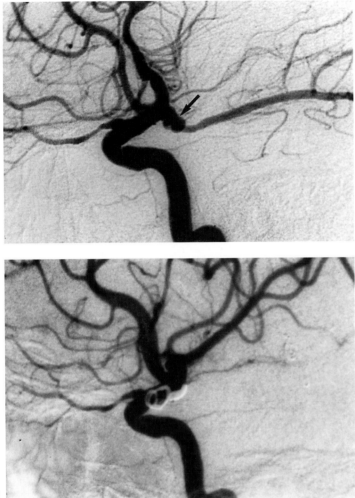

FIG. IA-10. Successful surgical clipping of an aneurysm in a 62-year-old woman with a posterior communicating artery aneurysm. **A:** Lateral view of a right internal carotid angiogram shows an aneurysm (*arrow*) near the origin of the posterior communicating artery. **B:** Lateral view of a right internal carotid angiogram shows successful clipping of the aneurysm. The posterior communicating artery filled from a posterior circulation (i.e., vertebral artery) injection (not shown).

number of factors, which include surgical manipulation leading to direct tissue trauma, vascular spasm leading to perfusion defects, impaired venous drainage during surgery, and water and electrolyte imbalance in the postoperative period. Usually, cerebral swelling begins 4 to 5 hr after surgery, reaches its maximum in about 2 to 3 days, and resolves slowly in the subacute postoperative period (2). Unenhanced CT usually confirms the diagnosis of edema, which often appears as a focal or diffuse hypodense area with mass effect. The mass effect is seen as sulcal and cisternal effacement, compressed ventricles, midline shift, and disruption of the gray–white matter interface. These changes may be present focally at the site of the surgical procedure or may be more diffuse, occasionally leading to postoperative external herniation of brain through the craniotomy site (Fig. IA-13) (64–67). Diffuse cerebral edema typically exhibits homogeneous, generalized decreased attenuation involving both the white and gray matter and loss of gray and white matter differentiation. The etiology of a low-attenuating focal lesion(s) early in the postoperative period on noncontrast CT or MR studies is a nonspecific finding. A contrast-enhanced study may be helpful in differentiating simple edema from the effects of surgical manipulation from infection, infarction, and residual tumor.

Patients with CT evidence of gross postoperative edema may have no or minimal neurologic impairment. However, in some patients, severely raised intracranial pressure may show transtentorial, tonsillar, and/or subfalcine internal cerebral herniation manifesting itself clinically as progressive neurologic deterioration and coma. Prompt correctional therapeutic measures and sequential CT scans may form part of the management in such cases (68).

Infection

Postoperative infection is an uncommon but life-threatening complication of a neurosurgical procedure. It is usually seen in the subacute postoperative period and is often associated with significant morbidity and mortality. Cerebritis is the initial stage of purulent brain infection, which will evolve if unchecked into frank abscess forma-

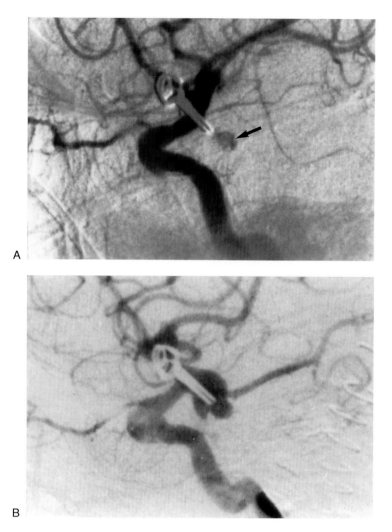

A

B

FIG. IA-11. Unsuccessful surgical clipping of an aneurysm in a 46-year-old woman with a posterior communicating artery aneurysm. **A:** Lateral projection of a left internal carotid angiogram obtained immediately after clipping of the aneurysm demonstrates filling of a small residual aneurysm lumen (*arrow*). **B:** Lateral projection of a left internal carotid angiogram obtained 2 weeks after surgery shows enlargement of the residual aneurysm lumen.

tion in 1 to 2 weeks. Both the cerebritis and brain abscess stages of cerebral infection are associated with surrounding edema and mass effect (Fig. IA-14). Corticosteroid administration may profoundly diminish the magnitude of surrounding edema as well as the degree of contrast enhancement (69–71). On the other hand, on appropriate medical therapy, inflammatory lesions may be seen on medical imaging to resolve over time (Fig. IA-15).

As noted in the foregoing, it is usually impossible on unenhenced CT or MR to differentiate cerebritis from sterile postoperative reaction, edema, infarction, or even residual tumor because they all appear as hypodense mass lesions in the region of prior surgery. On enhanced CT and MR, an area of early cerebritis may show faint, patchy enhancement within the first several days following surgery. If untreated, at the seventh postoperative day an area of relative hypodensity develops centrally as a result of cerebral necrosis. In this stage (i.e., late cerebritis), the lesion may show nodular or ring-like enhancement following i.v. contrast administration. On delay postcontrast imaging

(e.g., 60 to 90 min), contrast slowly "fills in" the center in some cases of later cerebritis. The surrounding edema is usually marked (72).

The late cerebritis stage lasts until approximately the end of the second postoperative week. During this period, the cerebritis evolves into an early capsular stage of abscess formation, consisting of a central core of liquefied necrotic and inflammatory debris surrounded by a thin capsule. On CT, the capsule appears as a thin ring with smooth inner margin, surrounding a center of low attenuation. Following i.v. contrast administration, there is ring enhancement of generally regular thickness. The ring enhancement is often thinner on the ventricular side of the developing abscess. As the abscess matures, mass effect and edema subside somewhat. The late capsular stage follows, which may last for weeks or months. During this stage, the abscess is well encapsulated and appears as a moderately thick, densely enhancing ring on enhanced CT imaging. With appropriate treatment, the cavity gradually shrinks as the abscess heals. A progressively decreasing diameter of the enhancing ring is believed by some to be the only reliable criterion for healing (73). A completely

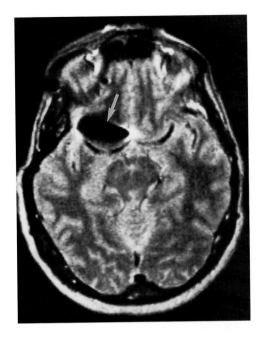

FIG. IA-12. Magnetic resonance image of a metallic artifact from a cerebral aneurysm clip in a 35-year-old man presenting with headache following prior cranial surgery of unknown type. Axial T_2-weighted (2000/80) CSE MR shows metallic artifact (*arrow*) in area of middle cerebral bifurcation aneurysm clip. This study was accidently performed because of an absence of history from the referring physician or patient of previous cranial aneurysm surgery.

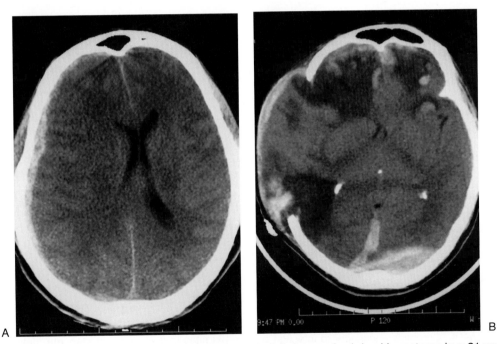

FIG. IA-13. External brain herniation following surgical drainage of subdural hematoma in a 21-year-old man who presented with loss of consciousness following a motor vehicle accident. **A:** Unenhanced axial CT scan shows a right subdural hematoma with mass effect and a shift of the midline structures to the left. The subdural hematoma was surgically evacuated after this scan. **B:** Axial CT scan obtained 6 days later, after the onset of coma, shows external brain herniation through the right craniectomy, intraparenchymal hemorrhages, collapse of the ventricular system, and interhemispheric and left occipital extraaxial hematomas.

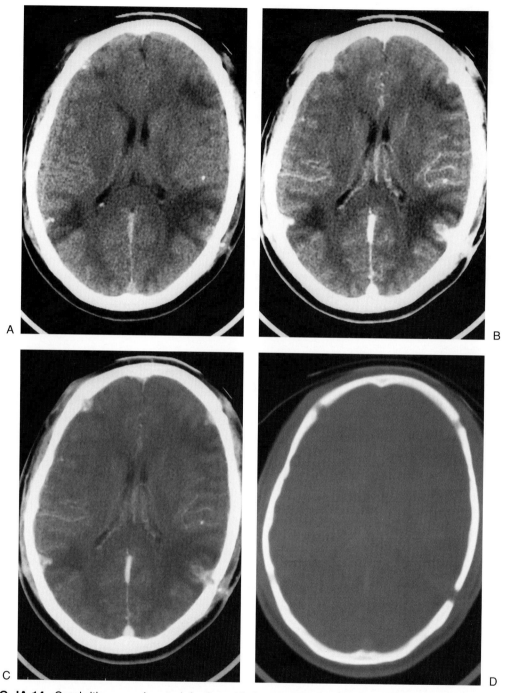

FIG. IA-14. Cerebritis secondary to infection of halo pin sites in a 29-year-old man who developed pain and swelling at the pin sites of his halo device. **A:** Unenhanced axial CT shows areas of white matter hypodensity in the areas of the halo pins. **B:** Enhanced axial CT at the same level as that of **A** shows nodular enhancement adjacent to the regions of the halo pin insertion. **C:** Axial CT filmed on soft tissue settings shows subgaleal swelling at the halo pin sites. **D:** Axial CT filmed on bone window settings shows the calvarial holes at the pin sites.

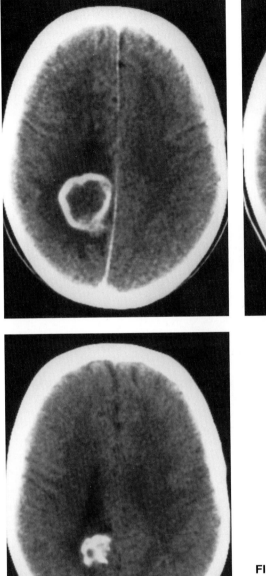

FIG. IA-15. Resolution of tuberculoma on medical therapy in a 35-year-old man from Saudi Arabia presenting with an episode of mental confusion. **A:** Enhanced CT scan shows a ring-enhancing right parietal lesion with surrounding edema. **B:** Enhanced CT scan obtained 6 months after initiation of antituberculous treatment shows that the lesion has decreased in size and now reveals solid nodular enhancement with surrounding edema. **C:** Unenhanced CT scan obtained 1.5 years after **A** shows a residual calcified lesion.

healed abscess will not enhance on enhanced CT or MR acquisitions. Some abscesses may calcify on healing.

The MR appearance of brain abscesses varies with time. Early cerebritis may appear as an ill-defined area of hyperintensity on T_2-weighted images. On T_1-weighted studies, cerebritis is iso- to hypointense and may enhance after i.v. Gd administration. In the late cerebritis stage, the central area of necrosis is hyperintense to the gray matter on T_2-weighted images and is surrounded by an irregular, thick, iso- to hypointense rim. When it is hypointense, the change is presumed to be caused by the presence of free radicals and fibrosis within and near the

developing capsule. This rim usually appears mildly hyperintense on T_1-weighted imaging and enhances following i.v. Gd administration. Edema and mass effect are invariably present. During the early and late capsule stages, the capsule wall is observed as a well-defined, thin hypointense ring on T_2-weighted sequences but continues to enhance intensely in a smooth ring fashion on T_1-weighted sequences. Edema and mass effect diminish as the abscess matures.

The use of steroids to reduce cerebral edema in the initial postoperative period profoundly diminishes the magnitude of inflammation-related contrast enhancement on enhanced CT or MR. This pathologic enhancement becomes less prominent after steroid administration in the cerebritis and early capsule stage; the late capsule stage is less affected by steroids (69–71). Sequential time-delayed enhanced scans may be useful in this setting. Importantly, the use of steroids and chemotherapeutic agents may also suppress the immune system, rendering patients prone to postoperative opportunistic infections (Fig. IA-16) (74–78).

Frequently, sequential enhanced CT or MR scans are required to make a definitive diagnosis of cerebral infection. In the first postoperative week, a densely enhancing nodular area that is adjacent or separate from the operative margin suggests residual tumor (5). Usually this enhancing area can be identified on the preoperative scan and remains unchanged on studies acquired soon after the surgery. A tumor-free operative margin enhances after 4 to 6 days and is not associated with edema. This self-limited enhancement persists for approximately a month. In the late postoperative period it is often difficult or impossible to differentiate a thick, ring-enhancing wall of an abscess from residual tumor, especially if the initial postoperative studies are not available (see Postoperative Site: Residual Tumor).

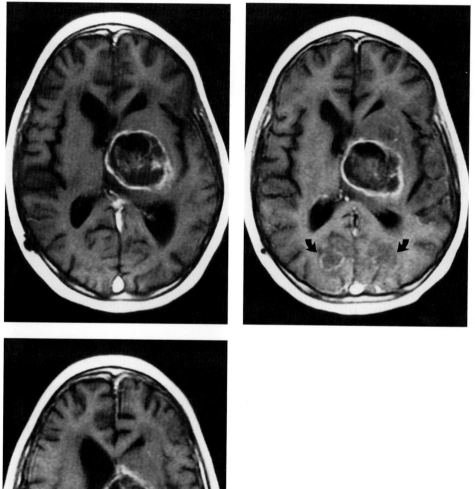

A

B

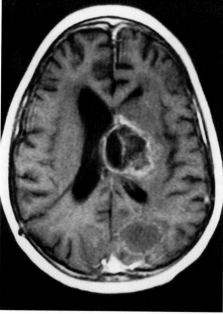

C

FIG. IA-16. Aspergillosis associated with steroid therapy for anaplastic astrocytoma in a 12-year-old boy presenting with a left thalamic anaplastic astrocytoma. **A:** Enhanced axial T$_1$-weighted (417/16) conventional spin-echo (CSE) MR demonstrates a ring-enhancing left thalamic mass (astrocytoma). **B:** Enhanced axial T$_1$-weighted (417/16) CSE MR obtained 20 days following **A** and after radiation, chemotherapy, and steroid therapy shows hypointense lesions (*curved arrows: Aspergillus*) in both occipital lobes. The lesion on the right reveals slight enhancement. The enhancing thalamic glioma is slightly smaller than on the prior examination (**A**). **C:** Enhanced axial T$_1$-weighted (417/16) CSE MR at a level above that of **B** shows the enhancing left thalamic tumor and slight enhancement of the lesion (*Aspergillus*) in the left occipital lobe.

Both CT and MR not only evaluate for the progression of disease but also can be an important guide in tailoring the treatment approach in cases of postoperative infection. Large and multifocal abscesses are prone to further complications. Abscesses less than 2.5 cm are usually treated medically, whereas those more than 2.5 cm require surgical drainage. If untreated, large abscesses tend to rupture into the adjacent cerebral ventricular system, producing ventriculitis (5). Rupture along the cortical surface leading to purulent leptomeningitis is also a reported complication.

Hemorrhage

Intracranial hemorrhage is one of the most serious complications to occur following surgery (Fig. IA-17). Advancements in the surgical techniques and perioperative management have substantially reduced the incidence of postoperative intraparenchymal, epidural, and subdural hematomas. Common causes of postoperative intracerebral hemorrhage include inadequate hemostasis, difficult tumor resection, direct vascular injury, venous thrombosis, perioperative systemic hypertension, rapid decompression of cranial hypertension, coagulation disorder (therapeutic anticoagulation, thrombocytopenia, complication of hepatic or neoplastic renal disease, disseminated intravascular coagulation), or surgery performed on vascular malformations or aneurysms (79). Although rare, such postoperative hemorrhage can occur in areas remote from the site of surgery. Hemorrhage after posterior fossa surgery, transsphenoidal surgery, and supratentorial craniotomy has been described that may or may not be associated with intracranial aneurysm, vascular malformation, or neoplasm (80–82).

Intracerebral hemorrhage can also develop after extracranial surgery. Fisher (83) implicated the use of vasopressors in the postoperative period as a cause of this hemorrhage. He observed that these hemorrhages were ''atypically located compared to chronic hypertensive hemorrhages'' and that only a ''modest'' rise in blood pressure seemed to precipitate hemorrhage (83).

Intracerebral hemorrhage is a well-documented complication of cardiac surgery (84,85). The proposed mechanisms to explain the hemorrhage include initial cerebrovascular embolism, cerebral hypoperfusion, transient ischemia, and infarction. The subsequent restoration of cerebral blood flow postoperatively might then lead to hemorrhage within the infarcted brain. Frequent changes in the coagulation state, the development of a consumption coagulopathy, and disseminated infection by such organisms as *Aspergillus fumigatus* (which displays propensity to vascular invasion) further predispose these patients to cerebral infarction and hemorrhage (85).

Intracerebral hemorrhage can be seen in patients with myocardial infarction following thrombolytic therapy (86–89). The risk of hemorrhage varies with the drug used (e.g., streptokinase, urokinase, t-PA), the dosage used and the coagulation profile of the patient after thrombolysis. Hemorrhage tends to occur within the first 24 hr after infusion of the thrombolytic agent. Hemorrhagic foci are often multiple and predominantly involve the cortical and subcortical white matter. These hemorrhages may coalesce to form a large hematoma. A layering of blood products within the hematoma may be observed on imaging. Because of an increase in the use of thrombolytic agents for other applications in medicine, secondary cerebral hemorrhage caused by these agents is expected to rise in the future.

A number of medical anticoagulation agents may lead to intracerebral hemorrhage (Fig. IA-18) (90–93). Anticoagulation agents commonly encountered in practice are heparin and coumadin. The hemorrhages may be unifocal or multifocal and can be massive. The use and abuse of sympathomimetic drugs can also cause intracranial bleeding. These include drugs such as amphetamines, phencyclidine (PCP), ephedrine, and pseudoephedrine. The cerebral vessels in these patients can appear greatly attenuated and beaded in appearance on cerebral angiography. Rupture of these friable vessels results in cerebral hemorrhage.

Spontaneous intracerebral hemorrhage has been observed as a late effect of radiotherapy in patients undergoing treatment for primary brain tumors (47–49). Recurrent neoplastic disease or radiation necrosis is the most likely cause of such hemorrhage when the bleed is in the original tumor site. On the other hand, when the CNS hemorrhage is distant from the site of the primary malignant tumor but still within the area irradiated, then radiation-induced vasculopathy should be considered as a potentially responsible factor. Radiation-induced fibrinoid vascular necrosis and postradiation telangiectasia of small cerebral vessels may be implicated in these cases of intracerebral hemorrhage (94).

On CT, acute hematomas generally appear as well-defined mass lesions of varying shape. The density of the hematoma depends on the hematocrit but also on its age, hemoconcentration, and protein content. When actively bleeding, the mass is fluid and may be hypo- to isodense to the brain on CT. As it evolves, the blood rapidly clots and becomes organized. Once clotted, the blood appears hyperdense in relation to the surrounding brain. Within 7 days, the breakdown of red blood cells and neovascularization result in a hypodense halo of edema around the hematoma. Neovascularization is seen on enhanced CT as a ring of enhancement surrounding the hematoma that disappears within weeks. During this period, the attenuation of the hematoma slowly changes from the periphery to the center, becoming isodense relative to brain parenchyma within a week and hypodense thereafter. Complete CT resolution may take a month or more, depending on the size.

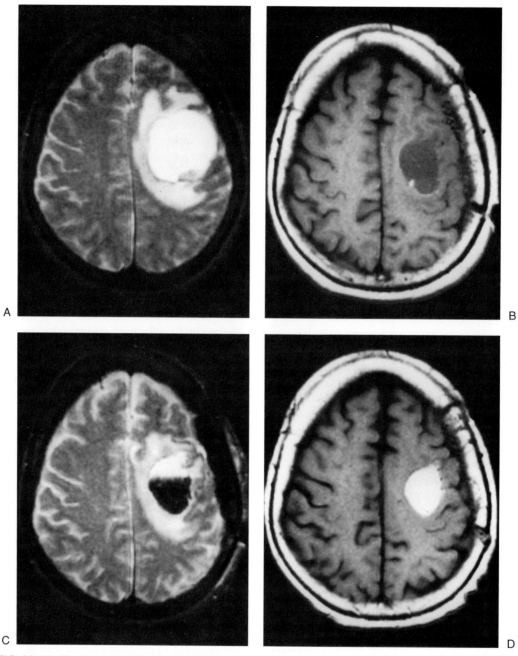

FIG. IA-17. Postoperative hemorrhage following resection of a glioblastoma in a 62-year-old woman.
A: Preoperative axial T$_2$-weighted (2000/80) CSE MR demonstrates a hyperintense left parietal lesion
with surrounding edema. Surgical resection revealed glioblastoma multiforme. **B:** Unenhanced axial
T$_1$-weighted (800/20) CSE MR obtained 6 days following surgery shows a left craniotomy associated
with a hypointense left parietal lesion with a thin hyperintense, irregular layer posteriorly. **C:** Axial T$_2$-
weighted (2000/80) CSE MR obtained at the same time as **B** shows a fluid−fluid level in the left
parietal lesion with a markedly hypointense dependent component corresponding to deoxyhemoglobin.
There is continuing perilesional edema. **D:** Unenhanced axial T$_1$-weighted (600/20) CSE MR obtained
20 days after **B** and **C** later shows homogeneous hyperintensity of the left parietal lesion. **E:** Axial T$_2$-
weighted (2000/80) CSE MR obtained at the same time as **D** shows that the center of the lesion is
also hyperintense on this sequence corresponding to methemoglobin. A thin hypointense rim (*arrow*)
represents a layer of hemosiderin in the wall of the hematoma. Note the reduction in the perilesional
edema (compare with **A** and **C**).

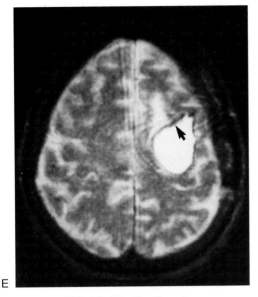

FIG. IA-17. *Continued.*

The majority of intracranial hemorrhages can be easily detected on CT, but small petechial hemorrhages and small clots adjacent to the cranial vault or base of the skull may be difficult to detect because of their similar density to the brain parenchyma and nearness to hyperdense bone, utilizing standard imaging techniques. Changing the viewing parameters (e.g., window level and width) may often be helpful. In addition, acute hematomas may appear isodense as compared to brain in patients with severe anemia (i.e., hemoglobin below 8 g/dl), and, therefore, they may be difficult or impossible visualize on CT in the absence of mass effect. Also, coagulopathy and rehemorrhaging can profoundly affect the appearance of the blood clot. For example, repeated hemorrhage not infrequently results in a friable clot of mixed density that may exhibit a fluid–fluid level(s).

The explanation for the signal characteristics of intracranial hemorrhages on MR is more complex and is still a subject of some debate. The MR signal from a hematoma is dramatically influenced by the oxidation state of the iron-containing hemoglobin, its water content, site and age of the blood clot, integrity of the red blood cells, hematocrit, and the protein content of the clot (20–26).

The ability of the MR to detect blood and blood products varies with the pulse sequence used and the field strength of the magnet (i.e., higher-field-strength magnets are more sensitive to some blood products). Gradient-recalled echo sequences are very sensitive to magnetically susceptible blood products, whereas fast spin-echo sequences are relatively insensitive in detecting blood and its breakdown products. The MR appearances of hemorrhage most commonly encountered in clinical practice utilizing a 1.5-Tesla magnet are discussed below (20–26).

Hyperacute hemorrhage (e.g., a few minutes to a few hours) still contains oxygenated hemoglobin within intact red blood cells. Oxyhemoglobin is diamagnetic and is not susceptible to the magnetic field. During this stage, the MR signal is mostly related to the high protein and water content of the hemorrhage. Therefore, hyperacute clot on T_1-weighted imaging appears isointense to gray matter while on T_2-weighted acquisitions it becomes relatively hyperintense.

In acute clot (e.g., 12 hr to 3 days), the oxyhemoglobin loses oxygen and slowly changes to deoxyhemoglobin. The red blood cells shrink, the clot retracts, and edema around the clot becomes evident. Deoxyhemoglobin, because of its profound magnetic susceptibility, produces T_2 shortening, leading to moderate loss of signal on T_2-weighted imaging. T_1 relaxation is largely unaffected. The clot remains relatively isointense or slightly hypointense on T_1-weighted imaging, while on T_2-weighted acquisitions it becomes hypointense compared to gray matter.

In subacute clot (e.g., 4 days to 1 month), two important changes take place. These alterations start from the periphery and spread to the center. The deoxyhemoglobin within the intact but crenated red blood cell is gradually converted into methemoglobin, which is profoundly paramagnetic. The intracellular methemoglobin is responsible for the signal change of the clot only in the early subacute phase. In the late subacute phase (e.g., 1 week to 1 month),

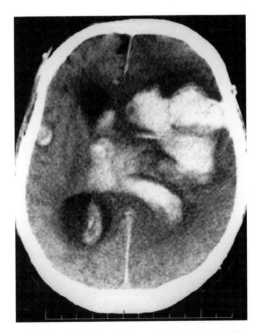

FIG. IA-18. Cerebral hemorrhage in a 42-year-old man on anticoagulant therapy (warfarin) presenting with sudden loss of consciousness. Unenhanced axial CT shows a large left hemispheric hemorrhage involving the basal ganglia and parietal and frontal lobes associated with marked mass effect. Hemorrhage is also present in the right parietal lobe and within the cerebral ventricles. Ventricular dilatation is present, indicating hydrocephalus.

the red blood cell disintegrates, releasing the methemoglobin into the interstitium (i.e., extracellular methemoglobin). Subsequently, a perivascular inflammatory reaction ensues that in part accounts for the ring enhancement observed on MR after i.v. contrast administration during this stage of the resolving hematoma. The paramagnetic methemoglobin produces a dramatic change in the MR signal characteristics of the blood clot. In the early subacute phase, the intracellular methemoglobin is hyperintense on T_1-weighted imaging, while on T_2-weighted acquisitions it is very hypointense. In the late subacute phase, the concentration of the extracellular methemoglobin increases from the periphery to the center of the hematoma. Extracellular methemoglobin appears hyperintense on both T_1- and T_2-weighted images. Over a period of time, edema around the clot also decreases.

In chronic hematomas (e.g., 1 month to 1 year or more), as the perivascular inflammatory response ensues, the activated macrophages and scavenger cells migrate into the blood clot. They engulf the extracellular methemoglobin from the hematoma and deposit it in the vascularized wall of the hematoma, converting it into ferritin and hemosiderin. Simultaneously, healing promotes the formation of a glial scar. The size of the hematoma and the edema also decrease significantly, until it eventually becomes a hemosiderin-laden scar. Hemosiderin and ferritin may persist in the scar for years. The presence of hemosiderin, beginning in the periphery of the hematoma, causes the MR signal to be hypointense on both T_1- and T_2-weighted imaging (20–26).

Postoperative Site: Residual Tumor

Postoperative CT frequently shows contrast enhancement in the surgical bed (3,4,95,96). This benign postoperative enhancement of the brain parenchyma may mimic residual enhancing tumor, making the interpretation of such lesions difficult. The presence of residual tumor has important therapeutic implications and may adversely affect the life expectancy of the patient. Thus, differentiation of surgically related alteration from residual tumor becomes important, both for the patient and for the surgeon. The mechanisms underlying nonneoplastic postoperative enhancement are not fully understood, but a breach in the blood–brain barrier, neovascularization, luxury perfusion, abnormal autoregulation, and granulation tissue have all been implicated (3,4,71,95,96). Computed tomographic studies performed to evaluate contrast enhancement of the brain after surgery in patients with brain tumor have demonstrated that tumor-free operative margins have enhanced as early as the fifth postoperative day (3,4,71,95,96). Thus, any mass-like, intense enhancement in the surgical bed prior to the fifth postoperative day may suggest unresected tumor. Benign enhancement becomes intense and ring-like at 2 to 4 weeks; this pattern

may persist for approximately 3 months or more after surgery. Persistence of parenchymal ring enhancement beyond 3 to 6 months should suggest a pathologic process other than benign postoperative change (4).

This being understood, it is recommended that a baseline enhanced CT scan should be performed within 3 to 4 days after surgery in order to assess for enhancing residual tumor (3,95,96). In the absence of such an early baseline study after surgery, it may be impossible to differentiate benign surgical change from residual tumor during the second postoperative week (5).

In addition to CT, MR has also been used to evaluate the postoperative brain. Because of its better spatial and contrast resolution, MR scans are more sensitive to the presence of Gd than CT is to iodinated contrast agents, and MR is capable of revealing minute enhancing lesions that may not be visible on CT. Unlike CT, acute postoperative blood at the surgical site can usually be differentiated from enhancing residual tumor on MR because of the MR signal characteristics of blood and its breakdown products during the first 4 days after surgery. However, subsequently, with conversion of oxyhemoglobin and deoxyhemoglobin to methemoglobin, this differentiation becomes extremely difficult. It has been suggested that early Gd-enhanced postoperative MR is the radiologic procedure of choice for evaluating for residual enhancing tumor. It is recommended that this baseline Gd-enhanced MR study should be performed within 3 to 4 days after surgery (5).

Recurrent Mass Lesion

A number of different mass lesions may be encountered on CT and MR in the late postoperative period. These lesions may be residual or recurrent, malignant or benign in nature. Intravenous Gd-enhanced MR is currently the investigation of choice for the evaluation of these masses (5). In the chronic phase, after surgery, in the absence of T_2-weighted abnormality in the brain surrounding the resection site and without evidence of gadolinium enhancement, the MR examination should be interpreted as showing no evidence of recurrence (Fig. IA-19). Although paramagnetic contrast enhancement can localize the site of a breach in the blood–brain barrier, it cannot differentiate the microscopic tumor margin from parenchymal necrosis and surrounding edema. Recurrent tumor arises most commonly from microscopic tumor cells left in situ beyond the surgically resected margin. Studies have shown that 80% of recurrent tumors grow within 2 cm of the original tumor bed (97). Recurrent tumor appears as a mass lesion with or without enhancement at the site of resection (see Figs. IA-8 and IA-23). Posttherapeutic CT scans of patients on corticosteroids should be interpreted with caution, as the reduced edema and decreased tumor enhancement may be misinterpreted as tumor ab-

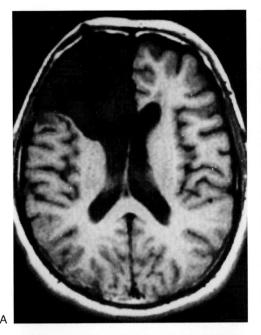

A

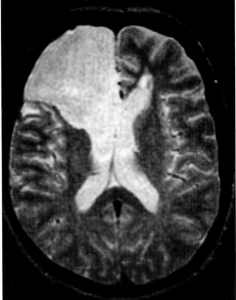

B

C

FIG. IA-19. No recurrence in a 43-year-old man presenting 6 months following resection of a right frontal glioblastoma multiforme. **A:** Unenhanced axial T$_1$-weighted (417/20) CSE MR shows the right frontal lobe resection site without mass effect. **B:** Axial T$_2$-weighted (2150/80) CSE MR demonstrates CSF-like signal in the right frontal surgical bed. **C:** Enhanced axial T$_1$-weighted (530/20) CSE MR shows no abnormal enhancement.

sence or regression (98). Some astrocytomas and many hemangioblastomas commonly regrow as cystic lesions with enhancing mural nodules. Usually the fluid in a cystic tumor has a somewhat higher attenuation than CSF on CT. Other primary CNS tumors with a propensity to recur are glioblastoma multiforme, pineal region tumors, choroid plexus tumors, meningioma, and epidermoid tumors. Besides CT and MR, angiography can be useful in the evaluation of highly vascular recurrent or residual lesions such as glioblastomas, hemangioblastomas, and meningiomas; PET with ^{18}F-FDG has also been found by some to be useful in differentiating metabolically active residual or recurrent tumor from benign postoperative changes (8).

Sequelae of Cranial Radiation and Chemotherapy

Diffuse Radiation-Induced Leukoencephalopathy

Radiation-induced leukoencephalopathy is a late clinical manifestation of diffuse white matter injury to the brain (6). The pathophysiology underlying the clinical encephalopathy includes parenchymal white matter demyelination and small vessel occlusion (99). After a latent period of several months to years following irradiation of a large volume of brain parenchyma, diffuse periventricular demyelination occurs that generally spares the compact subcortical "U" fibers (6). On MR, the periventricular white matter injury appears as symmetric, multifocal, or confluent scalloped bands of hyperintensity on proton density and T_2-weighted images. Corresponding T_1-weighted images reveal low signal within the white matter (99–110). These regions of abnormal signal extend from the frontal to the occipital region. The corpus callosum, internal capsule, basal ganglia, and posterior fossa are usually not affected. On CT, these CNS abnormalities appear as low attenuation within the hemispheric white matter (Fig. IA-20). Most patients with these MR and CT abnormalities are asymptomatic; however, if they are clinically affected, impairment of mental function is the most prominent feature (111). Remyelination and reversal of microvascular occlusion may occur in some patients, but in 60% to 66% of the cases, the white matter injury is associated with irreversible generalized cerebral atrophy (99,100,112).

Chemotherapy-Induced Leukoencephalopathy

Chemotherapy administered as an adjunct to radiotherapy seems to potentiate its neurotoxicity. Necrotizing leukoencephalopathy and mineralizing microangiopathy are commonly seen after intrathecal or systemic administration of methotrexate, used in the CNS prophylaxis of acute lymphocyhtic leukemia in children. On CT and MR, the diffuse white matter changes resemble those seen after cranial irradiation alone (113–123). In the acute phase, areas of gray–white matter junction enhancement may be seen in some cases following i.v. contrast agent administration (Fig. IA-21).

Radiation Necrosis

Focal or diffuse brain injury may occur as a complication of radiation therapy or interstitial brachytherapy of primary or secondary tumors of the brain or after radiation treatment for head and neck tumors and AVMs (6,55,100–110,124–126). Acute focal necrosis of the brain is a rare but delayed complication of irradiation. Seventy percent of cases occur within 2 years of the cranial radiation therapy (107). Radiation necrosis histologically represents coagulation necrosis of white matter. This is accompanied by fibrinoid necrosis of the vessels in the acute phase surrounded by neovascular proliferation in the late phase. Angiographically, radiation necrosis is seen as an avascular mass lesion at the site of the previously irradiated tumor; however, it can occur at a distance from the primary lesion in the same hemisphere or even on the contralateral side (108). On contrast-enhanced CT or MR, radiation necrosis appears as an irregular solid–nodular or ring-enhancing lesion with central low attenuation. Not uncommonly, the lesions of radiation necrosis may be multifocal (Fig. IA-22). In some cases, radiation necrosis will coexist with recurrent neoplasia (Fig. IA-23). Such lesions show prolongation of T_1 and T_2 relaxation times on unenhanced MR. The lesion of radiation necrosis is typically surrounded by considerable vasogenic edema. Histopathologic data are often required in order to confirm the diagnosis of radiation necrosis (104–109).

It has been suggested that PET imaging with ^{18}F-FDG may be able to differentiate a metabolically active tumor

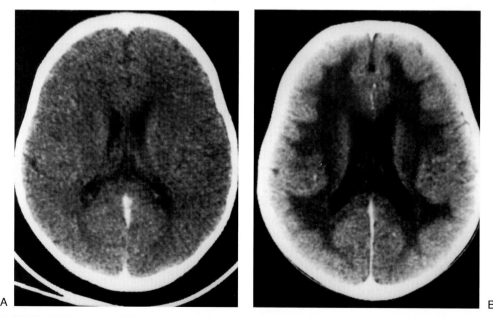

FIG. IA-20. Diffuse necrotizing leukoencephalopathy in a 5-year-old boy presenting after whole-brain radiotherapy for posterior fossa medulloblastoma. **A:** Preradiotherapy enhanced axial CT shows no abnormalities. **B:** Enhanced axial CT obtained 5 months following radiotherapy shows diffuse hypodensity of the hemispheric white matter bilaterally.

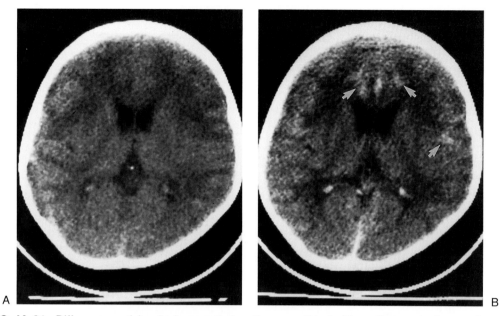

FIG. IA-21. Diffuse necrotizing leukoencephalopathy associated with methotrexate therapy in a 9-year-old boy with acute lymphocytic leukemia. **A:** Unenhanced axial CT shows diffuse hypodensity of the white matter. **B:** Enhanced axial CT shows scattered areas of gray–white matter junction enhancement (*arrows*).

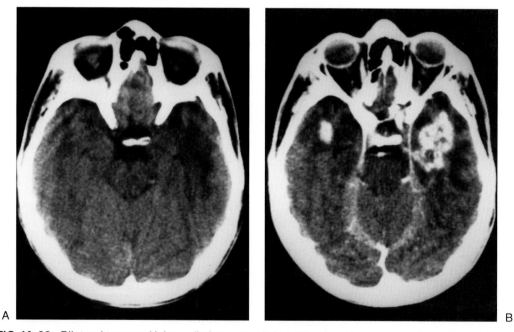

FIG. IA-22. Bilateral temporal lobe radiation necrosis in a 19-year-old man presenting with a history of radiation therapy 5 years earlier for nasopharyngeal carcinoma. **A:** Unenhanced axial CT demonstrates hypodense areas in both temporal lobes, larger on the left than the right. **B:** Enhanced axial CT demonstrates irregularly enhancing lesions in the right and left temporal lobes.

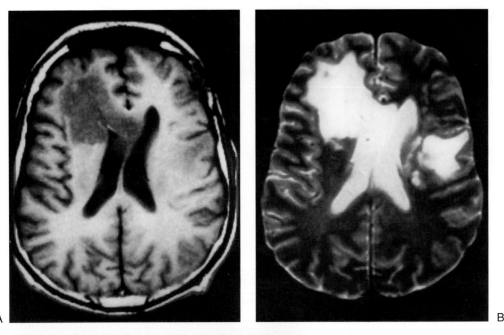

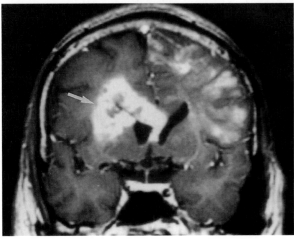

FIG. IA-23. Cerebral radiation necrosis and recurrent astrocytoma in a 40-year-old man presenting with progressive mental deterioration following radiation therapy 4 years earlier for cerebral astrocytoma. **A:** Unenhanced axial T_1-weighted (600/15) CSE MR shows a hypointense right frontal mass that extends to the left hemisphere through the corpus callosum. Note also compression of the anterior horn of the right lateral ventricle and sulcal effacement in the left parietal lobe. **B:** Axial T_2-weighted (2500/80) CSE MR shows the right frontal lesion to be hyperintense with surrounding perilesional edema. Note also a left parietal hyperintense area in the left parietal region. **C:** Enhanced coronal T_1-weighted (600/15) CSE MR shows marked enhancement of the right-sided mass (*arrow:* recurrent astrocytoma) and multifocal enhancement throughout the left parietal area (radiation necrosis).

from hypometabolic radiation necrosis. However, PET imaging is limited by its inability to distinguish radiation necrosis from other hypometabolic lesions such as hematomas or well-differentiated relatively metabolically inactive tumors (8,107,127).

Radiation-Induced Secondary Tumors

Radiation-induced neoplasms of the brain following therapeutic cranial irradiation are rare (88–92). Both benign and malignant tumors develop after cranial irradiation. Commonly encountered neoplasms include meningioma, fibrosarcoma, and glioma (128–132). Meningiomas have been reported to follow radiation treatment of the scalp for tinea capitis or vascular nevi (89), primary sarcomas have occurred after radiotherapy treatment of pituitary adenoma (88), and a histologic spectrum of gliomas have been observed after

irradiation of a number of primary brain tumors during childhood (127,130–132).

As would be expected, the radiation-induced tumor arises in the previously irradiated zone (Fig. IA-24). The age of the patient and site of these induced tumors have been found to be significantly different from those seen in the general population. They show rapid growth and aggressive histology and are histologically different from the previous tumor or lesion for which radiation was initially administered (130). For instance, radiation-induced meningiomas show high cellularity, numerous giant cells, and gross nuclear pleomorphism, which are not seen in meningiomas not related to prior radiation (128).

Osmotic Myelinolysis

White matter demyelination can occur as a complication of other forms of medical management. Osmotic my-

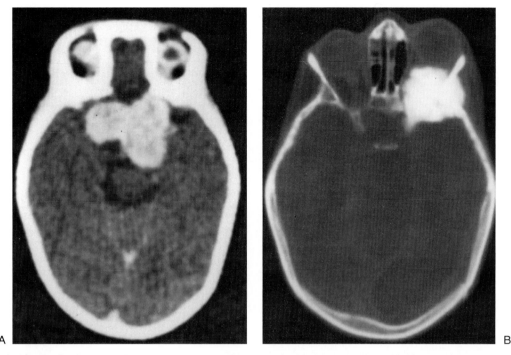

FIG. IA-24. Radiation-induced osteosarcoma in a 5-year-old girl presenting with history of optic glioma treated with radiotherapy. **A:** Pretreatment enhanced axial CT shows a markedly enhancing lobulated mass (optic glioma) in the suprasellar region. The lesion was subsequently treated with radiotherapy. **B:** Axial CT with bone window filming obtained 5 years after the study depicted in **A** shows a densely calcified spiculated mass (osteosarcoma) involving the sphenoid bone on the left.

elinolysis (OM), or central pontine myelinolysis, frequently occurs as a result of rapid correction of hyponatremia, although hypernatremia itself has also been implicated (133,134). The signs of OM develop after a delay of 1 to 6 days or more after rapid correction of the hyponatremic state (135). Osmotic demyelination commonly involves the ventral pons and may extend into the cerebellar peduncles symmetrically, with relative sparing of the descending corticospinal tracts. Extrapontine locations that may also be involved in this pathologic process include basal ganglia, thalamus, lateral geniculate body, subcortical white matter, and the white matter of the cerebellum (133,136,137). Myelinolysis appears as a hypodense area in the pons on unenhanced CT (138). An increase in the water content of the lesion is demonstrated as prolongation of T_1 and T_2 relaxation on MR. A typical "butterfly" or "bat-wing" pattern may be seen in the pons on T_2-weighted MR sequences (Fig. IA-25). Most of these lesions do not enhance after i.v. contrast administration, although there may be exceptions to this general rule (139). The signal abnormalities associated with OM are nonspecific and have also been demonstrated after radiotherapy, chemotherapy, infarction, multiple sclerosis, neoplasia, and encephalitis (140,141).

Focal Cerebral Atrophy

On CT and MR, cerebral atrophy consists of an increase in size of the cranial CSF spaces at the expense of a loss of brain parenchyma. These changes are more commonly generalized than focal. In addition to a number of degenerative diseases, chemotherapy, radiotherapy, and some drugs may also be responsible for the loss of brain parenchyma. Determining the cause of atrophy on the basis of imaging alone is usually difficult or impossible.

The atrophy may be more pronounced in one area than another. For example, moderate to marked cerebellar atrophy is known to occur after phenytoin (Dilantin) therapy (Fig. IA-26) (142–147). Furthermore, the atrophy caused by phenytoin spares the cerebral hemispheres. On imaging the sulcal spaces of the cerebellum and the superior cerebellar and cerebellopontine angle, cisterns enlarge. The fourth ventricle may also be passively expanded. Other posttherapeutic causes of regional or focal atrophy include focused cranial radiation, degeneration of the red nucleus after dentate nucleus resection, and encephalomalacia resulting from surgery on extraaxial tumors (Fig. IA-27) (148,149).

Diffuse Cerebral Atrophy

Slowly progressive neuronal degeneration and death are responsible for the loss of brain parenchyma in global cerebral atrophy. This is a "normal" part of aging. The onset of diffuse posttherapeutic atrophy is usually slow and is often detected long after the initial insult. The nonspecific irreversible injury accounts for enlarged cere-

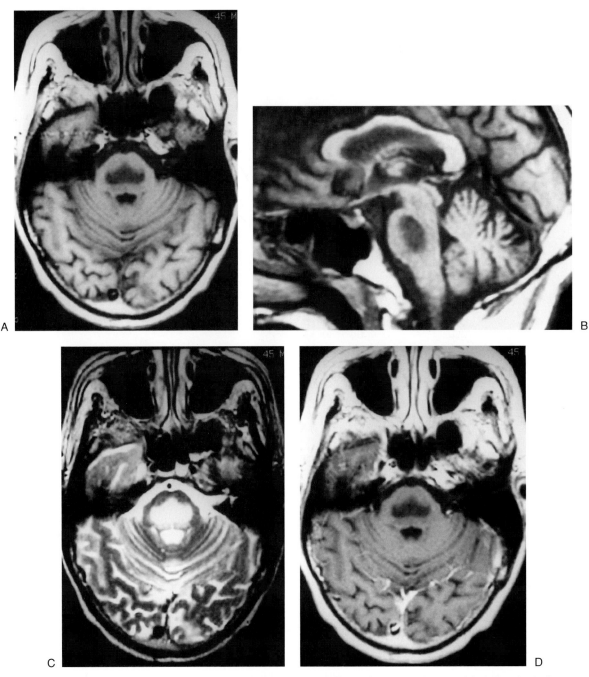

FIG. IA-25. Osmotic demyelination (central pontine myelinolysis) in a 45-year-old male alcoholic presenting with coma following rapid correction of hyponatremia. **A:** Unenhanced axial T₁-weighted (500/16) CSE MR demonstrates a well-circumscribed hypointense central pontine lesion. Note the "bat-wing" configuration of the pathologic process. **B:** Unenhanced sagittal T₁-weighted (600/11) CSE MR also shows the hypointense lesion in the pons. **C:** Axial T₂-weighted (3500/102) FSE MR shows the pontine lesion to be hyperintense. **D:** Enhanced axial T₁-weighted (600/11) demonstrates no enhancement of the pontine lesion.

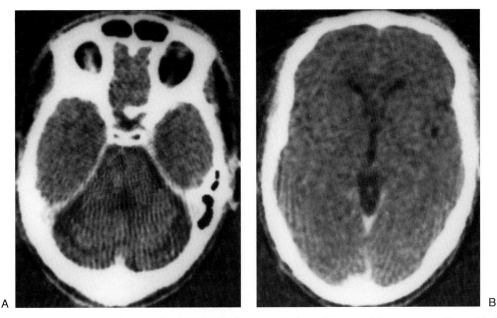

FIG. IA-26. Phenytoin-related selective cerebellar atrophy in a 38-year-old man presenting with 20-year history of seizures treated with phenytoin and phenobarbital. **A:** Enhanced axial CT through the posterior fossa shows cerebellar atrophy. **B:** Enhanced axial CT through the supratentorial region is normal.

bral ventricles, prominent cortical sulci, and dilated subarachnoid cisterns. Treatment-related atrophy is often caused by chemotherapy (e.g., methotrexate) and cranial irradiation, coupled with malnutrition and primary CNS disease. These factors operate singly or in combination to produce a spectrum of abnormalities ranging from reversible insult to irreversible atrophy (150,151).

Reversible Cerebral Shrinkage

Generalized loss of brain volume may not be associated with any absolute neuronal loss (152). A loss of brain water or protein catabolism, or both, is said to be responsible for this "reversible cerebral shrinkage" (153,154). Such shrinkage is commonly seen after steroid administration (Fig. IA-28). Besides exogenous steroid therapy, reversible cerebral shrinkage may be seen on imaging in patients with anorexia nervosa, childhood malnutrition, Cushing syndrome, patients on ACTH therapy, and, to a degree, in alcoholics following recent abstention. Reversible cerebral shrinkage has also been documented in the long term after radiation and chemotherapy (150,155).

Calcification

Mineralizing microangiopathy is seen in 25% to 30% of children who survive more than nine months following administration of intrathecal methotrexate and cranial irradiation (Fig. IA-9) (50,156). Dystrophic calcification is the hallmark of this microangiopathy. On CT, vascular calcification is seen in the basal ganglia, especially in the putamen, the subcortical gray and white matter junctions, and the cortical gray matter (6,7,157–160). These findings are frequently associated with white matter hypodensities and cerebral atrophy. Mineralization has a hyperintense signal on both T_1- and T_2-weighted MR sequences. T_1 shortening as a result of dystrophic calcification may potentially simulate hemorrhage in these cases on MR. Pontine calcification has also been documented after radiotherapy for suprasellar tumor (161), and extensive parenchymal calcifications have been reported in childhood survivors of medulloblastoma after surgery and radiotherapy (162). Finally, it is well known and expected that some successfully treated infectious granulomas will go on to calcify.

Hydrocephalus

Computed tomography has been very helpful in the evaluation of the postoperative course of hydrocephalus (163). A decrease in ventricular size, disappearance of periventricular lucency, and restoration of the cortical mantle are readily observed in children following successful shunting of hydrocephalus. However, the seemingly simple procedure of ventricular drainage is associated with a number of complications. In the acute postoperative phase following shunt placement, hemorrhage into the ventricles and parenchyma may be seen (Fig. IA-29). Malposition of the shunt tube intracranially requiring repositioning is easily demonstrated by CT.

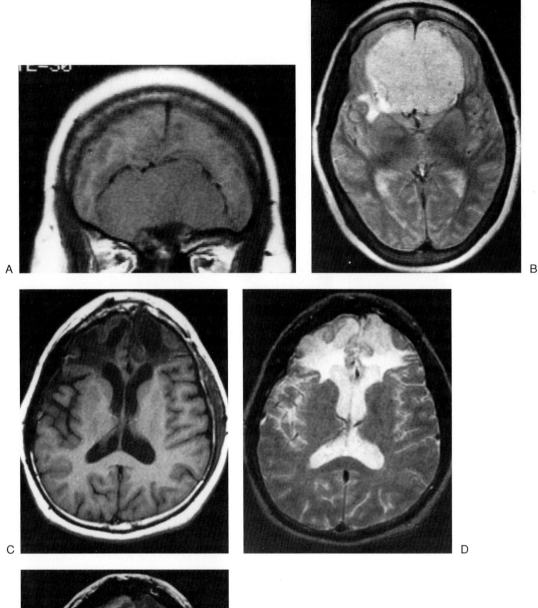

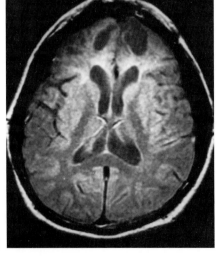

FIG. IA-27. Postsurgical encephalomalacia in a 60-year-old woman presenting with headache. **A:** Presurgical coronal T_1-weighted (500/30) CSE MR demonstrates an extraaxial midline frontal isointense mass. Surgical resection revealed meningioma. **B:** Presurgical axial T_2-weighted (2000/80) CSE MR shows the hyperintense midline frontal mass (meningioma). **C:** Unenhanced axial T_1-weighted (417/20) CSE MR obtained 5 years after surgical resection of the meningioma shows hypointense areas in the frontal lobes associated with thinning of the cortex representing encephalomalacia. **D:** Axial T_2-weighted (2200/80) CSE MR shows that both frontal lobes are hyperintense. **E:** Axial proton density (2200/30) CSE MR shows the central areas of the frontal lesion to be hypointense (macrocytic encephalomalacia) (*arrows*) surrounded by hyperintense signal (microcytic encephalomalacia and gliosis).

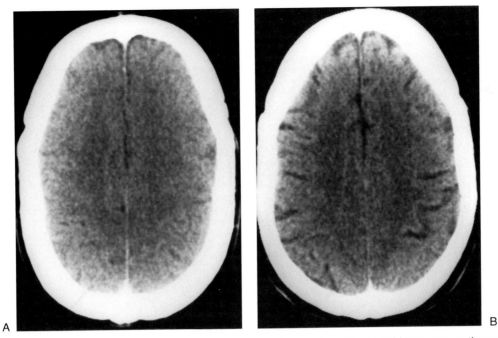

FIG. IA-28. Cerebral shrinkage on exogenous steroid therapy in a 45-year-old man presenting with recurrent headaches. **A:** Initial unenhanced axial CT shows no abnormality. **B:** Unenhanced axial CT acquired 1 month after **A** and following 1 month of exogenous steroid therapy shows diffuse enlargement of the cortical sulci compatible with cerebral shrinkage.

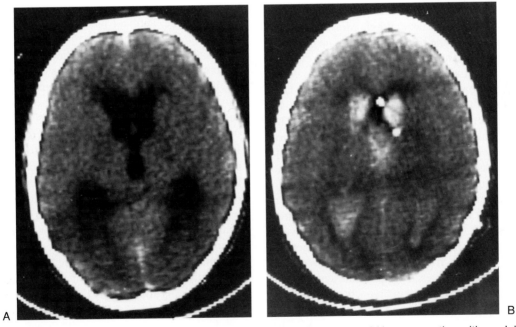

FIG. IA-29. Intraventricular hemorrhage following shunting in a 5-year-old boy presenting with medulloblastoma and hydrocephalus. **A:** Preshunting unenhanced axial CT demonstrates hydrocephalus. **B:** Unenhanced axial CT following shunt placement shows intraventricular hemorrhage. Two hyperdense shunt tubes are noted anteriorly.

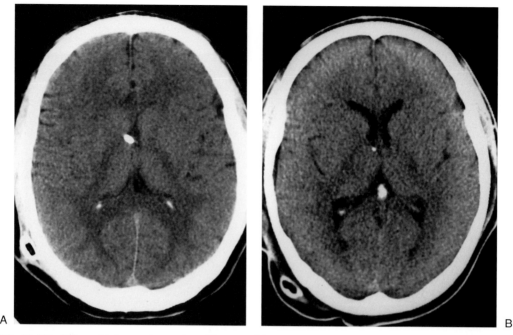

FIG. IA-30. Slit ventricle syndrome in a 28-year-old man with a chronically placed ventricular shunt who developed severe low-pressure headaches (when upright) followed by continuous headaches and dizziness. The headaches resolved following placement of a low-pressure valve and antisiphon device in the shunt line. **A:** Initial unenhanced axial CT shows very small ventricles (slit ventricles). **B:** Subsequent unenhanced axial CT shows normal-size ventricles following placement of low-pressure valve and antisiphon device in the shunt line.

On the other hand, slit-like ventricles can also be seen on CT in shunted hydrocephalic children. Most such cases are asymptomatic, but some patients present with the "slit ventricle syndrome." This is a poorly understood clinical entity that refers to the development of headache, vomiting, and some impairment of consciousness in the face of collapsed (i.e., "slit") ventricles (Fig. IA-30) (164). The ventricles in effect seem to be "over" shunted. The placement of a valve on the shunt drainage line that prevents excessively rapid emptying of ventricular fluid will often correct the clinical syndrome; at the same time, the ventricles gain slightly in volume. On the other hand, a too-rapid decompression of dilated ventricles can lead to the development of extracerebral collections (e.g., hygromas or hematomas) (17). Disappearance of the periventricular lucencies following correction of the hydrocephalus is believed to result from resorption of extracellular fluid. However, in some cases, these periventricular hypodensities observed on CT may remain unchanged or even increase after surgical intervention. This is thought to be an expression of irreversible cerebral damage. The hypodensity is attributed to axonal swelling, demyelination, atrophy, and gliosis (165). The CT may show ventricular asymmetry, septations, dilatation, entrapment, or compartmentalization following treatment of aseptic, chemical, or infectious ventriculitis (166,167).

CONCLUSIONS

Imaging of the posttherapeutic cranium requires a thorough and accurate knowledge of the original pathology as well as the surgical and/or medical treatment that a patient has undergone. The time elapsed since surgical intervention can alter the significance and interpretation of certain imaging findings such as contrast enhancement or air in and around the surgical bed. The use of steroids can reduce the sensitivity of contrast-enhanced CT or MR scans for the detection of breakdowns in the blood–brain barrier as well as predispose patients to opportunistic infections. The CT is usually sufficient for the evaluation of such acute postoperative complications as parenchymal hemorrhage, extraaxial collections, brain edema, and hydrocephalus. The MR is more useful in the evaluation of residual or recurrent tumor, infection, and white matter changes associated with radiation or chemotherapy. Although cerebral angiography in general has a more limited role than CT or MR, it is still the modality of choice for the posttherapeutic analysis of vascular pathology such as determining the success of an aneurysm clipping and identifying a residual AVM nidus after treatment.

REFERENCES

1. De La Paz RL, Davis KR: Postoperative imaging of the posterior fossa. In: Taveras JM, Ferrucci JT, eds. *Radiology Diagnosis, Imaging, Intervention Vol 3. Neuroradiology and Radiology of the Head and Neck* (Chapter 75). Philadelphia: JB Lippincott, 1988: 1–11.
2. Takahashi M, Korogi Y: Supratentorial neoplasms: post-operative changes. In: Taveras JM, Ferrucci JT, eds. *Radiology Diagnosis, Imaging, Intervention Vol 3. Neuroradiology and Radiology of the*

Head and Neck (Chapter 57). Philadelphia: JB Lippincott, 1988: 1–10.

3. Jeffries BF, Kishore PRS, Singh KS, Ghatak NR, Krempa J: Contrast enhancement in the postoperative brain. *Radiology* 1981; 139: 409–413.

4. Jeffries BF, Kishore PRS, Singh KS, Ghatak NR, Krempa J: Postoperative computed tomographic changes in the brain. An experimental study. *Radiology* 1980; 135: 751–753.

5. Forsting M, Albert FK, Kunze S, Adams HP, Zenner D, Sartor K: Extirpation of glioblastomas: MR and CT follow-up of residual tumor and regrowth patterns. *Am J Neuroradiol* 1993; 14: 77–87.

6. Boyko OB: Neuroimaging of radiation injury to the central nervous system. *Neuroimaging Clin North Am* 1993; 3: 803–816.

7. Valk PE, Dillon WP: Radiation injury of the brain. *Am J Neuroradiol* 1991; 12: 45–62.

8. Kim EE, Chung SK, Haynie TP, et al: Differentiation of residual or recurrent tumors from post-treatment changes with F-18 FDG PET. *RadioGraphics* 1992; 12: 269–279.

9. Elster AD, DiPersio DA: Cranial postoperative site: assessment with contrast-enhanced MR imaging. *Radiology* 1990; 174: 93–98.

10. Lanzieri CF, Larkins M, Mancall A, et al: Cranial postoperative site: MR imaging appearance. *Am J Neuroradiol* 1988; 9: 27–34.

11. Marion DW: Complications of head injury and their therapy. *Neurosurg Clin North Am* 1991; 2: 411–424.

12. Blomstedt GC: Craniotomy infections. *Neurosurg Clin North Am* 1992; 3: 375–385.

13. Gordon L, Buncke HJ, Alpert BS: Free latissimus dorsi muscle flap with split-thickness skin graft cover: A report of 16 cases. *Plast Reconstruct Surg* 1982; 70: 173–178.

14. Maxwell GP, Manson PN, Hoopes JE: Experience with 13 latissimus dorsi myocutaneous free flaps. *Plast Reconstruct Surg* 1979; 64: 1–8.

15. Tsuchiya K, Makita K, Furui S, Kusano S, Inoue Y: Contrast-enhanced magnetic resonance imaging of sub- and epidural empyemas. *Neuroradiology* 1992; 34: 494–496.

16. Kasdon DL, Magruder MR, Stevens EA, Paullus WS: Bilateral interhemispheric subdural hematomas. *Neurosurgery* 1979; 5: 57–59.

17. Tjan TG, Aarts NJM: Bifrontal epidural haematoma after shunt operation and posterior fossa exploration. Report of a case with survival. *Neuroradiology* 1980; 19: 51–53.

18. Nixon KT, Hudgins PA, Davis PC, O'Brien MS, Hudgins RJ, Hoffman JC: Delayed intracranial hemorrhage in children after suboccipital craniectomy. *Am J Roentgenol* 1994; 163: 897–900.

19. Iplikcioglu AC, Akkas O, Sungur R: Ossified chronic subdural hematoma: Case report. *J Trauma* 1991; 31: 272–295.

20. Taber KH, Ford JJ, Hayman LA. Magnetic resonance imaging appearance of hemorrhage: Sources of imaging contrast. *Neuro Clin North Am* 1992; 2: 61–74.

21. Hayman LA, Pagani JJ, Kirkpatrick JB, Hinck VC: Pathophysiology of acute intracerebral and subarachnoid hemorrhage: Applications to MR imaging. *Am J Neuroradiol* 1989; 10: 457–461.

22. Bradley WG: MR appearance of hemorrhage in the brain. *Radiology* 1993; 189: 15–26.

23. Barkovich AJ, Atlas SW: Magnetic resonance imaging of intracranial hemorrhage. *Radiol Clin North Am* 1988; 26: 801–820.

24. Gomori JM, Grossman RI, Steiner I: High-field magnetic resonance imaging of intracranial hematomas. *Isr J Med Sci* 1988; 24: 218–223.

25. Gomori JM, Grossman RI, Goldberg HI, Zimmerman RA, Bilaniuk LT: Intracranial hematomas: Imaging by high-field MR. *Radiology* 1985; 157: 87–93.

26. Zimmerman RD, Heier LA, Snow RB, Liu DPC, Kelly AB, Deck MDF: Acute intracranial hemorrhage: Intensity changes on sequential MR scans at 0.5T. *Am J Roentgenol* 1988; 150: 651–661.

27. Gomori JM, Grossman RI, Hackney DB, Goldbert HI, Zimmerman RA, Bilaniuk LT: Variable appearances of subacute intracranial hematomas on high-field spin-echo MR. *Am J Neuroradiol* 1987; 1019–1026.

28. Burke JW, Podrasky AE, Bradley WG: Meninges: Benign postoperative enhancement on MR images. *Radiology* 1990; 174: 99–102.

29. Natelson SE, Dyer ML, Harp DL: Delayed CSF seeding of benign oligodendroglioma. *South Med J* 1992; 85: 1011–1012.

30. Packer RJ, Allen J, Nielsen S, Petito C, Deck M, Jereb B: Brainstem glioma: Clinical manifestations of meningeal gliomatosis. *Am Neurol* 1983; 14: 177–182.

31. Kumar A, Aggarwal S, Willinsky R, TerBrugge KG: Posterior fossa surgery: An unusual cause of superficial siderosis. *Neurosurgery* 1993; 32: 455–457.

32. Janss AJ, Galetta SL, Freese A, et al: Superficial siderosis of the central nervous system: magnetic resonance imaging and pathological correlation. *J Neurosurg* 1993; 79: 756–760.

33. Fitz CR: Inflammatory diseases of the brain in childhood. *Am J Neuroradiol* 1992; 13: 551–567.

34. Finlayson AI, Penfield W: Acute postoperative aseptic leptomeningitis: Review of cases and discussion of pathogenesis. *Arch Neurol Psychiatry* 1941; 46: 250–276.

35. Arita N, Taneda M, Hayakawa T: Leptomeningeal dissemination of malignant gliomas. Incidence, diagnosis and outcome. *Acta Neurochir (Wien)* 1994; 126: 84–92.

36. Davis PC, Friedman NC, Fry SM, Malko JA, Hoffmann JC, Braun IF: Leptomeningeal metastasis: MR imaging. *Radiology* 1987; 163: 449–454.

37. Renaudin JW, DiTullio MV, Brown WJ: Seeding of intracranial ependymomas in children. *Child's Brain* 1979; 5: 408–412.

38. Rippe DJ, Boyko OB, Friedman HS, et al: Gd-DTPA-enhanced MR imaging of leptomeningeal spread of primary intracranial CNS tumor in children. *Am J Neuroradiol* 1990; 11: 329–332.

39. Stanley P, Senac MO, Segall HD: Intraspinal seeding from intracranial tumors in children. *Am J Neuroradiol* 1984; 5: 805–809.

40. Yousem DM, Patrone PM, Grossman RI. Leptomeningeal metastases: MR evaluation. *J Comput Assist Tomogr* 1990; 14: 255–261.

41. Conomy JP, Kellermeyer RW: Delayed cerebrovascular consequences of therapeutic radiation. *Cancer* 1975; 36: 1702–1708.

42. Darmody WR, Thomas LM, Gurdjian ES: Postirradiation vascular insufficiency syndrome. *Neurology* 1967; 17: 1190–1192.

43. Painter MJ, Chutorian AM, Hilal SK: Cerebrovasculopathy following irradiation in childhood. *Neurology* 1975; 25: 189–194.

44. Werner MH, Burger PC, Heinz ER, Friedman AH, Halperin EC, Schold SC: Intracranial atherosclerosis following radiotherapy. *Neurology* 1988; 38: 1158–1160.

45. Kagan AR, Bruce DW, Di Chiro G: Fatal foam cell arteritis of the brain after irradiation for Hodgkin's disease: Angiography and pathology. *Stroke* 1971; 2: 232–238.

46. Brant-Zawadzki M, Anderson M, DeArmond SJ, Conley FK, Jahnke RW: Radiation-induced large intracranial vessel occlusive vasculopathy. *Am J Roentgenol* 1980; 134: 51–55.

47. Tamura M, Ono N, Zama A, Fujimaki H, Ohye C: Delayed brain hemorrhage associated with prophylactic whole brain irradiation for pediatric malignant brain tumor: a case report. *Child's Nerv Syst* 1993; 9: 300–301.

48. Allen JC, Miller DC, Budzilovich GN, Epstein FJ: Brain and spinal cord hemorrhage in long-term survivors of malignant pediatric brain tumors: A possible late effect of therapy. *Neurology* 1991; 41: 148–150.

49. Chung E, Bodensteiner J, Hogg JP: Spontaneous intracerebral hemorrhage: A very late delayed effect of radiation therapy. *J Child Neurol* 1992; 7: 259–263.

50. Davis PC, Hoffman JC, Pearl GS, Braun IF: CT evaluation of effects of cranial radiation therapy in children. *Am J Neuroradiol* 1986; 7: 639–644.

51. Marks MP, Delapaz RL, Fabrikant JI, et al: Intracranial vascular malformations: Imaging of charged-particle radiosurgery. Part I. Results of therapy. *Radiology* 1988; 168: 447–455.

52. Marks MP, Delapaz RL, Fabrikant JI, et al: Intracranial vascular malformations: Imaging of charged-particle radiosurgery. Part II. Complications. *Radiology* 1988; 168: 457–462.

53. Yamamoto M, Jimbo M, Lindquist C: Radiation-induced edema after radiosurgery for pontine arteriovenous malformation. A case report and detection by magnetic resonance imaging. *Surg Neurol* 1992; 237: 15–21.

54. Flickinger JC, Lunsford LD, Kondziolka D, et al: Radiosurgery and brain tolerance: An analysis of neurodiagnostic imaging changes after gamma knife radiosurgery for arteriovenous malformations. *Int J Radiat Oncol Biol Phys* 1992; 23: 19–26.

55. Guo WY: Radiological aspects of gamma knife radiosurgery for arteriovenous malformations and other non-tumoural disorders of the brain. *Acta Radiol [Suppl]* 1993; 388: 1–34.

56. Little JR, Awad IA: Intracranial aneurysms. In: Little JR, Awad AD, eds. *Reoperative Neurosurgery.* Baltimore: Williams & Wilkins, 1992:211–218.

57. New PFJ, Rosen BR, Brady TJ: Potential hazards and artifacts of ferromagnetic and nonferromagnetic surgical and dental materials and devices in nuclear magnetic resonance imaging. *Radiology* 1983;147:139–148.

58. Dujovny M, Kossovsky N, Kossowsky R, et al: Aneurysm clip motion during magnetic resonance imaging: *In vivo* experimental study with metallurgical factor analysis. *Neurosurgery* 1985;17:543–548.

59. Becker RL, Norfray JF, Teitelbaum GP, et al: MR imaging in patients with intracranial aneurysm clips. *Am J Neuroradiol* 1988;9:885–889.

60. Shellock FG, Curtis JS: MR imaging and biomedical implants, materials, and devices: an updated review. *Radiology* 1991;180:541–550.

61. Shellock FG: MR imaging of metallic implants and materials: a compilation of the literature. *Am J Roentgenol* 1988;151:811–814.

62. Klucznik RP, Carrier DA, Pyka R, Haid RW: Placement of a ferromagnetic intracerebral aneurysm clip in a magnetic field with a fatal outcome. *Radiology* 1993;187:855–856.

63. Kanal E, Shellock FG, Talagala L: Safety considerations in MR imaging. *Radiology* 1990;176:593–606.

64. Bruce DA, Alavi A, Bilaniuk L, Dolinskas C, Obrist W, Uzzel B: Diffuse cerebral swelling following head injuries in children: The syndrome of "malignant brain edema." *J Neurosurg* 1981;65:170–178.

65. Zimmerman RA, Bilaniuk LT, Bruce D, Dolinskas C, Obrist W, Kuhl D: Computed tomography of pediatric head trauma: Acute general cerebral swelling. *Radiology* 1978;126:403–408.

66. Veiga-Pires JA, Von Nieuwenhuizen O, Kaiser MC: Brainstem compression in a child with acute progressive brain edema following trauma. *J Comput Assist Tomogr* 1980;4:121–123.

67. Brant-Zawadzki M, Pitts LH: The role of CT in evaluation of head trauma. In: Federle MP, Brant-Zawadzki M, eds. *Computed Tomography in the Evaluation of Trauma.* Baltimore: Williams & Wilkins, 1982:1–59.

68. Spiegelmann R, Hadani M, Ram Z, Faibel M, Shacked I: Upward transtentorial herniation: A complication of postoperative edema at the cervicomedullary junction. *Neurosurgery* 1989;24:284–288.

69. Enzmann DR, Britt RH, Placone R: Staging of human brain abscess by computed tomography. *Radiology* 1983;146:703–708.

70. Britt RH, Enzmann DR: Clinical stages of human brain abscesses on serial CT scans after contrast infusion. *J Neurosurg* 1983;59:972–989.

71. Rao CVGK, Kishore PRS, Bartlett J, Brennan TG: Computed tomography in the postoperative patient. *Neuroradiology* 1980;19:257–263.

72. Enzmann DR, Britt RH, Yeager AS: Experimental brain abscess evaluation: computed tomographic and neuropathologic correlation. *Radiology* 1979;133:113–122.

73. Enzmann DR, Britt RH, Lyons B, Carroll B, Wilson DA, Buxton J: High-resolution ultrasound evaluation of experimental brain abscess evolution: comparison with computed tomography and neuropathology. *Radiology* 1982;142:95–102.

74. Torack RM: Fungus infections associated with antibiotic and steroid therapy. *Am J Med* 1957;22:872–882.

75. Parker JC, Dyer ML: Neurologic infections due to bacteria, fungi, and parasites. In: Davis RL, Robertson DM, eds. *Textbook of Neuropathology.* Baltimore: Williams & Wilkins, 1985:632–703.

76. Sepkowitz K, Armstrong D: Space-occupying fungal lesions of the central nervous system. In: Scheld WM, Whitley RJ, Durack DT, eds. *Infections of the Central Nervous System.* New York: Raven Press, 1991:741–764.

77. Patchell RA, White CL, Clark AW, Beschorner WE, Santos GW: Neurologic complications of bone marrow transplantation. *Neurology* 1985;35:300–306.

78. Hooper DC, Pruitt AA, Rubin RH: Central nervous system infection in the chronically immunosuppressed. *Medicine* 1982;61:166–188.

79. Osborn AG: Intracranial hemorrhage. In: *Diagnostic Neuroradiology.* (Chapter 7). St. Louis: Mosby YearBook, 1974:154–198.

80. Haines SJ, Maroon JC, Jannetta PJ: Supratentorial intracerebral hemorrhage following posterior fossa surgery. *J Neurosurg* 1978;49:881–886.

81. van Calenbergh F, Goffin J, Plets C: Cerebellar hemorrhage complicating supratentorial craniotomy: report of two cases. *Surg Neurol* 1993;40:336–338.

82. Furuya K, Segawa H, Shiokawa Y, Ide K, Sano K: Brain stem haemorrhage during transsphenoidal surgery. *Acta Neurochir (Wien)* 1993;125:188–191.

83. Fisher CM: The pathology and pathogenesis of intracerebral hemorrhage. In: Fields WS, ed. *Pathogenesis and Treatment of Cerebrovascular Disease.* Springfield, IL: Charles C Thomas, 1961:295–311.

84. Smith JL, Cross SA: Occipital lobe infarction after open heart surgery. *J Clin Neuroophthalmol* 1983;3:23–30.

85. Adair JC, Call GK, O'Connell JB, Baringer JR: Cerebrovascular syndromes following cardiac transplantation. *Neurology* 1992;42:819–823.

86. Kaufman HH, McAllister P, Taylor H, Schmidt S: Intracerebral hematoma related to thrombolysis for myocardial infarction. *Neurosurgery* 1993;33:898–900.

87. DaSilva VF, Bormanis J: Intracerebral hemorrhage after combined anticoagulant–thrombolytic therapy for myocardial infarction: Two case reports and a short review. *Neurosurgery* 1992;30:943–945.

88. Gore JM, Sloan M, Price TR, et al: Intracerebral hemorrhage, cerebral infarction, and subdural hematoma after acute myocardial infarction and thrombolytic therapy in the Thrombolysis in Myocardial Infarction Study. *Circulation* 1991;83:448–459.

89. Kase CS, O'Neal AM, Fisher M, Girgis GN, Ordia JL: Intracranial hemorrhage after use of tissue plasminogen activator for coronary thrombolysis. *Ann Intern Med* 1990;112:17–21.

90. Kase CS, Robinson RK, Stein RW, et al: Anticoagulant-related intracerebral hemorrhage. *Neurology* 1985;35:943–948.

91. Walenga JM, Mamon JF: Coagulopathies associated with intracranial hemorrhage. *Neuroimag Clin North Am* 1992;2:137–152.

92. Franke CL, dJonge J, van Swieten JC, Op de Coul AAW, Van Gijn J: Intracerebral hematomas during antigoagulatn treatment. *Stroke* 1990;21:726–730.

93. Landefeld CS, Goldman L: Major bleeding in outpatients treated with warfarin: Incidence and prediction by factors known at the start of outpatient therapy. *Am J Med* 1989;87:144–152.

94. Mitomo M, Kawai R, Miura T, Kozuka T: Radiation necrosis of the brain and radiation-induced cerebrovasculopathy. *Acta Radiol* 1986;369:227–280.

95. Cairncross JG, Pexman JHW, Rathbone MP, DelMaestro RF: Postoperative contrast enhancement in patients with brain tumor. *Ann Neurol* 1985;17:570–572.

96. Laohaprasit V, Silbergeld DL, Ojemann GA, Eskridge JM, Winn HR: Postoperative CT contrast enhancement following lobectomy for epilepsy. *J Neurosurg* 1990;73:392–395.

97. Burger PC, Heinz ER, Shibata T, Kleihues P: Topographic anatomy and CT correlations in the untreated glioblastoma multiforme. *J Neurosurg* 1988;68:698–704.

98. Brown SB, Brant-Zawadzki M, Eifel P, Coleman CN, Enzmann DR: CT of irradiated solid tumor metastases to the brain. *Neuroradiology* 1982;23:127–131.

99. Constine LS, Konski A, Ekholm S, McDonald S, Rubin P: Adverse effects of brain irradiation correlated with MR and CT imaging. *J Radiat Oncol Biol Phys* 1988;15:319–330.

100. Curnes JT, Laster DW, Ball MR, Moody DM, Witcofski RL: Magnetic resonance imaging of radiation injury to the brain. *Am J Neuroradiol* 1986;7:389–394.

101. Wang A-M, Skias DD, Rumbaugh CL, Schoene WC, Zamani A: Central nervous system changes after radiation therapy and/or chemotherapy: Correlation of CT and autopsy. *Am J Neuroradiol* 1983;4:466–471.

102. Kingsley DPE, Kendall BE: CT of the adverse effects of therapeutic radiation of the central nervous system. *Am J Neuroradiol* 1981;2:453–460.

103. Deck MDF: Imaging techniques in the diagnosis of radiation damage to the central nervous system. In: Gilbert HA, Kagan AR, eds. *Radiation Damage to the Nervous System.* New York: Raven Press, 1980:107–127.

104. Batnitzky S, Halleran WJ, McMillan JH, Price HI, Kalsbeck JE: Radiologic manifestations of delayed radiation necrosis of the brain. *Acta Radiol* 1986;369:231–234.

105. Gh HS, Fuentes J-M, Dubois J-B, Alirezai M, Castan P, Vlahobich B: Radiation necrosis of the brain: Time of onset and incidence related to total dose and fractionation of radiation. *Neuroradiology* 1985;27:44–47.

106. Lee AWM, Cheng LOC, Ng SH, et al: Magnetic resonance imaging in the clinical diagnosis of late temporal lobe necrosis following radiotherapy for nasopharyngeal carcinoma. *Clin Radiol* 1990;42:24–31.

107. Sheline GE, Wara WM, Smith V: Therapeutic irradiation and brain injury. *Int J Radiat Oncol Biol Phys* 1980;6:1215–1228.

108. Marks JE, Baglan RJ, Prassad SC, Blank WF: Cerebral radionecrosis: Incidence and risk in relation to dose, time, fractionation and volume. *Int J Radiat Oncol Biol Phys* 1981;7:243–252.

109. Mikhael MA: Radiation necrosis of the brain: correlation between computed tomography, pathology, and dose distribution. *J Comput Assist Tomogr* 1978;2:71–80.

110. Tsuruda JS, Kortman KE, Bradley WG, Wheeler DC, Dalsem WV, Bradley TP: Radiation effects on cerebral white matter: MR evaluation. *Am J Neuroradiol* 1987;8:431–437.

111. Packer RJ, Zimmerman RA, Bilaniuk LT: Magnetic resonance imaging in the evaluation of treatment-related central nervous system damage. *Cancer* 1986;58:635–640.

112. Groothuis DR, Vick N: Radionecrosis of the central nervous system: the perspective of the clinical neurologist and neuropathologist. In: Gilbert HA, Kagan AR, eds. *Radiation Damage to the Nervous System*. New York: Raven Press, 1980:93–106.

113. Shalen PR, Ostrow PT, Glass PJ: Enhancement of the white matter following prophylactic therapy of the central nervous system for leukemia: Radiation effects and methotrexate leukoencephalopathy. *Radiology* 1981;140:409–412.

114. Price RA, Birdwell DA: The central nervous system in childhood leukemia. *Cancer* 1978;42:717–728.

115. Jankovic M, Scotti G, De Grandi C, et al: Correlation between cranial computed tomographic scans at diagnosis in children with acute lymphoblastic leukaemia and central nervous system relapse. *Lancet* 1988;2:1212–1214.

116. Peylan-Ramu N, Poplack DG, Pizzo PA, Adornato BT, Di Chiro G: Abnormal CT scans of the brain in asymptomatic children with acute lymphocytic leukemia after prophylactic treatment of the central nervous system with radiation and intrathecal chemotherapy. *N Engl J Med* 1978;298:815–818.

117. Esselteine DW, Freeman CR, Chevalier LM, et al: Computed tomography brain scans in long term survivors of childhood acute lymphoblastic leukemia. *Med Pediatr Oncol* 1981;9:429–438.

118. Liang DC, Lin JCT, Shih SL, et al: Cranial computed tomography in children with acute lymphoblastic leukemia after prophylactic treatment with cranial radiation therapy and intrathecal methotrexate. *Cancer* 1993;71:2105–2108.

119. Pääkkö E, Vainionpää L, Lanning M, Laitinen J, Pyhtinen J: White matter changes in children treated for acute lymphoblastic leukemia. *Cancer* 1992;70:2728–2733.

120. Wilson DA, Nitschke R, Bowman ME, Chaffin MJ, Sexauer CL, Prince JR: Transient white matter changes on MR images in children undergoing chemotherapy for acute lymphocytic leukemia: correlation with neuropsychologic deficiencies. *Radiology* 1991; 180:205–209.

121. Vainionpää L, Laitinen J, Lanning M: Cranial computed tomographic findings in children with newly diagnosed acute lymphoblastic leukemia: a prospective follow-up study during treatment. *Med Pediatr Oncol* 1992;20:273–278.

122. Kolmannskog S, Moe PJ, Anke JM: Computed tomographic findings of the brain in children with acute lymphocytic leukemia after central nervous system prophylaxis without cranial irradiation. *Acta Paediatr Scand* 1979;68:875–877.

123. Frytak S, Earnest F, O'Neill BP, Lee RE, Creagan ET, Trautmann JC: Magnetic resonance imaging for neurotoxicity in long-term survivors of carcinoma. *Mayo Clin Proc* 1985;60:803–812.

124. Oppenheimer JH, Levy ML, Sinha U, et al: Radionecrosis secondary to interstitial brachytherapy: Correlation of magnetic resonance imaging and histopathology. *Neurosurgery* 1992;31:336–343.

125. Glass JP, Hwang T, Leavens ME, Libshitz HI: Cerebral radiation necrosis following treatment of extracranial malignancies. *Cancer* 1984;54:1966–1972.

126. Dooms GC, Hecht S, Brant-Zawadzki M, Berthiaume Y, Norman D, Newton TH: Brain radiation lesions: MR imaging. *Radiology* 1986;158:149–155.

127. Ron E, Modan B, Boice JD, et al: Tumors of the brain and nervous system after radiotherapy in childhood. *N Engl J Med* 1988;319: 1033–1039.

128. Kumar PP, Good RR, Skultety FM, Leibrock LG, Severson GS: Radiation-induced neoplasms of the brain. *Cancer* 1987;59:1274–1282.

129. Munk J, Peyser E, Gruszkiewicz J: Radiation induced intracranial meningiomas. *Clin Radiol* 1969;20:90–94.

130. Liwnicz BH, Bergia TS, Liwnicz RG, Aaron BS: Radiation-associated gliomas: A report of four cases and analysis of postradiation tumors of the central nervous system. *Neurosurgery* 1985; 17:436–445.

131. Raffel C, Edwards MSB, Davis RL, Ablin AR: Postirradiation cerebellar glioma. *J Neurosurg* 1985;62:300–303.

132. Fontana M, Stanton C, Pompili A, et al: Late multifocal gliomas in adolescents previously treated for acute lymphoblastic leukemia. *Cancer* 1987;60:1510–1518.

133. Wright DG, Laureno R, Victor M: Pontine and extrapontine myelinolysis. *Brain* 1979;102:361–385.

134. Dickoff DJ, Raps M, Yahr MD: Striatal syndrome following hyponatremia and its rapid correction. *Arch Neurol* 1988;45:112–114.

135. Weissman JD, Weissman BM: Pontine myelinolysis and delayed encephalopathy following the rapid correction of acute hyponatremia. *Ann Neurol* 1989;46:926–927.

136. Tien R, Arieff AI, Kucharczyk W, Wasik A, Kucharczyk J: Hyponatremic encephalopathy: Is central pontine myelinolysis a component? *Am J Med* 1992;92:513–522.

137. Maraganore DM, Folger WN, Swanson JW, Ahlskog JE: Movement disorders as sequelae of central pontine myelinolysis: report of three cases. *Movement Dis* 1992;7:142–148.

138. Rosenbloom S, Buchholz D, Kumar AJ, Kaplan RA, Moses H, Rosenbaum AE: Evolution of central pontine myelinolysis on CT. *Am J Roentgenol* 1984;5:110–112.

139. Miller GM, Baker HL, Okazaki H, Whisnant JP: Central pontine myelinolysis and its imitators: MR findings. *Radiology* 1988;168: 795–802.

140. Korogi Y, Takahashi M, Shinzato J, et al: MR findings in two presumed cases of mild central pontine myelinolysis. *Am J Neuroradiol* 1993;14:651–654.

141. Breuer AC, Blank NK, Schoene WC: Multifocal pontine lesions in cancer patients treated with chemotherapy and CNS radiotherapy. *Cancer* 1978;41:2112–2120.

142. Bittencourt PRM, Perucca E, Crema A: Cerebellar toxicity of antiepileptic drugs. In: Blum K, Manzo L, Dekker M, eds. *Neurotoxicology*. New York: Marcel Decker, 1985;233–250.

143. Koller WC, Glatt SL, Perlik S, Huckman MS, Fox JH: Cerebellar atrophy demonstrated by computed tomography. *Neurology* 1981; 31:405–412.

144. Selhorst JB, Kaufman B, Horwitz SJ: Diphenylhydantoin-induced cerebellar degeneration. *Arch Neurol* 1972;27:453–456.

145. Ghatak NR, Santoso RA, McKinney WM: Cerebellar degeneration following long-term phenytoin therapy. *Neurology* 1976;26:818–820.

146. McLain LW, Martin JT, Allen JH: Cerebellar degeneration due to chronic phenytoin therapy. *Ann Neurol* 1980;7:18–23.

147. Rapport RL, Shaw C-M: Phenytoin-related cerebellar degeneration without seizures. *Ann Neurol* 1977;2:437–439.

148. Jacoby CG, Tewfik HH, Blackwelder JT: Cerebellar atrophy developing after cranial irradiation. *J Comput Assist Tomogr* 1982;6: 159–162.

149. Bontozoglou NP, Chakeres DW, Martin GF, Brogan MA, McGhee RB: Cerebellorubral degeneration after resection of cerebellar dentate nucleus neoplasms: Evaluation with MR imaging. *Radiology* 1991;180:223–228.

150. Wang AM, Skias DD, Rumbaugh CL, Schoene WC, Zamani A: Central nervous system changes after radiation therapy and/or chemotherapy: Correlation of CT and autopsy findings. *Am J Neuroradiol* 1983;4:466–471.

151. Clausen N, Pedersen H: Cranial computed tomography during

treatment of childhood lymphocytic leukemia. *Acta Paediatr Scand* 1982;71:257–262.

152. Bentson J, Reza M, Winter J, Wilson G: Steroids and apparent cerebral atrophy on computed tomography scans. *J Comput Assist Tomogr* 1978;2:16–23.

153. Bashir R, Lewall DB, Al-Kawi MZ: Reversible brain shrinkage documented by computerized tomography. *King Faisal Specialist Hosp Med J* 1984;4:217–222.

154. Lagenstein I, Willig RP, Kühne D: Reversible cerebral atrophy caused by corticotrophin. *Lancet* 1979;1:1246–1247.

155. Enzmann DR, Lane B: Enlargement of subarachnoid spaces and lateral ventricles in pediatric patients undergoing chemotherapy. *J Pediatr* 1978;92:535–539.

156. Bleyer WA, Griffin TW: White matter necrosis, mineralizing microangiopathy, and intellectual abilities in survivors of childhood leukemia. In: Gilbert HA, Kagan AR, eds. *Radiation Damage to the Nervous System: A Delayed Therapeutic Hazard.* New York: Raven Press, 1980:155–174.

157. Peylan-Ramu N, Poplack DG, Blei CL, Herdt JR, Vermess M, Di Chiro G: Computer assisted tomography in methotrexate encephalopathy. *J Comput Assist Tomogr* 1977;1:216–221.

158. Graham JD, Owens C, Godlee JN: Case of the month: A calcified brain. *Br J Radiol* 1993;66:1065–1066.

159. Davis PC, Hoffman JC, Pearl GS, Braun IF: CT evaluation of effects of cranial radiation therapy in children. *Am J Roentgenol* 1986;147:587–592.

160. Harwood-Nash DCF, Reilly BJ: Calcification of the basal ganglia following radiation therapy. *Am J Roentgenol Radium Ther Nucl Med* 1970;108:392–395.

161. Price DB, Hotson GC, Loh JP: Pontine calcification following radiotherapy: CT demonstration. *J Comput Assist Tomogr* 1988; 12:45–46.

162. Pearson ADJ, Campbell AN, McAllister VL, Pearson GL: Intracranial calcification in survivors of childhood medulloblastoma. *Arch Dis Child* 1983;58:133–136.

163. Harwood-Nash DC, Fitz CR: Computed tomography. In: Harwood-Nash DC, Fitz CR, eds. *Neuroradiology in Infants and Children, Vol 2* (Chapter 8). St. Louis: CV Mosby, 1976:461–504.

164. Di Rocco C: Is the slit ventricle syndrome always a slit ventricle syndrome? *Child's Nerv Syst* 1994;10:49–58.

165. Palmieri A, del Vecchio E, Ambrosio A, Pasquini U, Menichelli F, Salvolini U: Immediate and late effects of ventricular shunting in infantile hydrocephalus. *Neuroradiology* 1982;23:203–205.

166. Lourie H, Shende MC, Krawchenko J, Stewart DH: Trapped fourth ventricle: A report of two unusual cases. *Neurosurgery* 1980;7:279–282.

167. Welch K: Selected topics relating to hydrocephalus. *Exp Eye Res* 1977;25(Suppl):345–375.

PART II

The Head and Neck

Posttherapeutic Neurodiagnostic Imaging,
edited by J.R. Jinkins,
Published by Lippincott-Raven Publishers, New York 1997.

CHAPTER **IIA**

The Posttherapeutic Orbit

Darryl J. Ainbinder, Robert A. Mazzoli, Mahmood F. Mafee, Ava Huchun, and Barrett G. Haik

Interpretation of posttherapeutic orbital imaging is a challenge. In addition to a standard interpretation, there are new demands raised by clinical queries specific to the therapeutic intervention. Within the orbit, clinicians may request imaging to assess such topics as vascularization of a porous orbital implant, recurrence of tumor, or evaluation of an unexpected posttherapeutic finding or complication. Recognition of familiar posttherapeutic radiographic patterns, combined with an appreciation of common surgical and nonsurgical treatments, should improve our interpretation of posttherapeutic imaging.

There are a number of modalities available for imaging the posttherapeutic orbit. Many techniques have both a historical and a contemporary role. These imaging techniques include conventional radiography, ultrasonography, dacryocystography, computed tomography (CT), and magnetic resonance (MR) imaging. In addition, radionuclide studies may be requested, such as technetium-99 bone scan to assess orbital implant vascularization, or gallium scans to follow-up histiocytic lesions.

Both old and new imaging modalities are often used. As an example, conventional radiography retains an important role in evaluating the overall shape and configuration of radiopaque material within the orbit, and MR imaging after i.v. gadolinium administration coupled with fat suppression provides superb soft tissue imaging within the orbital apex and base of the skull. Overall, a range of imaging techniques plays a role in posttherapeutic imaging of the orbit.

Ultrasonography functions as an extension of the physical examination. The technique is dependent on the acoustic interface and the absorptive properties of ocular tissues. A-mode ultrasonography provides data regarding one-dimensional amplitude modulation of a reflecting interface. B-mode ultrasonography provides a two-dimensional section, with excellent detail regarding intraocular and anterior orbital anatomic relationships. In combination, both modes provide echographic data regarding anatomy and acoustic tissue properties (1).

Computed tomography provides excellent detail of the eye, orbital soft tissues, and bony orbit; it has an established role in the evaluation of the posttraumatic orbit (2). Technological advances including spiral CT will continue to expand the use of CT in posttherapeutic imaging. As with any imaging tool, there are limitations that require clinical pathologic correlation. For example, the absence of bone destruction in a patient with invasive eyelid carcinoma does not exclude neoplastic bone invasion (3).

Magnetic resonance imaging provides remarkable soft tissue contrast and spatial resolution. It is not subject to the bony artifacts and beam hardening that limit CT visualization of the soft tissues of the orbital apex and optic nerve within the optic canal. MR has multiplanar capability. Images may be obtained in the axial, sagittal, and coronal planes directly, without the need to move the patient. In addition, MR imaging provides information on the flow within vascular structures and on the biochemical structure of the imaged tissues. Surface coils may further improve the spatial and contrast resolution of MR imaging of the orbit (4). A broad array of clinical questions may be addressed with MR, including: concerns of orbital implant vascularization, tumor regression, and tumor recurrence patterns (5). Computed tomography and MR are complementary studies: CT offers the advantage of imaging calcified and bony lesions, while MR imaging provides superb tissue contrast, spatial resolution, and visualization of areas previously limited by bony artifact.

D. J. Ainbinder, R. A. Mazzoli: Department of Ophthalmology, Madigan Army Medical Center, Fort Lewis, Washington 98431.

M. F. Mafee: Department of Radiology, The University of Illinois at Chicago, Chicago, Illinois 60612.

A. Huchun: Department of Ophthalmology, Walter Reed Army Medical Center, Washington, D.C. 20306.

B. G. Haik: Department of Ophthalmology, University of Tennessee, Memphis, Tennessee 38103.

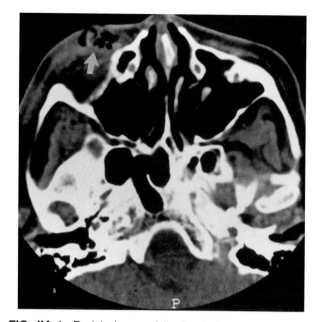

FIG. IIA-1. Facial abscess following incision and drainage. Axial CT demonstrates incisionally induced air in the edematous soft tissue (*arrow*) without evidence of bone disruption. This 65-year-old diabetic patient sustained blunt facial trauma in a motor vehicle accident 4 days prior to development of a deep facial abscess. Following incision and drainage, she achieved an excellent outcome with oral antibiotic therapy. The CT delineation of the limited soft tissue trauma provided critical input into the formation of a management plan.

In the following discussion, we have organized the images within broad ophthalmic regions, including (a) eyelid and ocular surface, (b) the eye, (c) orbit, and (d) periorbital structures and systemic disorders with orbital manifestations. Familiarity with the common therapeutic procedures within each location allows for maximizing selection and interpretation of images in the posttherapeutic patient.

EYELID AND OCULAR SURFACE

Eyelid

Patients with partially treated preseptal cellulitis often have associated paranasal sinusitis or facial trauma. Computed tomography is very useful in detecting the cause and extent of the underlying disease process, providing critical input into the formation of management strategies (Fig. IIA-1).

Ptosis

Within the eyelid, the septum forms a contiguous tissue plane with the periorbita, envelops the preaponeurotic fat pad anterior to the levator aponeurosis, and serves as a

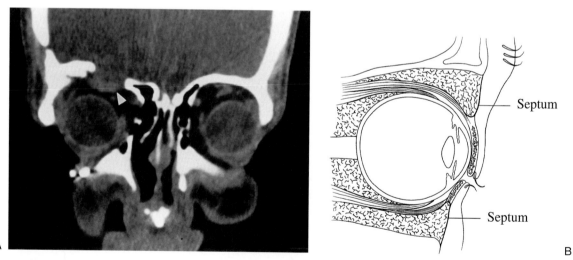

FIG. IIA-2. Levator ptosis following craniofacial trauma. **A:** Coronal CT demonstrates dura, which is adjacent to the levator aponeurosis (*arrowhead*). This patient, who requested ptosis correction, was not able to provide an accurate history of his previous head trauma or the surgical therapy. Correction of his eyelid ptosis would have involved a levator aponeurosis repair. However, CT confirmed that the tissue plane immediately posterior to the levator aponeurosis was dura; thus, surgery was deferred. **B:** Illustration of a sagittal section of the orbit. The septum, a fine connective tissue reflection of the periorbita, separates the anterior lamella of the eyelid from the deeper orbital contents. The preaponeurotic fat pad, which is just posterior to the septum, is a key landmark in identification of the levator aponeurosis. These anatomic relationships are particularly important following previous surgery or trauma.

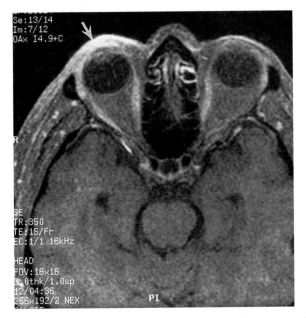

FIG. IIA-3. Postbuccal mucosa and conjunctiva autograft for conjunctival carcinoma *in situ.* Enhanced axial, fat-suppressed, T_1-weighted (TR/TE: 350/15) MR shows diffuse gadolinium enhancement of the conjunctival surface that was consistent with the pathology on multiple biopsies demonstrating chronic inflammation and granulation tissue (*arrow*). This 50-year-old patient presented with large surface feeding vessels and a gelatinous thickened epithelium 4 years after a total conjunctival resection with placement of buccal mucosa autografts. The MR was obtained to confirm that the surface biopsies were representative and that there was not a deeper orbital component of the disease process.

delineation between the anterior lamella of the eyelid and deeper orbital tissues. The periorbita is the periosteum of the orbit, which has unique reflections including the septum at the arcus marginalis (Fig. IIA-2). The levator aponeurosis is a key structure in the repair of ptosis. Following previous surgical and traumatic disturbance of the normal anatomy, imaging may provide vital structural information.

Imaging may be crucial in patients with previous craniofacial trauma and secondary ptosis; CT can provide firm data regarding defects in the regional anatomy, with attention to the anterior cranial fossa, frontal sinus, and levator aponeurosis. Direct thin-section coronal CT provides an optimal image (Fig. IIA-2).

Conjunctiva and Ocular Surface

Posttherapeutic imaging following resection of conjunctival and ocular surface tumors raises a different set of problems, including the range of findings consistent with the surgical intervention and possible evidence of a more invasive disease process. Patients with primary acquired conjunctival melanosis with severe atypia, or carcinoma *in situ,* may have broad areas of conjunctival resection with mucosal grafting. Following extensive surgery, aberrant wound healing may mimic recurrent disease. This clinical concern for recurrent disease can be alleviated by a combined clinical, biopsy, and imaging evaluation of the patient (Fig. IIA-3).

THE EYE

Ocular surgery can be divided into anterior segment surgery, such as a corneal transplant and cataract extraction, or posterior segment vitreoretinal surgery. There are a number of unique therapeutic interventions, such as radiation plaque therapy for intraocular tumors, that may initiate a need for posttherapeutic imaging. Familiarity with common procedures and the potential clinical questions that may arise provide a foundation for imaging interpretation.

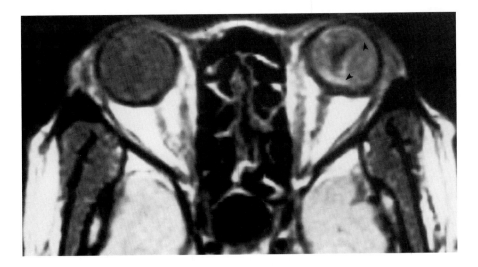

FIG. IIA-4. Serous choroidal detachment following anterior segment surgery. Proton-density-weighted (2500/30) axial MR depicts the choroidal detachment anatomic boundaries of the ciliary body and the vortex veins (*arrowheads*).

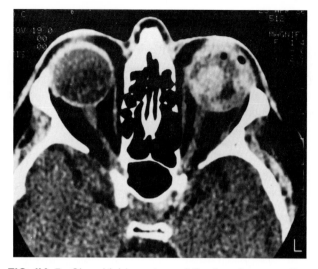

FIG. IIA-5. Choroidal hematoma following glaucoma filtration surgery. Axial CT shows a bullous choroidal density compatible with blood.

Anterior Segment Surgery

Hypotony, a profound state of low intraocular pressure, may occur during penetrating keratoplasty (corneal transplant), glaucoma filtration surgery, and briefly with cataract extraction. Effusions within the choroidal vascular coat of the eye may develop as a result of hypotony.

Usually these effusions are recognized clinically by their anatomic configuration with bullous attachments to the ciliary body and the vortex veins (Fig. IIA-4). A suprachoroidal hemorrhage has the same attachments but is associated clinically with pain and more catastrophic forward displacement of intraocular contents (Figs. IIA-5 and IIA-6). Both MR and CT can help differentiate hemorrhagic and inflammatory diseases of the choroid from uveal tumors (6).

Vitreoretinal Surgery

Patients may undergo imaging following posterior segment surgery as part of a staged multitrauma therapeutic plan (Fig. IIA-7) (7). The boundaries of the retina include the optic nerve posteriorly and the ora serrata anteriorly. Treatment of a rhegmatogenous (i.e., tear) retinal detachment may involve scleral buckling or pars plana vitrectomy with air–fluid exchange. The key surgical goal is to seal all retinal breaks against the underlying retinal pigment epithelium (RPE). A scleral buckle imbricates the sclera, providing external support for the torn retina. An air–fluid exchange provides internal support for the torn retina. (Fig. IIA-7) The half-life of the intraocular gas ranges from days to weeks, based on the mixture of gases utilized.

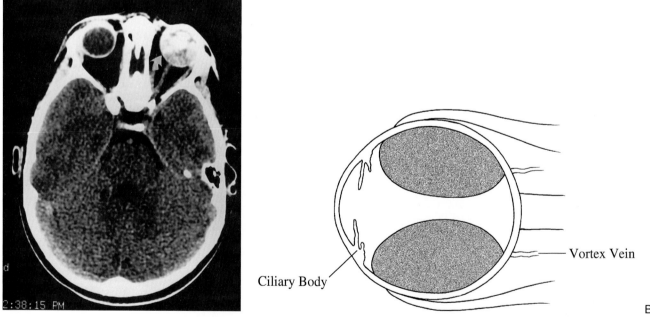

FIG. IIA-6. Suprachoroidal hemorrhage following cataract extraction. **A:** Postcontrast axial head CT demonstrates the boundaries of a suprachoroidal hemorrhage at the ciliary body anteriorly and the vortex veins posteriorly (*arrow*). A large pigmented choroidal mass was identified in this patient following cataract surgery. The CT was requested to evaluate a choroidal melanoma. A CT interpretation of a suprachoroidal hemorrhage as the etiology of the pigmented mass spared the patient from a planned enucleation. **B:** Illustration of a choroidal detachment caused by a suprachoroidal hemorrhage. The anatomic boundaries include the ciliary body anteriorly and the vortex veins posteriorly.

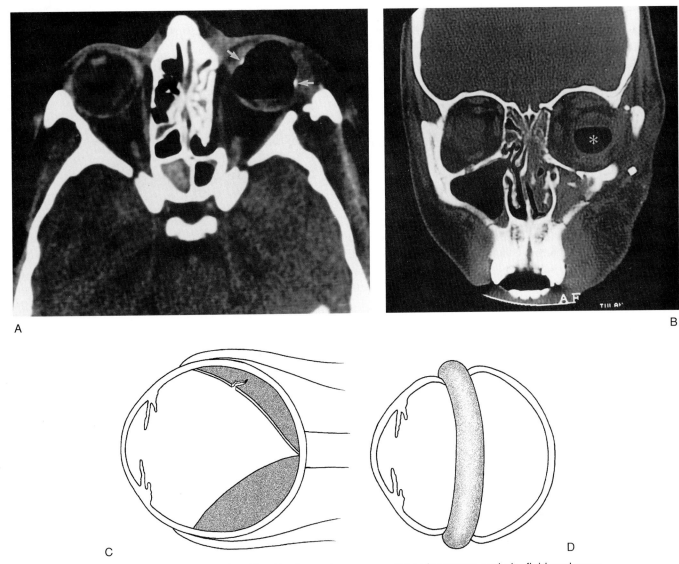

FIG. IIA-7. Postoperative scleral buckle, lensectomy, pars plana vitrectomy, and air–fluid exchange for a traumatic retinal detachment. Primary repair of an open globe in a patient with major craniofacial trauma. **A:** Axial CT demonstrates intraocular air, aphakia, an encircling band (*arrows*), and fractures of the medial wall and zygoma. **B:** Direct coronal CT demonstrates an air–fluid level within the vitreous space, acting as a tompanode for the torn retina. Multiple facial and orbital fractures are evident prior to repair. This patient sustained craniofacial and penetrating ocular trauma and was imaged following primary repair of a macula-threatening retinal detachment. The CT was obtained in preparation for staged repair of the patient's Lefort II and III fractures. In this thoughtful process, she achieved an excellent outcome including 20/30 visual acuity. **C,D:** Illustrations of a retinal detachment (**C**) and scleral buckle (**D**) depict a rhegmatogenous (i.e., tear) retinal detachment with a peripheral retinal tear. The boundaries of the retina include the ora serrata anteriorly and the optic nerve head posteriorly. A scleral buckle effectively closes the retinal break against the retinal pigment epithelium (RPE). The residual subretinal fluid is absorbed by the RPE.

Silicone oil and other dense vitreous substitutes may be used in the repair of complex retinal detachments. On imaging, it is critical to ascertain that these vitreous substitutes are present in the vitreous space and not in the subretinal space, where these agents actually impede retinal attachment and inhibit the metabolic support to the neurosensory retina by the RPE and choroid (Fig. IIA-8).

Phthisis bulbi is a common final pathologic result of failed eyes. Phthisic eyes may contain clues regarding the underlying disease process as well as complications from previous therapy. The entire spectrum of ophthalmic disease, from retinoblastoma to cataract extraction, can result in this common final pathway. (Figs. IIA-9 and IIA-10). In phthisis bulbi, the eye is hypotonous from ciliary body shutdown and appears cuboidal in configuration with thickening of the sclera (>1 mm). The ocular contents are disorganized, often containing osseous metaplasia of the retinal pigment epithelium.

Radiation Plaque Therapy

Computed tomography accurately determines the location and size of uveal melanomas, while echography is frequently utilized in the diagnosis and in monitoring the response following radiation plaque therapy (1,8–11). Magnetic resonance has been shown to be a superb imaging modality for the evaluation of uveal melanoma and simulating lesions; MR is superior at differentiating simulating lesions such as choroidal hemangioma and choroidal detachment from uveal melanoma (12,13). Simulating lesions, including metastatic uveal tumors, require vigi-

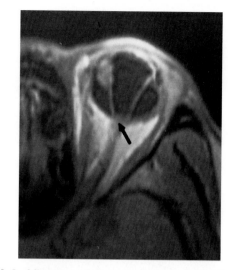

FIG. IIA-8. Migration of silicone oil into the subretinal space following attempted repair of a complex retinal detachment. T_1-weighted (500/15) axial MR demonstrates a V-shaped detached retina firmly adherent at the optic nerve head (*arrow*) and ora serrata. A signal intensity consistent with silicone oil is present in the subretinal space. Any substance in the subretinal space will inhibit nutritional support of the overlying neurosensory retina.

lance regarding their diagnosis and response to therapy (Fig. IIA-11).

Imaging is very important in some patients with retinoblastoma previously treated with enucleation, cryotherapy, or radiation therapy (Figs. IIA-12, IIA-13, and IIA-14). These patients undergo frequent examinations

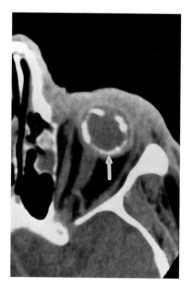

FIG. IIA-9. Phthisis bulbi following complicated cataract and retinal surgery. Axial CT demonstrates a shrunken, disorganized eye with a ring of calcification (*arrow*) caused by osseous metaplasia of the retinal pigment epithelium.

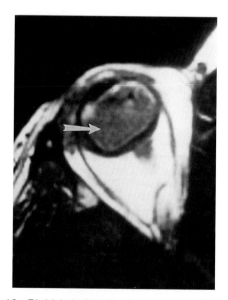

FIG. IIA-10. Phthisis bulbi following unsuccessful retinal detachment repair including intravitreal injection of silicone oil. T_1-weighted (550/15) axial MR demonstrates a cuboidal disorganized eye with thickened sclera. A signal intensity consistent with silicone oil is present in the vitreous space (*arrow*).

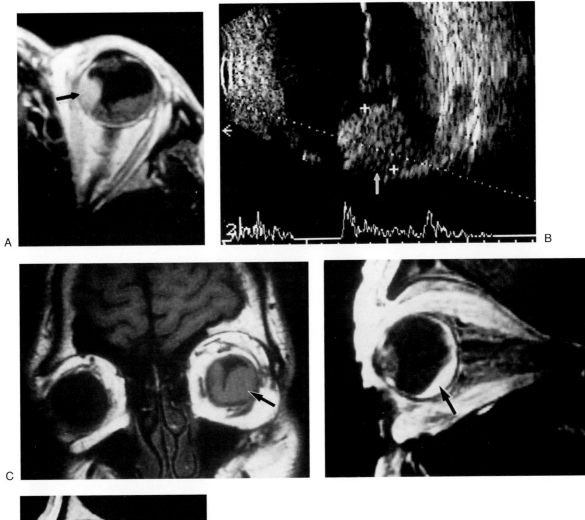

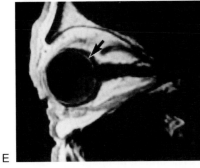

FIG. IIA-11. Metastatic carcinoid tumor to the choroid. A uveal melanoma-simulating tumor prior to and following radiation plaque therapy. **A:** Preradiation enhanced T$_1$-weighted (550/15) axial MR demonstrates a mushroom-shaped hyperintense lesion (*arrow*) and adjacent subretinal exudate. This pattern is more commonly indicative of a choroidal melanoma. **B:** Preradiation combined A- and B-mode axial ultrasound demonstrates a mushroom-shaped choroidal mass with low internal reflectivity and an adjacent exudative retinal detachment (*arrow*). **C:** Preradiation enhanced T$_1$-weighted (550/15) coronal MR demonstrates extensive subretinal exudate involving the macula temporally (*arrowhead*). **D:** Preradiation enhanced, fat-suppressed T$_1$-weighted (550/15) sagittal MR demonstrates significant gadolinium enhancement of this uveal metastatic tumor. **E:** Postradiation enhanced T$_1$-weighted MR obtained 6 weeks following iodine-125 plaque therapy demonstrates marked reduction in the tumor mass. This 60-year-old white man presented with a symptomatic choroidal mass with many features suggestive of a uveal melanoma on clinical, ultrasound, and orbital MR evaluation. Painless decrease in vision secondary to the shifting subretinal exudate brought attention to this mushroom-shaped pigmented uveal tumor. On MR, the lesion appeared hyperintense on T$_1$-weighted images, with significant gadolinium enhancement, and was hypointense on T$_2$-weighted images, characteristics suggestive of a choroidal melanoma. However, MR of the brain demonstrated multiple round enhancing lesions at the gray–white interface with peritumoral edema, suggesting a uveal metastasis, not a primary melanoma. An oncology work-up demonstrated a primary carcinoid tumor of the ileum with tissue confirmation of broad metastatic disease. Iodine-125 plaque therapy provided a brisk reduction in tumor size and exudate, with restoration of his vision. The apical dose was 4500 rads, approximately one-half of the usual melanoma dose. The rapid response was very characteristic of a metastatic choroidal tumor.

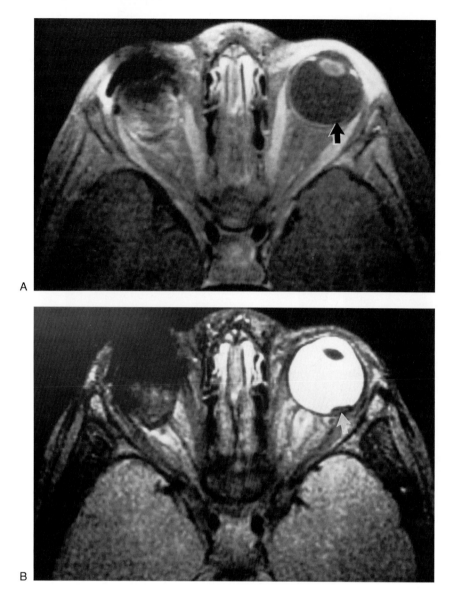

FIG. IIA-12. Bilateral retinoblastoma following enucleation of the right eye and iodine-125 plaque therapy of the left eye. **A:** Enhanced fat-suppressed T_1-weighted (550/15) axial MR demonstrates gadolinium enhancement of the hydroxyapatite orbital implant on the right and minimal enhancement of the regressed lesion in the left eye (*arrow*). **B:** T_2-weighted (2500/80) axial MR demonstrates the hypointense signal of the regressed retinoblastoma in the left eye (*arrow*). This MR was obtained to detect vascularization of the hydroxyapatite orbital implant and for tumor surveillance. Prior to radiation, the tumor in the left eye was moderately hyperintense on T_1-weighted images, demonstrated gadolinium enhancement, and was hypointense on T_2-weighted images. It is of radiographic and clinical interest how the imaging characteristics of the retinoblastoma in the left eye changed following radiation plaque therapy. The tumor is much smaller and demonstrates markedly less gadolinium enhancement.

under anesthesia to assess the response to therapy and maintain surveillance for new tumors. Imaging confirmation of appropriate regression patterns can provide additional reassurance (Fig. IIA-12). Enhanced T_1-weighted fat-suppressed MR would be the author's choice of image for detecting optic nerve extension.

ORBITAL SURGERY

The separation between ocular and orbital disease is sometimes difficult because of their intimate relationships. There are a number of imaging considerations pertaining to the orbit following enucleation. The clinical questions may include vascularization of porous orbital implants or orbital dermis fat grafts, anatomic preservation of extraocular muscles, implant migration, or recur-

rence of tumor. The choice of imaging modality is guided by the clinical aspects of individual case.

Enucleation

Retinoblastoma is the most common intraocular tumor of childhood that results in the need for enucleation (Figs. IIA-13 and IIA-14). Trauma is a leading cause of enucleation among all ages. Patients who undergo primary repair of a ruptured globe may need further imaging studies in order to proceed to enucleation combined with orbital and facial reconstruction (Fig. IIA-15).

At the time of enucleation, an orbital implant is typically positioned within the muscular cone. An ocular prosthesis is custom formed and painted when the conjunctival surface is healed. Figure IIA-13B provides an illustration of these

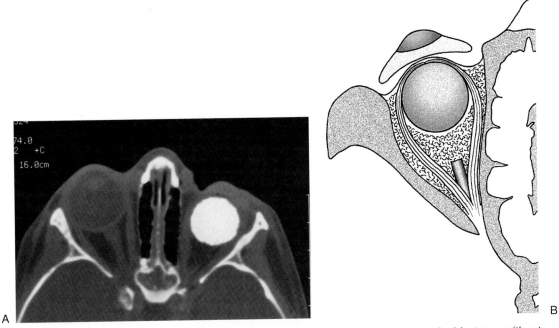

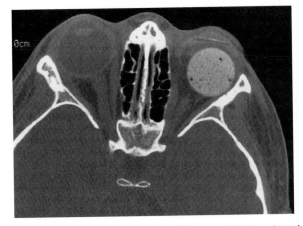

FIG. IIA-13. Enucleation with a hydroxyapatite orbital implant for a unilateral retinoblastoma without optic nerve extension. **A:** Axial CT shows the coarse surface of a bare hydroxyapatite orbital implant. **B:** Illustration of an enucleation. An orbital implant is sutured within the muscular cone. Tenons capsule and conjunctiva provide additional anterior soft tissue support. An ocular prosthesis is custom made when the conjunctival surface has healed.

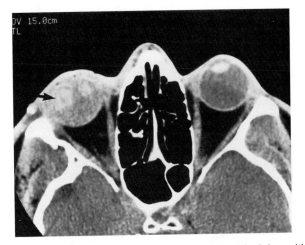

FIG. IIA-14. Enucleation with a silicone orbital implant for a unilateral retinoblastoma with optic nerve involvement and subarachnoid seeding of the brain. Axial CT demonstrates a smooth silicone orbital implant and an overlying ocular prosthesis. Although the optic nerve involvement was less than a few millimeters in this 5-month-old child, subarachnoid seeding resulted in his eventual death.

FIG. IIA-15. Postsurgical repair of a ruptured globe with loss of intraocular contents and extensive intraocular hemorrhage in a multitrauma patient. Axial CT demonstrates air and intraocular hemorrhage (*arrow*) within the disorganized right eye. The zygoma is fractured and rotated, and there is evidence of a lateral canthal orbital foreign body.

components, which are clearly visible by CT in Fig. IIA-14. There are many types of orbital implants, including nonporous implants such as silicone, polymethylmethacrylate (PMMA), and, in older patients, hand-blown glass implants. Porous orbital implants include polyethylene and hydroxyapatite. Porous implants provide the advantage of potential fibrovascular ingrowth into the implant, which helps prevent migration. Hydroxyapatite has a coarse texture, which may be wrapped in donor sclera or fascia by many surgeons to prevent erosion along the rough surface (14). Following enucleation, computed tomography is well suited for evaluating the orbital anatomy surrounding an implant as well as assessing possible implant migration (Figs. IIA-16 and IIA-17) (15).

Mobility of an ocular prosthesis involves the translation of movement from the extraocular muscles to the orbital implant, which then conforms to and provides movement for the overlying ocular prosthesis. Good ocular prosthesis mobility can be obtained if the shape of the orbital implant and overlying soft tissues configures well to the posterior surface of the ocular prosthesis. Thus, it is clear why patients with orbital implant migration may have problems with the fit and function of their ocular prosthesis (Figs. IIA-16 and IIA-17).

Some surgeons integrate hydroxyapatite orbital implants directly to the prosthesis by drilling the vascularized implant. A well-vascularized implant will support the desired conjunctival lining of the drill cavity. A peg may then be fixed to the ocular prosthesis and placed in the drillhole, resulting in increased natural movement of the prosthesis. Surgeons may request a gadolinium-enhanced MR to assess vascularization prior to drilling

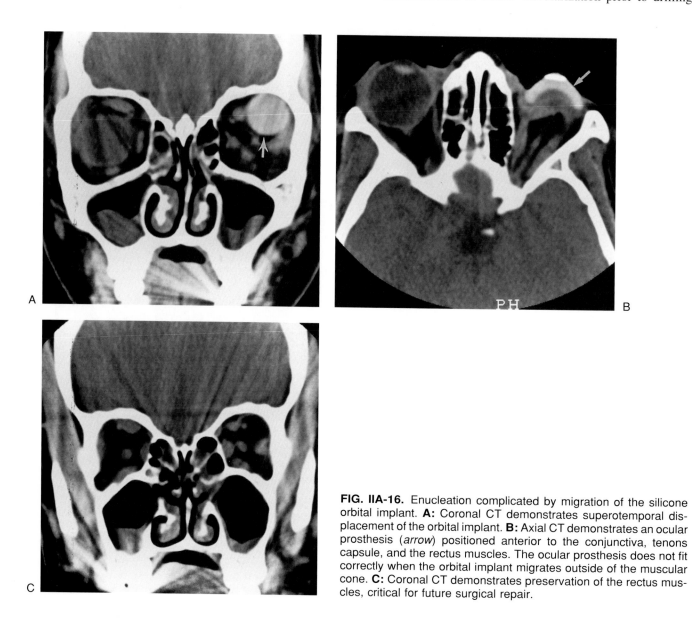

FIG. IIA-16. Enucleation complicated by migration of the silicone orbital implant. **A:** Coronal CT demonstrates superotemporal displacement of the orbital implant. **B:** Axial CT demonstrates an ocular prosthesis (*arrow*) positioned anterior to the conjunctiva, tenons capsule, and the rectus muscles. The ocular prosthesis does not fit correctly when the orbital implant migrates outside of the muscular cone. **C:** Coronal CT demonstrates preservation of the rectus muscles, critical for future surgical repair.

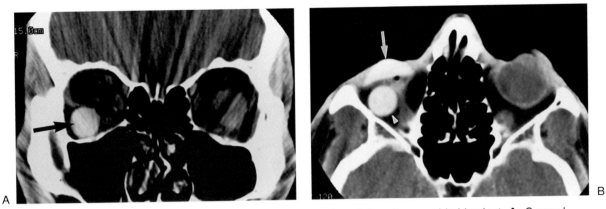

FIG. IIA-17. Enucleation complicated by inferior migration of the silicone orbital implant. **A:** Coronal CT demonstrates migration of a polymethylmethacrylate (PMMA) orbital implant (*arrow*). **B:** Axial CT shows malposition of the ocular prosthesis (*arrow*) in relation to the orbital implant (*arrowhead*).

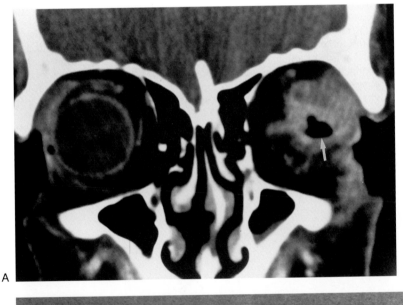

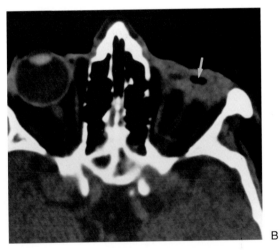

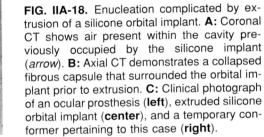

FIG. IIA-18. Enucleation complicated by extrusion of a silicone orbital implant. **A:** Coronal CT shows air present within the cavity previously occupied by the silicone implant (*arrow*). **B:** Axial CT demonstrates a collapsed fibrous capsule that surrounded the orbital implant prior to extrusion. **C:** Clinical photograph of an ocular prosthesis (**left**), extruded silicone orbital implant (**center**), and a temporary conformer pertaining to this case (**right**).

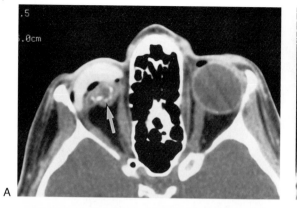

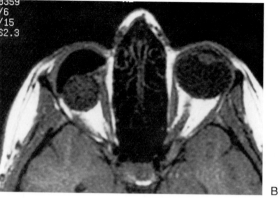

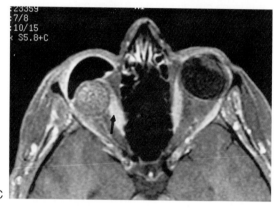

FIG. IIA-19. Impending extrusion of a porous polyethylene orbital implant after enucleation of a severely traumatized phthisical eye. **A:** Preenucleation axial CT showing a shrunken eye with a ring of osseous metaplasia. The orbital volume is markedly reduced, which is poorly compensated for by a thick ocular prosthesis. **B:** Postenucleation nonenhanced T₁-weighted (450/17) axial MR demonstrates reduced orbital volume and impending extrusion of the porous polyethylene orbital implant. **C:** Postenucleation enhanced, fat-suppressed T₁-weighted (466/15) axial MR demonstrates significant gadolinium enhancement of the medial rectus muscle (*arrow*), with modest enhancement of the porous orbital implant. MR evidence of a reasonable vascular supply is critical to the planning and success of a future dermis fat graft reconstruction. Dermis fat grafts can provide conjunctival surface and orbital volume. They remain viable when positioned over a vascularized porous orbital implant as noted in Fig. IIA-20.

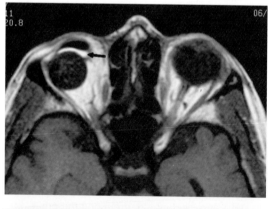

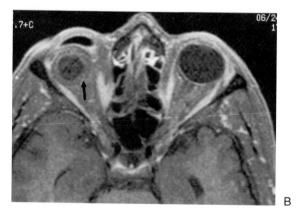

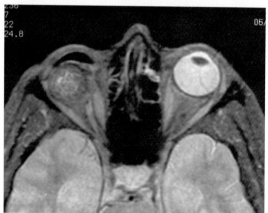

FIG. IIA-20. Enucleation with a porous polyethylene orbital implant, overlying dermis fat graft, and an ocular prosthesis. **A:** T₁-weighted (500/15) axial MR demonstrates the hyperintense signal characteristics of a dermis fat graft (*arrow*) anterior to the orbital implant. The orbital volume is very good, resulting in a thin overlying ocular prosthesis. **B:** Enhanced fat-suppressed T₁-weighted (400/15) axial MR demonstrates gadolinium enhancement of the periphery of the porous implant (*arrow*), consistent with excellent fibrovascular ingrowth. **C:** Enhanced proton-weighted (2500/40) axial MR as well as T₂-weighted sequences are less useful in evaluating orbital implant vascularization.

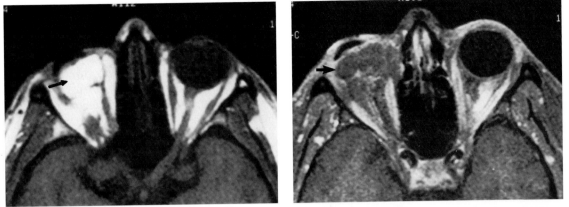

FIG. IIA-21. Orbital reconstruction with a dermis fat graft. **A:** T₁-weighted (350/15) axial MR shows the hyperintense signal of a dermis fat graft (*arrow*). **B:** Enhanced fat-suppressed T₁-weighted (350/12) axial MR demonstrates significant gadolinium enhancement of the medial and lateral rectus muscles as well as the fibrovascular septa within the dermis fat graft. The orbital volume is symmetric with the fellow orbit. The thin hypointense ocular prosthesis is displaced laterally. This 18-year-old patient had an enucleation at age 2 with multiple surgeries to provide normal expansion of his orbital volume. However, contracture of the conjunctival fornix has resulted in a poorly fitting ocular prosthesis. An MR was obtained to evaluate the status of the orbital vascular supply prior to reformation of the fornix with a buccal mucosal graft. Enhanced fat-suppressed T₁-weighted MR is the important sequence in assessing the orbital blood supply.

(5,15,16). Vascularization is determined by the extent and uniformity of gadolinium enhancement within the orbital implant.

Orbital Reconstruction

Computed tomography is very helpful prior to and following orbital reconstruction. In patients with orbital implant extrusion, CT demonstrates the status of the extraocular muscles and connective tissue planes critical for reconstruction (Fig. IIA-18).

Enhanced fat-suppressed T₁-weighted MR provides exquisite data regarding the orbital vascular supply. Extraocular muscles provide a vital blood supply, which will show gadolinium enhancement when viable. Vascularized porous implants demonstrate similar enhancement. Fibrovascular ingrowth into porous orbital implants proceeds from the periphery to the center (Fig. IIA-20). Enhanced MR correlates with the periphery-to-center fibrovascular ingrowth pattern documented on histopathologic evaluation (17–19). A viable blood supply provides the cornerstone of orbital autograft reconstruction (Figs. IIA-19, IIA-20, and IIA-21).

The choice of imaging modality is dependent on the clinical question. Combined axial and coronal CT can help define postsurgical anatomic configuration. Enhanced MR can address issues of vascular support in patients with severely traumatized or postradiation orbits in which the blood supply is tenuous.

There are many indications for imaging following orbital reconstruction. Posttherapeutic pain, infection, nasolacrimal obstruction, and ocular motility disturbance are some of the concerns that may prompt a study. The CT may help identify subtotal reduction, one potential cause of postoperative orbital pain (Fig. IIA-22).

Motility disturbance following orbital reconstruction is a troubling occurrence. Patients may have diplopia from extraocular muscle paresis, bony restriction, or scarring. When the motility disturbance does not follow an expected

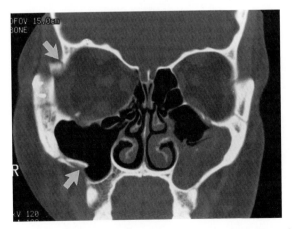

FIG. IIA-22. Zygomatic–maxillary–frontal fracture with subtotal reduction and chronic pain. Coronal CT demonstrates persistent displacement of the fracture (*arrow*).

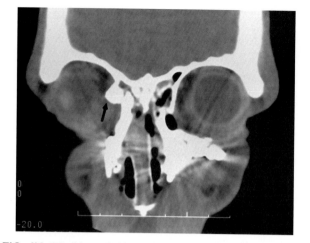

FIG. IIA-23. Naso-Orbital-Ethmoidal (N.O.E.) fracture following surgical repair, with telescoping of the bone fragments. Coronal CT shows bony telescoping (*arrow*) into the right orbit. The trochlea of the superior oblique muscle is distorted by the displaced fracture. This patient developed diploplia from an acquired superior oblique restriction following attempted repair of the nasoethmoidal fracture.

pattern, axial and direct coronal CT may provide critical etiologic insight. Making the correct diagnosis is important. In patients with restrictive motility caused by surgical telescoping of orbital fractures, correction of the bony relationships is important (Fig. IIA-23). Patients with enophthalmos

and extraocular muscle paresis may require orbital volume support and strabismus surgery (Fig. IIA-24).

The types of materials utilized in orbital reconstruction are nearly as numerous as the clinical questions that may arise following repair. Silicone sheet, titanium, porous implants, and autogenous bone are just a few of the potential materials utilized in orbital reconstruction. Surgeons may request imaging to evaluate the bone and soft tissue relationships to the implant or vascularization of porous implants (Figs. IIA-25 and IIA-26).

Dacryocystorhinostomy and Dacryocystectomy

The inferior extent of the cribiform plate and the anterior ethmoid air cells are important landmarks for dacryocystorhinostomy (DCR) surgery (Figs. IIA-27 through IIA-30). There is considerable interpatient variability of these landmarks. Craniofacial repair or resection of midline tumors such as esthesioneuroblastoma induce additional anatomic variability (Fig. IIA-27) (20). The surgeon applies CT data to avoid violation of the cribriform plate and to be aware of the ethmoid air cells in the region of the dacryocystorhinostomy. Direct coronal CT provides the best view of the cribriform plate, and axial CT provides evaluation of the anterior ethmoid air cells.

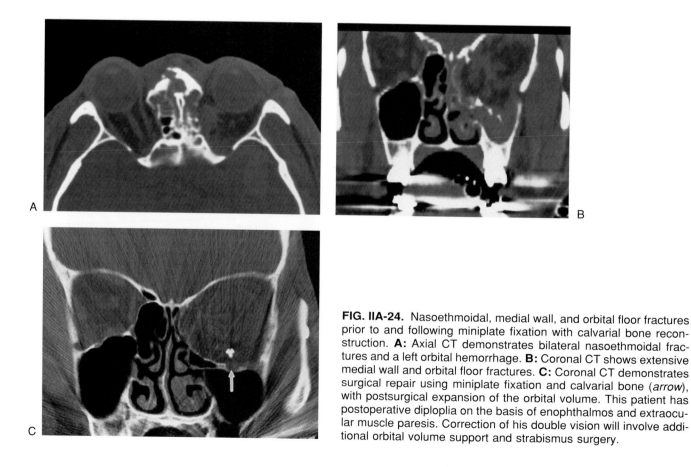

FIG. IIA-24. Nasoethmoidal, medial wall, and orbital floor fractures prior to and following miniplate fixation with calvarial bone reconstruction. **A:** Axial CT demonstrates bilateral nasoethmoidal fractures and a left orbital hemorrhage. **B:** Coronal CT shows extensive medial wall and orbital floor fractures. **C:** Coronal CT demonstrates surgical repair using miniplate fixation and calvarial bone (*arrow*), with postsurgical expansion of the orbital volume. This patient has postoperative diploplia on the basis of enophthalmos and extraocular muscle paresis. Correction of his double vision will involve additional orbital volume support and strabismus surgery.

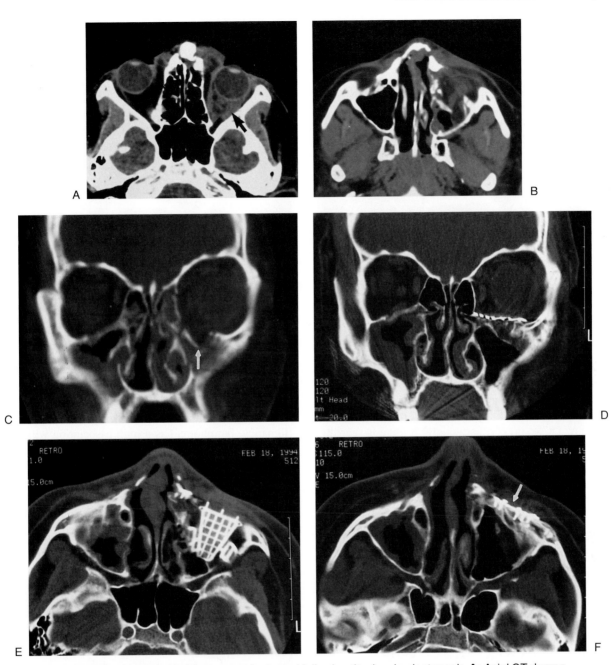

FIG. IIA-25. Multiple orbital fractures prior to and following titanium implant repair. **A:** Axial CT demonstrates a left orbital hemorrhage (*arrow*). **B:** Axial CT demonstrates fractures of the orbital floor and anterior maxillary table. **C:** Coronal CT shows the medial wall, orbital rim (*arrow*), and maxillary fractures. **D:** Coronal CT shows a titanium floor implant. **E:** Axial CT demonstrates a titanium floor implant. **F:** Axial CT demonstrates miniplate titanium fixation of the orbital rim (*arrow*).

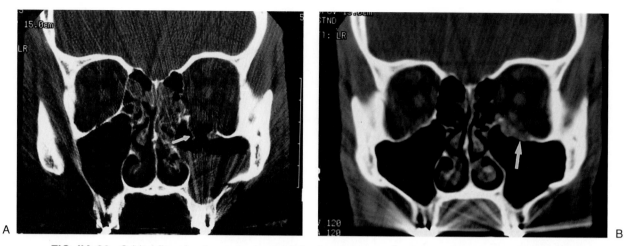

FIG. IIA-26. Orbital floor fracture prior to and following porous polyethylene sheet repair. **A:** Coronal CT demonstrates the orbital floor (*arrow*) and maxillary fractures. **B:** Coronal CT following porous polyethylene sheet repair of the orbital floor (*arrow*). Porous polyethylene can support fibrovascular ingrowth. Surgeons may request imaging to evaluate vascularization or soft tissue relationship to the implant.

Nasolacrimal obstruction is a common sequel of midfacial and paranasal sinus surgery (Fig. IIA-27). However, it is possible for the reverse to occur, given the variability of paranasal sinus anatomy. Paranasal sinus obstruction may follow DCR surgery, particularly if there is scarring of the paranasal sinus ostia (Fig. IIA-28).

Dacryocystography (DCG), produced by radiographic filming during the nasolacrimal injection of contrast media, can provide information regarding the dynamic state of drainage. Filling defects, commonly caused by dacryoliths or neoplasia, may also be detected. Dacryocysto-graphic examinations are often obtained because of recurrent obstruction or clinical suspicion of a primary or recurrent tumor (Fig. IIA-29).

Among all patients with known systemic or orbital malignancy, lymphoma has a high association with dacryocystitis. These patients may have already been treated with systemic chemotherapy or local radiation. The midfacial infection of dacryocystitis poses additional risks in these immunocompromised patients. A CT may be requested to confirm the diagnosis and prepare for surgery (Fig. IIA-30) (21–23).

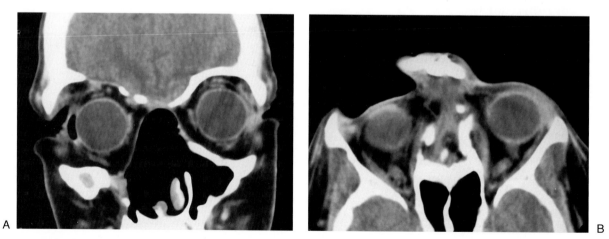

FIG. IIA-27. Extensive midline and cribiform resection for an esthesioneuroblastoma. **A:** Coronal CT demonstrates an extensive midline and cribriform resection. Dura and a skin graft are at the only barrier where the cribriform plate has been resected. The nasolacrimal ducts and lacrimal sacs were also compromised by resection of the tumor, resulting in chronic dacryocystitis. The inferior extent of the soft tissue reformation of the cribriform plate and the stability of the midfacial reconstruction were critical imaging features prior to a modified DCR. **B:** Axial CT demonstrates the region of nasal bone graft reconstruction and marked orbital volume displacement on the right greater than left.

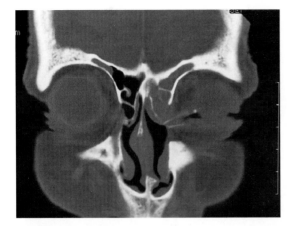

FIG. IIA-28. Frontoethmoidal sinus obstruction following a DCR. Coronal CT demonstrating sinus obstruction at the site of the dacryocystorhinostomy. Following surgery, the patient's dacryocystitis resolved; however, she developed frontal–ethmoidal sinusitis caused by scarring of the sinus ostium.

Orbitotomy

Neurodiagnostic imaging is a critical tool in the management of patients with recurrent vascular lesions of the orbit, such as lymphangioma. Patients with a known tissue diagnosis of orbital lymphangioma may return with acute proptosis as a result of lymphoid hyperplasia concurrent with an upper respiratory infection or following hemorrhage. Both etiologies of acute proptosis can threaten sight. Lymphoid hyperplasia is treated with steroids, but hemorrhage may require surgical drainage and debulking of the lesion. Imaging helps evaluate previous therapy

and provides a framework for future management (Figs. IIA-31 and IIA-32).

Ultrasonography functions as an extension of the physical examination, particularly for patients with lymphangioma and acute proptosis. The walls of a hemorrhagic cyst demonstrate a moderate spike with variable internal reflectivity. Lymphangioma cysts transmits sound well into the posterior orbit with little acoustic shadowing (Fig. IIA-31).

When debulking is considered, or there is diagnostic confusion, MR provides a superb study of orbital lymphangioma (Fig. IIA-32). Lymphangioma demonstrates infiltration of the orbit with multiple cystic spaces. There may be expansion of the orbital volume suggestive of a chronic childhood lesion. The bone is characteristically intact. Fluid layering within a multicystic infiltrative orbital lesion is most supportive of lymphangioma. Lymphangioma provides an excellent model of hemorrhage, with age-dependent MR imaging characteristics (24). Evidence of previous surgical debulking may be subtle, including a slight increase in fibrosis.

Well-differentiated orbital lymphoma tends to mold to the surrounding globe and orbit without bone destruction (21–23). Lymphoid tumors of the orbit are common, may recur following treatment, and have a biological overlap with some inflammatory and connective tissue diseases. Imaging provides meaningful data throughout the course of disease in these patients (Figs. IIA-33 and IIA-34).

Exenteration

Exenteration surgery removes the orbital contents. Orbital periosteum provides the dissection plane unless the

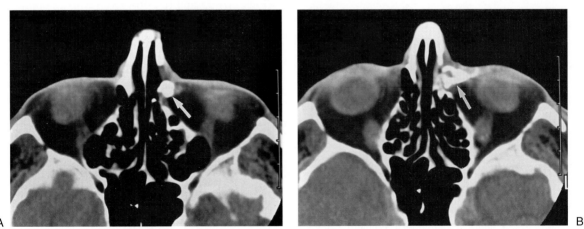

A   B

FIG. IIA-29. Recurrent squamous papilloma of the lacrimal sac following a previous DCR. **A:** This CT dacryocystogram shows contrast within the sac (*arrow*) and the bony ostomy following the previous DCR. **B:** The CT dacryocystogram demonstrates a central filling defect (*arrow*) caused by a recurrent squamous papilloma of the lacrimal sac. This patient had a combined DCR and resection of a lacrimal sac squamous papilloma 7 years previously. The CT dacryocystogram was obtained because of progressive nasolacrimal obstruction and clinical suspicion of a recurrent tumor. Based on imaging data, dacryocystectomy, resection of the entire nasolacrimal sac, was performed and confirmed the diagnosis of recurrent squamous papilloma.

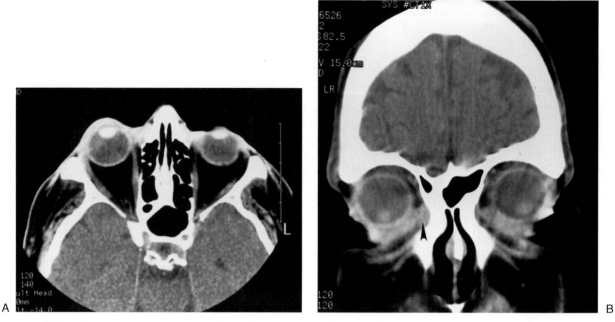

FIG. IIA-30. Postchemotherapy and antibiotic management of a patient with disseminated lymphoma and chronic dacryocystitis. **A:** Axial CT demonstrates bilateral anteromedial, soft tissue lesions that mold to the surrounding structures without evidence of bone destruction. **B:** Coronal CT demonstrates involvement of the lacrimal sac on the right greater than the left (*arrowhead*). This patient was a 60-year-old woman with widespread lymphoma. She developed recurrent right dacryocystitis, improving only while on antibiotics. Lymphoma involving both orbits was suspected based on the CT appearance of a soft tissue mass with molding to the surrounding structures. Lymphoma of the sac was confirmed at DCR, which was successful in treating her dacryocystitis.

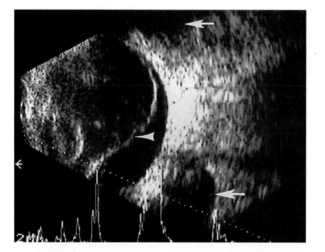

FIG. IIA-31. Orbital lymphangioma with multiple hemorrhagic cysts and an associated exudative retinal detachment. Ophthalmic ultrasound demonstrates multiple cystic spaces posterior to the sclera with low internal reflectivity (*arrows*) and a retinal detachment (*arrowhead*). This patient is a 36-year-old woman with a long-standing history including lymphangioma, marked proptosis, amblyopia, and uveitis with a chronic exudative retinal detachment. She has had several debulking surgeries.

surgery is extended to include an orbital wall for infiltrative tumors such as adenoid cystic carcinoma (ACC) (Figs. IIA-35 and IIA-36). Even with an optimal surgical resection, concern for recurrent ACC is warranted because of its notorious pattern of perineural spread beyond the surgical margin. On follow-up imaging, prosthetic devices should be removed to limit potential artifact (Fig. IIA-37) (25). In contrast to ACC, many invasive lesions such as basal cell carcinomas are cured by exenteration (Fig. IIA-38).

PERIORBITAL STRUCTURES AND SYSTEMIC DISORDERS WITH ORBITAL MANIFESTATIONS

Paranasal Sinus Surgery

Imaging plays a critical role in the evaluation of regional disease with orbital manifestations (26). This is true in patients with prior paranasal sinus disease and surgery who present with orbital findings. Mucoceles, dacryocystitis, orbital cellulitis, cranial nerve deficits, optic neuropathy, and blindness are just a few of the potential

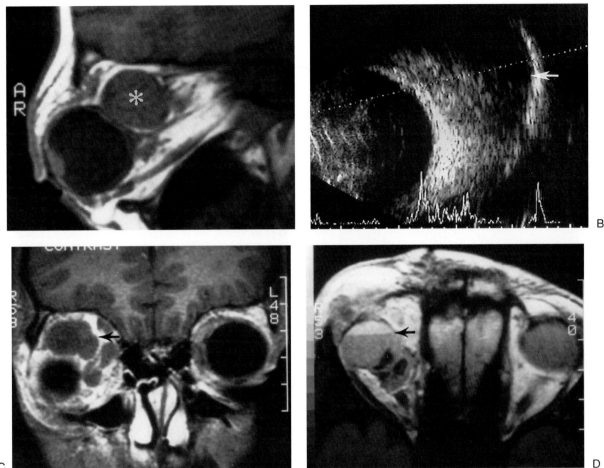

FIG. IIA-32. Progressive orbital lymphangioma with hemorrhagic cysts. A prior incisional biopsy was interpreted as an orbital hemangioma. **A:** T$_1$-weighted (350/17) sagittal MR demonstrates an isointense circumscribed hemorrhagic cyst (*asterisk*) with deformation of the superior globe. **B:** Sagittal ophthalmic ultrasound demonstrates the corresponding superior hemorrhagic cyst (*arrow*) with moderate internal reflectivity caused by fine septa and blood. **C:** Enhanced T$_1$-weighted (500/13) coronal MR demonstrates a multicystic infiltrative orbital lesion (*arrow*). Orbital volume expansion suggests a progressive childhood lesion. **D:** Proton-density (2450/20) axial MR demonstrates multiple cysts with layering of blood and blood breakdown products (*arrow*). This 8-year-old boy was referred for acute proptosis. At age 6 he had a similar presentation and underwent an anterior orbitotomy to exclude the diagnosis of rhabdomyosarcoma. He carried a tissue diagnosis of "orbital hemangioma." Hemorrhage into the cystic spaces may confuse the true pathologic diagnosis of lymphangioma. The MR was pathognomonic of orbital lymphangioma with hemorrhage. Debulking surgery was performed.

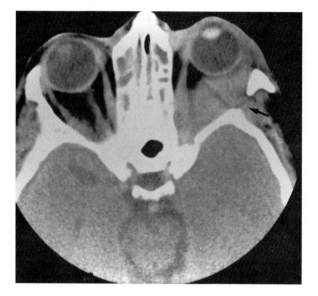

FIG. IIA-33. Orbital lymphoma with evidence of a previous lateral orbitotomy. Axial CT demonstrates a previous lateral orbitotomy (*arrow*). A soft tissue mass fills the orbit, molding to the soft tissues and bone. This 70-year-old patient presented with a 3-month history of painless, well-tolerated proptosis. A biopsy confirmed the radiologic diagnosis of a well-differentiated orbital lymphoma. At the age of 62, she developed acute painful orbital inflammation, proptosis, and diffuse ophthalmoplegia. Rheumatologic and oncologic evaluations were negative. The CT, incisional biopsy obtained via a lateral orbitotomy, and brisk response to steroid therapy were all diagnostic of orbital pseudotumor. There is a biologic overlap of lymphoid cell lines between these two diseases, which in this case transformed into a malignant lymphoid lesion. CT provided valuable imaging data throughout the course of her disease.

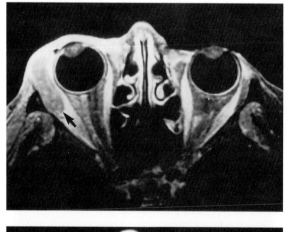

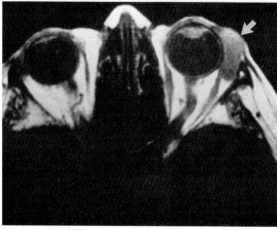

FIG. IIA-34. Bilateral progressive lacrimal gland lymphoma prior to and following radiation therapy. **A:** Preradiation enhanced fat-suppressed T₁-weighted (500/15) axial MR demonstrates an enhancing mass of the right lacrimal gland (*arrow*). Patient was aged 90 years. **B:** Preradiation coronal CT demonstrates a right lacrimal gland mass that molds to the orbit and globe (*arrow*). **C:** After radiation to the right orbit, enhanced T₁-weighted (500/15) axial MR demonstrates regression of the right lacrimal gland lesion. Now, at age 92, there is progression of disease involving the left lacrimal gland (*arrow*).

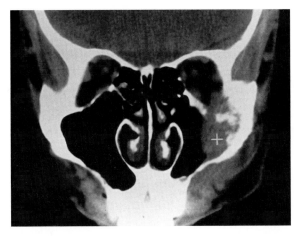

FIG. IIA-35. Recurrent adenoid cystic carcinoma following excision of minor salivary gland. Coronal CT demonstrates an infiltrative, destructive soft tissue mass with invasion of the orbit.

orbital complications that may stimulate radiographic evaluation (Figs. IIA-39, IIA-40, and IIA-41). In each case, imaging may be obtained to answer specific concerns. For example, in patients with orbital and preseptal cellulitis, CT plays an important role in evaluating the severity of associated sinus disease and in monitoring the response to therapy.

A subperiosteal hematoma may form a cholesterol granuloma and overlap some of the imaging features of a mucocele. (Fig. IIA-40) However, with a subperiosteal granuloma, one would expect a history of previous trauma, and the cystic cavity is not contiguous with the sinus, as it is with a mucocele.

Head and Neck Surgery

Concerning the management of regional tumors, imaging can play an important role in the surveillance of many problems, including recurrent head and neck tumors such as parotid gland epithelial and lymphoid tumors, delayed malignancy within the radiation field such as basal cell carcinoma, and nonneoplastic sequelae of therapy (Figs. IIA-42 and IIA-43). Patients treated with radiation adjacent to the orbit are at risk for severely dry eyes from lacrimal gland and conjunctival goblet cell injury. When these terribly dry eyes develop radiation keratitis and progress to enucleation, there is the additional surgical problem of a compromised orbital blood supply.

Neurosurgery

Posttherapeutic neuroophthalmologic imaging is particularly important in evaluating such tumors as sphenoid wing meningioma (27). Computed tomography may document involvement of the optic nerve, confirming the cause of optic nerve atrophy and decline in vision (Fig. IIA-44).

Imaging continues to play a key role in the posttherapeutic evaluation of patients with neurosurgical trauma. Orbital CT obtained to evaluate the orbital component of a multitrauma patient may provide evidence of neurosurgical disease. Proptosis with gross engorgement of the

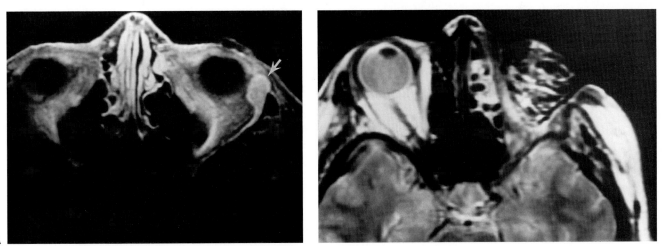

A   B

FIG. IIA-36. Infiltrative adenoid cystic carcinoma of the lacrimal gland prior to and following exenteration. **A:** Enhanced T_1-weighted (500/15) axial MR shows a rounded lacrimal gland mass with an advancing margin along the lateral wall (*arrow*). **B:** Proton-weighted (2500/30) axial MR 2 weeks following exenteration. The lateral wall has been removed, and packing material fills the orbit.

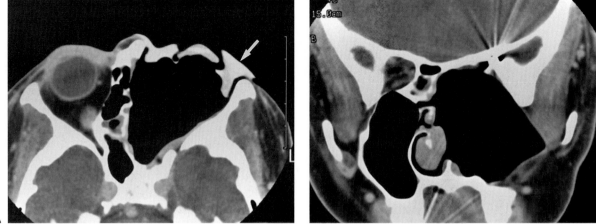

FIG. IIA-37. Exenteration, ethmoidectomy, and maxillectomy for adenoid cystic carcinoma of the lacrimal sac. **A:** Enhanced axial CT demonstrates the extensive resection. The patient is wearing a silicone–latex maxillofacial prosthesis (*arrow*). **B:** Coronal CT shows the extent of surgical resection.

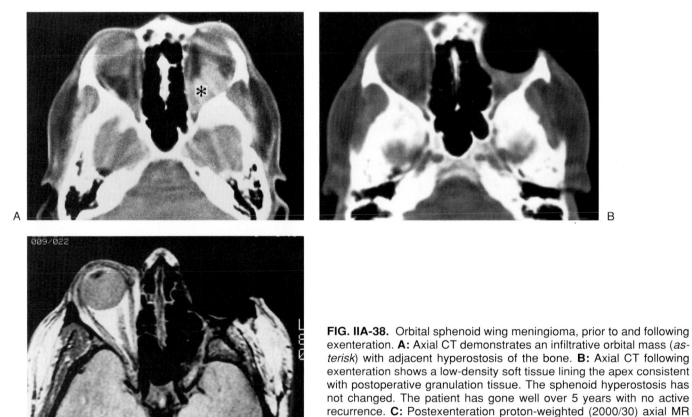

FIG. IIA-38. Orbital sphenoid wing meningioma, prior to and following exenteration. **A:** Axial CT demonstrates an infiltrative orbital mass (*asterisk*) with adjacent hyperostosis of the bone. **B:** Axial CT following exenteration shows a low-density soft tissue lining the apex consistent with postoperative granulation tissue. The sphenoid hyperostosis has not changed. The patient has gone well over 5 years with no active recurrence. **C:** Postexenteration proton-weighted (2000/30) axial MR shows the soft tissue surgical defect.

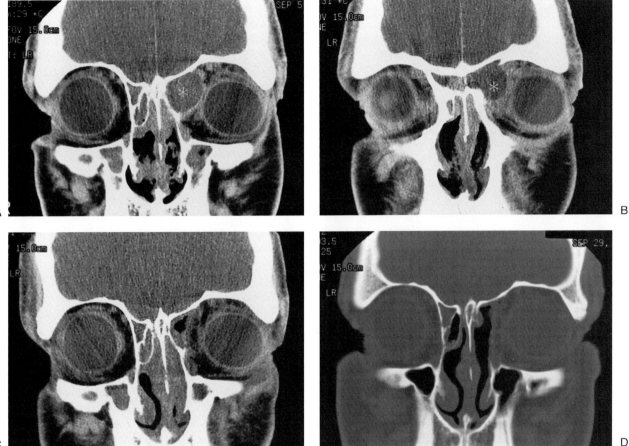

FIG. IIA-39. Mucopyocele following sinonasal surgery. **A:** Coronal CT demonstrates a frontoethmoidal recess and cystic lesion (*asterisk*) with a thin rim of overlying bone. **B:** Coronal CT demonstrates the contiguous nature of the cystic lesion with the frontal sinus (*asterisk*). **C:** Coronal CT demonstrates decompression of the cystic cavity, which now contains air following endoscopic drainage. **D:** Coronal CT following excision of the mucopyocele shows excellent drainage and no residual obstruction. This 26-year-old patient presented with a painful medial orbital mass suggestive of a mucopyocele by history and exam. There was a history of recurrent nasal polyps, previous ethmoidectomy, and antrostomy (**A**). Endoscopic drainage and intravenous clindamycin provided rapid temporizing improvement (**C**). Extirpation and obliteration of the frontal sinuses combined with excision of the mucopyocele was performed 1 week later with a successful outcome (**D**).

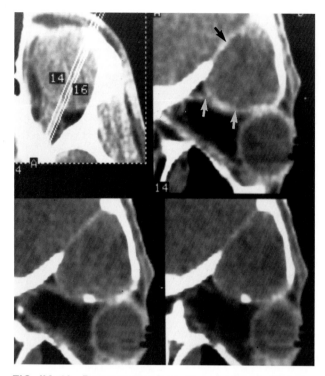

FIG. IIA-40. Postoperative formation of subperiosteal cholesterol granuloma. Serial sagittal reformatted CT demonstrating a cystic lesion. There is thinning of the orbital roof (*black arrow*) and expansion within the subperiosteal space (*white arrows*). In comparison with a mucopyocele (Fig. IIA-39B), a cholesterol granuloma is not contiguous with the paranasal sinuses.

rectus muscles and enlargement of the superior ophthalmic vein may prompt arteriography in suspected cases of a carotid–cavernous sinus fistula (Fig. IIA-45). In addition, CT is well suited for the detection of orbital and CNS hemorrhage following both surgical and nonsurgical trauma (Fig. IIA-46).

Systemic Disorders with Orbital Manifestations

Atypical orbital relationships may prompt imaging that vastly expands the diagnostic information pertaining to a patient (28). Diseases such as neurofibromatosis or craniofacial developmental anomalies may first present with orbital manifestations. Follow-up imaging after primary treatment of a limited aspect of the overall disease may shed light on the full syndrome (Figs. IIA-47 and IIA-48).

Patients with granulomatous diseases may require multiple imaging modalities to monitor disease progression and response to systemic therapy. Relentless disease may require more aggressive management. Although clinical findings such as progressive cranial nerve deficits, nasolacrimal obstruction, or uveitis are key indicators, objective radiographic data help all involved physicians to appreciate the same results (Figs. IIA-49, IIA-50, and IIA-51). Smoldering granulomatous diseases may require imaging surveillance when prompted by a change in the clinical presentation.

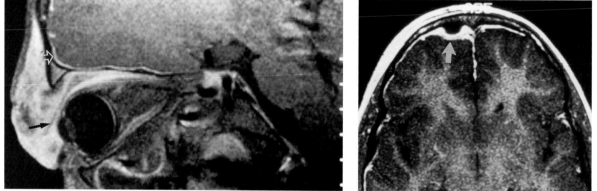

A B

FIG. IIA-41. Epidural abscess following attempted endoscopic management of sinusitis associated with severe preseptal cellulitis. **A:** Enhanced fat-suppressed T_1-weighted (500/15) sagittal MR demonstrates the septum, which is firmly adherent to the periorbita (*arrow*). The thickened preseptal eyelid demonstrates nonhomogeneous gadolinium enhancement. There is gadolinium enhancement of the dura (*arrowhead*). **B:** Enhanced T_1-weighted (500/15) axial MR of the brain obtained 3 days later demonstrates an epidural abscess (*arrow*). This 14-year-old previously healthy patient presented with severe preseptal cellulitis unresponsive to oral antibiotics. The MR demonstrated frontal–ethmoidal sinusitis, a lid abscess, and gadolinium enhancement of the dura, indicating pachymeningitis. The patient underwent endoscopic sinus surgery with intravenous antibiotic therapy including grampositive, gram-negative, and anaerobic coverage. However, effective sinus drainage was not achieved. On the third day of admission, she developed meningismus and an epidural abscess. She responded briskly to a craniotomy and external sinus surgery. The cultures at this time grew a mixture of aerobic and anaerobic *Streptococcus* from the CSF, dura, and sinuses.

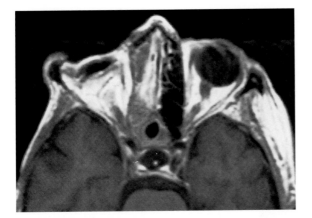

FIG. IIA-42. Radiation keratitis resulting in enucleation following therapy of a parotid gland carcinoma. Enhanced T$_1$-weighted (500/15) axial MR shows a contracted anophthalmic orbit following enucleation. This patient was treated with 6000 rads for a parotid carcinoma. An indolent neurotropic corneal ulcer in a severely dry eye resulted in enucleation. Conjunctival contracture and radiation vasculitis precluded placement of an orbital implant.

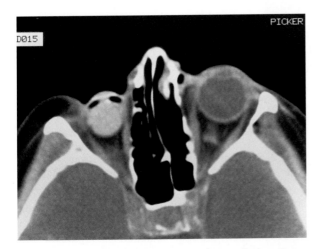

FIG. IIA-43. Enucleation 50 years after radiation therapy of an orbital sarcoma. Enhanced CT demonstrates marked orbital volume loss and conjunctival contracture. This patient had a history of childhood radiation for an orbital sarcoma. She has had multiple basal cell carcinomas within the radiation field. Deep orbital pain prompted this study to exclude an orbital mass.

CONCLUSIONS

Imaging has tremendous application in the posttherapeutic orbit. Conventional radiography details the overall shape and configuration of retained metallic foreign bodies and orbital fixation devices. Ultrasonography plays an important role in the monitoring of ocular and orbital pathology. CT is a key imaging modality: following primary repair of ocular and orbital trauma, CT provides excellent ocular, orbital soft tissue, and bony detail. Enhanced MR provides an excellent evaluation of the orbital blood supply and soft tissue characteristics.

A broad array of posttherapeutic concerns can involve the anatomic landscape from the ocular surface to the neuroophthalmic pathways of the brain. Several core questions may be addressed. Is the porous orbital implant vascularized? Is there a structural abnormality following reconstruction that could account for a motility disturbance? What are the anatomic relationships of the orbit following previous surgery? Is there an adequate orbital blood supply? Is there a recurrence of disease? Multiple imaging modalities provide the necessary diversity to address such a broad spectrum of posttherapeutic concerns. A sound understanding of common posttherapeutic imaging patterns, combined with a full surgical and clinical history, should help optimize effective patient therapy.

ACKNOWLEDGMENT

This work was supported in part by a grant from the St. Giles Foundation of New York.

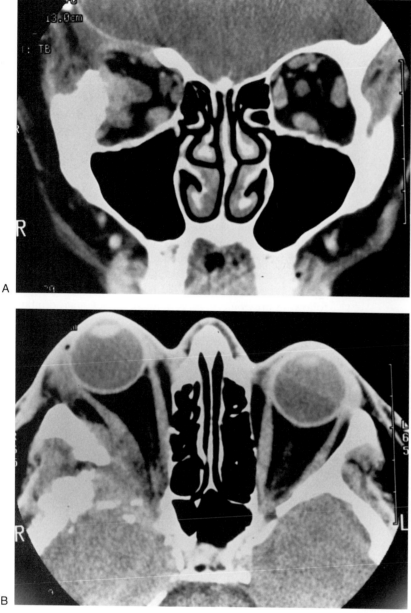

FIG. IIA-44. Sphenoid wing meningioma recurrence after prior resection. **A:** Coronal CT demonstrates a prior sphenoid wing resection. The lateral wall shows hyperostosis and an infiltrative soft tissue mass with involvement of the lateral rectus muscles. **B:** Axial CT demonstrates proptosis, bone infiltration, and a recurrent soft tissue mass with encroachment into the orbit apex. The CT documentation of involvement within the orbital apex provided information regarding the cause of the patient's optic nerve atrophy and decline in vision.

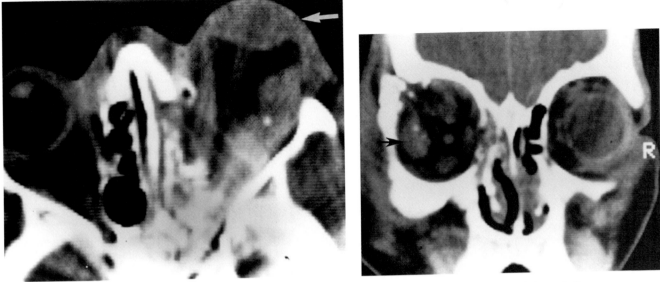

FIG. IIA-45. Carotid–cavernous sinus arteriovenous fistula following a gunshot wound through the globe traversing the orbital apex and impaling on the clivus. **A:** After primary neurosurgical stabilization, axial CT demonstrates the pathway of the bullet through the globe (*arrow*) traversing the orbital apex. The rectus muscles are engorged. The globe is flattened and disorganized. **B:** Coronal CT demonstrates enlargement of the rectus muscles (*arrow*) and the lateral wall entrance wound. Proptosis with gross engorgement of the rectus muscles on CT prompted arteriography and subsequent treatment of a carotid–cavernous sinus arteriovenous fistula.

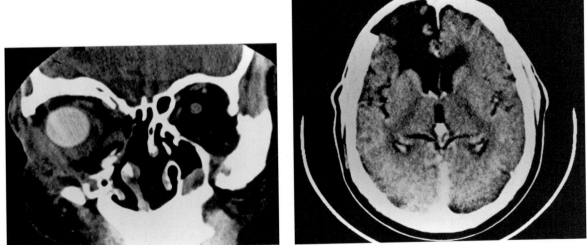

FIG. IIA-46. Enucleation for absolute traumatic glaucoma with a distant history of treatment for massive craniofacial trauma. **A:** Coronal CT demonstrates a silicone orbital implant with evidence of midface to cranium malalignment. **B:** Axial CT of the brain shows chronic posttraumatic encephalomalacia. This 60-year-old patient developed pain and echymosis 2 days after enucleation. Previous massive craniofacial trauma, including a defect in the orbital roof, raised the concern for a postoperative orbital hemorrhage with the potential to dissect along the epidural space; CT was able to exclude this diagnosis.

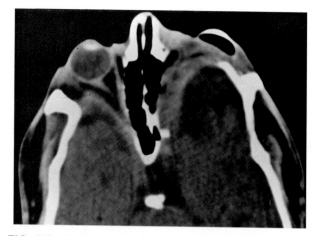

FIG. IIA-47. Neurofibromatosis 1 with bilateral sphenoid wing hypoplasia following enucleation of the left eye. Axial CT demonstrates bilateral sphenoid wing hypoplasia. An ocular prosthesis is present on the left. Brain tissue fills the posterior orbit. This patient presented at 2 years of age with a blind, exposed, and painful eye. At the time of enucleation, the orbital anatomy was noted to be markedly abnormal, resulting in a request for an immediate postoperative tomogram. This CT, obtained many years later, shows the subsequent neuroradiographic evidence of neurofibromatosis 1, including sphenoid wing hypoplasia.

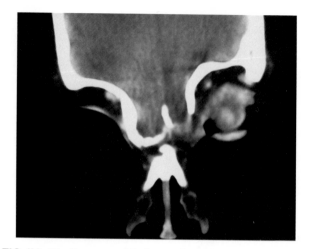

FIG. IIA-48. Dacryocystitis in a patient with a prior encephalocele repair. Coronal CT demonstrates the vulnerable position of the CNS tissues within a DCR surgical field.

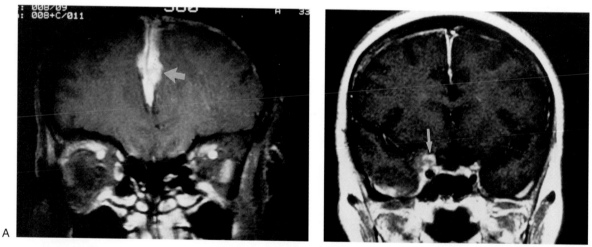

FIG. IIA-49. Leptomeningeal sarcoidosis in a 50-year-old black patient previously treated with low-dose pulse corticosteroid management for pulmonary sarcoidosis. **A:** Enhanced fat-suppressed T_1-weighted (500/15) coronal MR demonstrates leptomeningeal enhancement. **B:** Enhanced fat-suppressed T_1-weighted (500/15) MR demonstrates cavernous sinus and base of the brain gadolinium enhancement greater on the right than the left. The patient presented with cranial nerve 5 and 6 deficits on the right and a confirmed history of sarcoidosis. The primary care physician's evaluation of pulmonary parameters suggested stability despite complaints of occasional double vision and abnormal facial sensation. The MR provided sufficient corroborative data to prompt a multisystem reevaluation of her therapy.

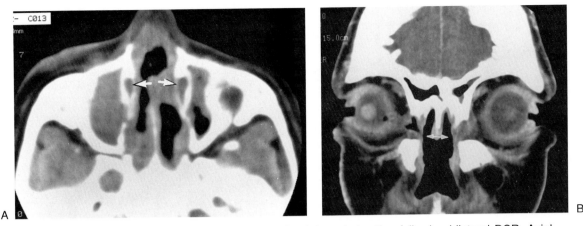

FIG. IIA-50. Sarcoidosis with recurrent nasolacrimal duct obstruction following bilateral DCR. Axial (**A**) and coronal (**B**) CTs demonstrate soft tissue occlusion of the dacryocystorhinostomies (*arrows*).

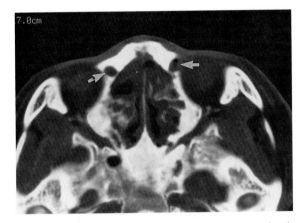

FIG. IIA-51. Wegener's granulomatosis with nasolacrimal duct obstruction following immunosuppressive therapy. Axial CT demonstrates bilateral soft tissue nasolacrimal duct obstruction (*arrows*).

REFERENCES

1. Coleman DJ: Reliability of ocular tumor diagnosis with ultrasound. *Trans Am Acad Ophthalmol Otol* 1973;77:677–683.
2. Koornneef L, Zonneveld FW: The role of direct multiplanar high resolution CT in the assessment and management of orbital trauma. *Radiol Clin North Am* 1987;25:753–765.
3. Glover AT, Grove AS Jr: Orbital invasion by malignant eyelid tumors. *Ophthal Plast Reconstruct Surg* 1989;5:1–12.
4. Bilaniuk LT, Schenck JF, Zimmerman RA, et al: Ocular and orbital lesions: Surface coil MR imaging. *Radiology* 1985;156:669–674.
5. De Potter P, Shields CL, Shields JA, et al: Role of magnetic resonance imaging in the evaluation of the hydroxyapatite orbital implant. *Ophthalmology* 1992;99:824–830.
6. Mafee MF, Peyman GA: Retinal and choroidal detachments: Role of magnetic resonance imaging and computed tomography. *Radiol Clin North Am* 1987;25:487–507.
7. Maguire AM, Enger C, Eliott D, et al: Computerized tomography in the evaluation of penetrating ocular injuries. *Retina* 1991;11:405–411.

8. Peyster RG, Augsburger JJ, Shields JA, et al: Choroidal melanoma: Comparison of CT, fundoscopy, and US. *Radiology* 1985;156:675–680.
9. Peyman GA, Mafee MF: Uveal melanoma and similar lesions: The role of magnetic resonance imaging and computed tomography. *Radiol Clin North Am* 1987;25:471–486.
10. Mafee MF, Peyman GA, McKusick MA: Malignant uveal melanoma and similar lesions studied by computed tomography. *Radiology* 1985;156:403–408.
11. Coleman DJ, Silverman RH, Rondeau MJ, et al: Ultrasonic tissue characterization of uveal melanoma and prediction of patient survival after enucleation and brachytherapy. *Am J Ophthalmol* 1991;112:682–688.
12. Mafee MF, Ainbinder DA, Hidayaat AA, et al: Magnetic resonance imaging and computed tomography in the evaluation of choroidal hemangioma. *Int J Neuroradiol* 1995;1:67–77.
13. Mafee MF, Peyman GA, Grisolano JE, et al: Malignant uveal melanoma and simulating lesions: MR imaging evaluation. *Radiology* 1986;160:773–780.
14. Perry AC: Integrated orbital implants. *Adv Ophthalmic Plast Reconstruct Surg* 1990;8:75–81.
15. Smit TJ, Koorneef L, Zonneveld FW, et al: Primary and secondary implants in the anophthalmic orbit: Preoperative and postoperative computed tomographic appearance. *Ophthalmology* 1991;98:106–110.
16. Hamilton HE, Christianson MD, Williams JP, et al: Evaluation of vascularization of coralline hydroxyapatite ocular implants by magnetic resonance imaging. *Clin Imaging* 1992;16:243–246.
17. Shields CL, Shields JA, Eagle RC Jr, DePotter P: Histopathologic evidence of fibrovascular ingrowth four weeks after placement of the hydroxyapatite orbital implant. *Am J Ophthalmol* 1991;111:363–366.
18. Ainbinder DJ, Haik BG, Tellado M: Hydroxyapatite orbital implant abscess: Histopathologic correlation of an infected implant following evisceration. *Ophthalmic Plast Reconstruct Surg* 1994;10:267–270.
19. Nunery WR, Heinz GW, Bonin JM, et al: Exposure rate of hydroxyapatite spheres in an anophthalmic socket: Histopathologic correlation and comparison with silicone sphere implants. *Ophthalmic Plast Reconstruct Surg* 1993;9:96–104.
20. Burke DP, Gabrielsen To, Knake JE, et al: Radiology of olfactory neuroblastoma. *Radiology* 1980;137:367–372.
21. Peyster RG, Shapiro MD, Haik BG: Orbital metastasis: Role of magnetic resonance imaging and computed tomography. *Radiol Clin North Am* 1987;25:647–662.
22. Mafee MF, Haik BG: Lacrimal gland and fossa lesions: role of computed tomography. *Radiol Clin North Am* 1987;25:767–779.
23. Hesselink JR, Davis KR, Dallow RL, et al: Computed tomography

of masses in the lacrimal gland region. *Radiology* 1979;131:143–147.

24. Bond JB, Haik BG, Taveras JL, et al: Magnetic resonance imaging of orbital lymphangioma with and without gadolinium contrast enhancement. *Ophthalmology* 1992;99:1318–1324.

25. Fry CL, Haik BG: Magnetic resonance imaging artifacts induced by ocular prosthesis. *Am J Ophthalmol* 1994;118:262–263.

26. Weber AL, Mikulis DK: Inflammatory disorders of the paraorbital sinuses and their complications. *Radiol Clin North Am* 1987;25:615–630.

27. Wilbur AC, Dobben GD, Linder B: Paraorbital tumors and tumor-like conditions: Role of CT and MRI. *Radiol Clin North Am* 1987;25:631–646.

28. Zimmerman RA, Bilaniuk LT, Metzger RA, et al: Computed tomography of orbital–facial neurofibromatosis 1. *Radiology* 1983;146:113–116.

Posttherapeutic Neurodiagnostic Imaging,
edited by J.R. Jinkins,
Lippincott-Raven Publishers, New York © 1997.

CHAPTER **IIB**

The Posttherapeutic Pituitary Gland

Gregory J. McGinn and Blake M. McClarty

The pituitary gland is one of the most challenging areas of the body to image. The gland, which measures only a few millimeters in size, lies at the center of the skull base and is almost completely encircled by bone. Imaging studies must be able to detect pituitary adenomas as small as 2 to 3 mm in size. The posttherapeutic pituitary is an even more difficult area to examine. The normal anatomy of the pituitary gland and surrounding structures is frequently altered following treatment. The radiologist must be thoroughly familiar with the normal or expected appearance of the posttherapeutic pituitary. In addition, the radiologist must be aware of potential complications that may arise during the course of treatment. The purpose of this chapter is to review the appearance of the pituitary gland on magnetic resonance (MR) and computed tomography (CT) following the treatment of pituitary adenomas.

Magnetic resonance has emerged as the imaging procedure of choice in the evaluation of the pituitary gland. It is more sensitive than CT in the detection of pituitary adenomas and is also more sensitive in the detection of intratumoral hemorrhage (1–3) (Fig. IIB-1). In addition, MR is superior to CT in demonstrating the relationship of the pituitary adenoma to its surrounding structures such as the optic chiasm (4) (Fig. IIB-2). Perhaps the only significant advantage of CT over MR is its ability to image bone, which has direct significance to the neurosurgeon who is planning transsphenoidal resection of a pituitary tumor (4).

Standard MR sequences for imaging the pituitary gland include thin section (3 mm) coronal T_1-weighted (e.g., TR = 500 msec, TE = 20 msec) spin-echo images before and after gadolinium contrast agent administration. In general, sagittal T_1-weighted images are useful for imaging the posterior lobe of the pituitary, and T_2-weighted (e.g., TR = 2000 msec, TE = 90 msec) spin-echo images may be used to help characterize areas of intratumoral hemorrhage and necrosis.

Computed tomographic scans are performed in a direct coronal position using a thin-slice technique (e.g., 1 to 1.5 mm thick, contiguous cuts) following rapid bolus i.v. iodinated contrast agent administration. Dynamic CT and MR studies of the pituitary have been reported in the literature, but the value of these techniques in the posttherapeutic pituitary has not been determined (5–8).

Pituitary adenomas are classified according to size as microadenomas (less than 10 mm) or macroadenomas (greater than 10 mm). Either type may be functioning (hormone-secreting) or nonfunctioning (non-hormone-secreting).

Small nonfunctioning pituitary microadenomas are a common finding in autopsy series of asymptomatic patients. Teramoto et al. found pituitary lesions greater than 2 mm in size in 6.1% of 1000 nonselected autopsy specimens (9). These small lesions consisted of microadenomas, Rathke's cleft cysts, and focal areas of gland hyperplasia.

On MR imaging studies, small, incidental hypointensities within the pituitary gland are not uncommon. Chong et al. found small, 2- to 5-mm hypointensities in the pituitary gland in 40% of 52 asymptomatic volunteers on unenhanced T_1-weighted spin-echo images (10). Another study by Hall et al. found 3- to 6-mm areas of decreased signal intensity in 10% of normal volunteers on T_1-weighted gadolinium-enhanced MR images (11). Many of these so-called "incidentalomas" discovered on MR imaging are felt to represent nonfunctioning microadenomas. Because these nonfunctioning adenomas are a frequent incidental finding, and because they are asymptomatic, treatment is considered unnecessary. Because of the high incidence of small asymptomatic pituitary lesions in the general population, the results of MR and CT scans should always be correlated with the serum hormone level and clinical findings in order to provide a meaningful interpretation.

MEDICAL THERAPY

Functioning pituitary microadenomas present with clinical signs and symptoms related to an elevated serum

G. J. McGinn, B. M. McClarty: Department of Radiology, St. Boniface General Hospital, University of Manitoba, Winnipeg, Manitoba R2H 2A6, Canada.

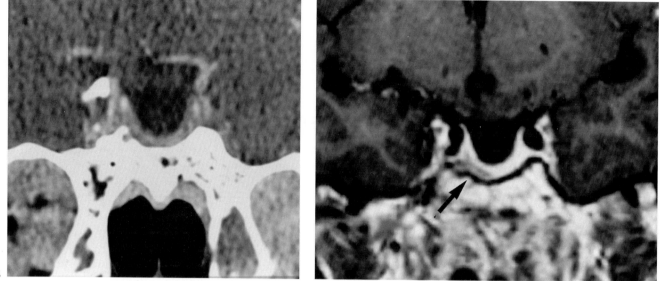

FIG. IIB-1. Comparative imaging by CT and MR in a 61-year-old woman presenting with acromegaly and elevated serum growth hormone level. **A:** Coronal contrast-enhanced CT fails to demonstrate the pituitary adenoma. **B:** Coronal T₁-weighted (TR = 500 msec, TE = 20 msec) gadolinium-enhanced MR image shows small, relatively nonenhancing right-sided microadenoma (*arrow*).

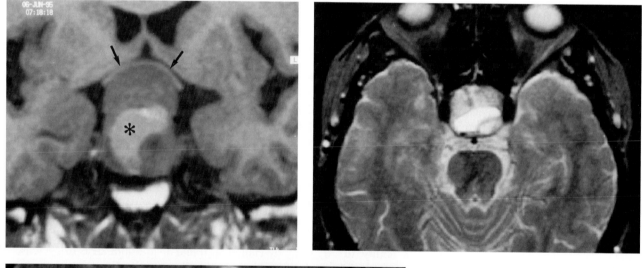

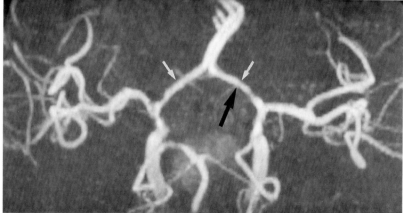

FIG. IIB-2. Relationship of pituitary adenoma to regional structures in a 62-year-old woman presenting with vomiting, sensory deficit, and a visual field defect. **A:** Coronal T₁-weighted (TR = 500 msec, TE = 20 msec) MR image shows pituitary macroadenoma elevating and compressing optic chiasm (*arrows*). Note intratumoral hemorrhage (*asterisk*). **B:** Axial T₂-weighted (TR = 2000 msec, TE = 90 msec) MR image confirms the intratumoral hemorrhage (i.e., extracellular methemaglobin). **C:** Three-dimensional time-of-flight MRA reveals elevation of anterior cerebral arteries (*arrows*).

hormone level. Prolactinomas represent the most common type of functioning microadenoma (12). Prolactinomas are unusual in that effective medical therapy is available in the form of bromocriptine. Numerous publications have described a reduction in size of prolactinomas following bromocriptine therapy (Fig. IIB-3). In the series of Kaplan et al. (12), only 33% of the microprolactinomas that were treated with bromocriptine prior to surgery could be identified on preoperative CT. However, in this same series, 75% of microprolactinomas that were not treated with bromocriptine prior to surgery could be identified on preoperative CT. The authors attribute this difference to a reduction in size and, therefore, detectability of the prolactinomas following bromocriptine therapy. Based on these observations, the authors recommended routine CT localization of microprolactinomas prior to beginning bromocriptine therapy in the event that future surgical therapy is required.

Prolactin-secreting macroadenomas have also been observed to decrease in size following bromocriptine therapy. Scotti et al. (13) performed serial CT scans on 30 patients with known macroprolactinomas who were being treated with dopaminergic drugs (bromocriptine or lisuride) over a period of 4 months to 6 years. They observed a reduction in size of the adenomas in 20 of the 30 patients. A rapid reduction in tumor size was observed in five patients within the first month of treatment. In 13 patients, tumor shrinkage was slower and was first observed after several months. Complete tumor regression as judged by imaging studies was not seen in any patient. Serum prolactin levels also decreased in 28 of the 30 patients.

Lundin et al. (14) demonstrated a reduction in size of all 13 macroprolactinomas in their series following bromocriptine therapy. The size reduction became statistically significant as early as 1 week, and the shrinkage continued for up to several years in some cases. The maximum tumor reduction ranged from 37% to 88% (mean 61.2%). The serum prolactin level returned to normal in 10 of 13 patients in their series after 18 months of treatment. The reduction in serum prolactin level always preceded the reduction in tumor volume on imaging in their series.

The shrinkage of macroadenomas following bromocriptine treatment has been attributed to cell involution and/or tumor necrosis (15,16). An increase in connective tissue stroma within prolactinomas has also been observed (15,17).

Hemorrhage within prolactinomas has also been observed during bromocriptine therapy (Fig. IIB-4). In our experience, hemorrhage within pituitary adenomas demonstrates a somewhat variable signal intensity on MR imaging. In the medical literature, acute hemorrhage (i.e., intracellular methemoglobin) has been described as an area of increased signal intensity on T_1-weighted spin-echo images with corresponding decreased signal intensity on T_2-weighted spin-echo sequences (18). Subacute to chronic hemorrhage (i.e., extracellular methemoglobin)

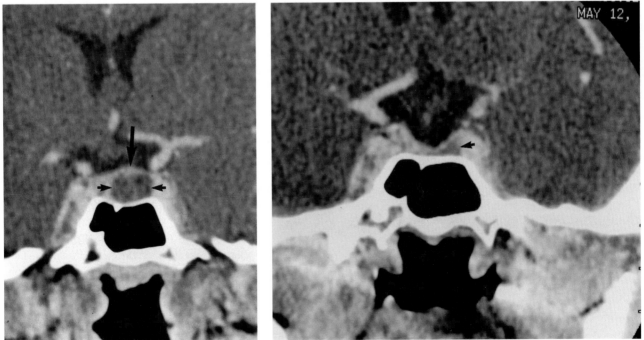

FIG. IIB-3. Effect of bromocriptine therapy on pituitary adenoma in a 37-year-old woman presenting with infertility. **A:** Coronal contrast-enhanced CT reveals a relatively nonenhancing left-sided prolactinoma (*arrows*). **B:** Following 2 years of bromocriptine therapy, CT shows significant reduction in size of the adenoma (*arrow*).

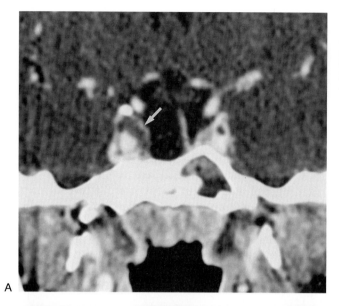

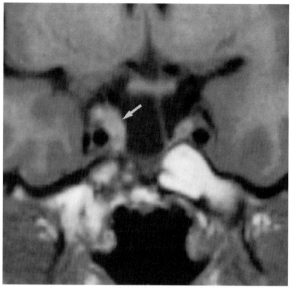

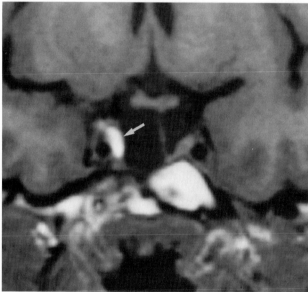

FIG. IIB-4. Effect of combined therapy on pituitary adenoma: hemorrhage related to bromocriptine treatment in a 25-year-old woman with recurrent hyperprolactinemia following surgery and radiotherapy for macroprolactinoma. Coronal contrast-enhanced CT (**A**) and unenhanced T_1-weighted (TR = 500 msec, TE = 20 msec) (**B**) MR show residual or recurrent right lateral adenoma (*arrows*). Bromocriptine therapy was initiated at this time. **C:** Six months later, coronal unenhanced T_1-weighted (TR = 500 msec, TE = 20 msec) MR image reveals decrease in size of adenoma with intratumoral hemorrhage (*arrow*) likely related to the bromocriptine therapy.

manifests as increased signal intensity on both T_1-weighted and T_2-weighted spin-echo sequences (19,20) (Figs. IIB-2 and IIB-4). Intratumoral hemorrhage is more difficult to identify on CT, but acute hemorrhage appears as an area of increased attenuation on unenhanced scans. Following i.v. contrast infusion, both acute and chronic hemorrhage may appear as an area of relatively decreased attenuation as compared to the adjacent normally enhancing pituitary gland.

In the series of Scotti et al. (13), an increase in tumor size was observed in two of the 30 macroprolactinomas that were being treated with bromocriptine. Both of these patients presented clinically with worsening visual field defects. Computed tomography demonstrated an increase in tumor volume and attenuation in both patients. Intratumoral hemorrhage and necrosis were confirmed surgically in one patient. The authors concluded that the increase

in tumor size in both patients was most likely a result of hemorrhage. Based on this experience, the authors suggested that when a sudden enlargement of a pituitary gland tumor occurs during medical treatment, intratumoral hemorrhage is the most likely etiology.

In a serial MR study of 13 macroprolactinomas during bromocriptine therapy, Lundin et al. (14) observed nine small new hemorrhages in seven different adenomas. Two of these hemorrhages resulted in slight tumor expansion, and none of the hemorrhages was symptomatic.

Yousem et al. (21) performed a retrospective evaluation of 68 pituitary adenomas. Intratumoral hemorrhage was diagnosed in 18 adenomas based on increased signal intensity within the adenoma on T_1-weighted and T_2-weighted spin-echo MR images. Surgical confirmation was available in five of the patients. In total, 13 of 29 (45%) patients receiving bromocriptine experienced intratumoral hemorrhage, whereas only five of 39 (13%) patients not receiving bromocriptine had intratumoral hemorrhage. The difference was statistically significant. Hemorrhage occurred in both micro- and macroadenomas. Ten of the 18 hemorrhages were asymptomatic. The authors concluded that bromocriptine therapy may result in intratumoral hemorrhage within pituitary adenomas.

Other, nonhemorrhagic structural changes have been observed within pituitary macroadenomas following bromocriptine therapy: CT studies have demonstrated the development of new areas of decreased attenuation within macroadenomas, presumably representing focal areas of edema or necrosis (12,22).

A recent MR study by Lundin et al. (14) also detected nonhemorrhagic signal changes within medically treated macroprolactinomas (14). Seven of 13 patients in their series revealed small intratumoral areas of decreased and increased signal intensity on T_1- and T_2-weighted MR images, respectively, consistent with cyst formation. In three patients, small areas of isointensity on T_1-weighted images and hyperintensity on T_2-weighted MR images were identified and were felt to represent necrosis or cysts. A trend toward increasing T_2 values over time within medically treated macroprolactinomas was also observed, suggesting a general increase in water content.

Asymptomatic herniation of the optic chiasm into the sella turcica has been observed following bromocriptine treatment and shrinkage of macroadenomas (14). Increased signal intensity has also been observed within the herniated optic chiasm on T_2-weighted spin-echo images (14). Because the chiasm was not biopsied in these patients, the cause of this T_2 signal alteration is unknown.

SURGICAL THERAPY

Microprolactinomas that fail medical therapy, other types of functioning microadenomas (e.g., growth-hormone- and ACTH-secreting tumors), and macroadenomas are usually treated surgically. Transsphenoidal resection has become the standard surgical approach for treating pituitary adenomas (23) (Fig. IIB-5). However, macroadenomas that involve the brain, cavernous sinus, or middle cranial fossa are best approached transcranially (24–27) (Fig. IIB-6). The transcranial approach has also been recommended for dumbbell-shaped tumors constricted at the diaphragma sella (24,28). Incomplete pneumatization of the sphenoid sinus as well as previous transsphenoidal surgery are relative contraindications to the transsphenoidal approach (24,25,27). Active sphenoid sinusitis represents another contraindication (28).

Following transsphenoidal resection, the surgical defect in the bony sellar floor is easily recognized on CT (4). However, the bony defect may be more difficult to appreciate on MR because both cortical bone in the sellar floor and air in the sphenoid sinus lack mobile protons

and therefore appear dark (signal void) on MR images (4). Postsurgical packing of the sellar floor is commonly performed to control hemorrhage and to prevent postoperative CSF leakage (29) (Figs. IIB-6 and IIB-7). Packing materials are varied and included Gelfoam, fat, fascia, and muscle. Grafts such as nasal septum, cartilage, or acrylic bone cement may be used to reconstruct the sellar floor.

There are relatively few studies in the medical literature that describe the normal radiologic appearance of postsurgical packing materials (1,12,30–34). On postoperative CT and MR, surgical packing materials have a highly variable appearance that may be confused with residual or recurrent tumor. Familiarity with the normal appearance of postsurgical packing material is, therefore, important for accurate scan interpretation.

Postoperative CT studies suggest that the septal bone graft used to reconstruct the sellar floor is visible in almost all patients (12). Kaplan et al. (12) observed the disappearance of the bony graft in one patient on a 13-month follow-up scan, presumably because of resorption of the bone fragment. Dolinkas and Simeone (32) described the migration of bony fragments into the suprasellar cistern in two patients. In one of these patients, the bony fragments produced symptomatic compression of the optic chiasm necessitating reoperation. Not surprisingly, Steiner et al. (31) were able to identify the bone grafts on MR in only one of 11 patients.

Postsurgical fat packing is easily recognized as an area of markedly decreased attenuation on CT (Fig. IIB-8). On T_1-weighted spin-echo MR images, the fat appears as an area of increased signal intensity with associated chemical shift artifact in the direction of the frequency-encoding gradient (Fig. IIB-9). Fat packing may persist indefinitely, but in some patients the fat packing has been observed to decrease in size or disappear over time, presumably as a result of resorption (30,32).

In the CT series of Kaplan et al. (12), the muscle grafts ranged from isodense to hyperdense on early postoperative unenhanced scans. Following i.v. contrast infusion, 11% of muscle grafts enhanced consistent with an inflammatory response to the tissue. Repeat surgery in two of these patients confirmed the presence of fibrosis and inflammation within the muscle grafts.

Gelfoam (gelatin sponge) is another commonly used packing material. On early postoperative CT scans performed within 3 weeks following surgery, Gelfoam appears as an area of decreased attenuation (12). Later postoperative scans almost always demonstrate complete resorption of the Gelfoam. A recent study by Steiner et al. (31) reviewed the MR appearance of gelatin foam (Spongostan) implants in 22 postoperative patients. The gelatin foam was identified as an intrasellar mass in seven of 22 patients on MR studies performed within 4 months of surgery. On T_1-weighted spin-echo images, the gelatin foam appeared isointense with gray matter in five of seven

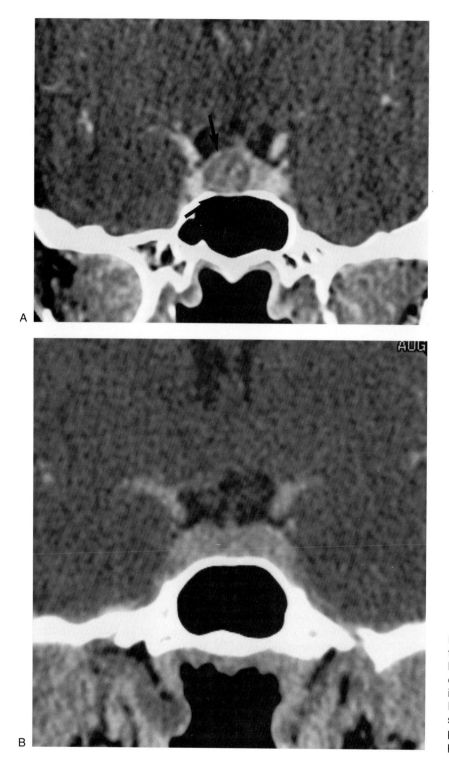

FIG. IIB-5. Successful surgical therapy of pituitary adenoma in a 26-year-old woman with hyperprolactinemia. **A:** Coronal contrast-enhanced CT reveals a relatively nonenhancing right-sided macroadenoma (*arrows*). **B:** Postoperative enhanced CT following transsphenoidal surgery shows successful, complete resection of adenoma with normal appearance of the pituitary gland.

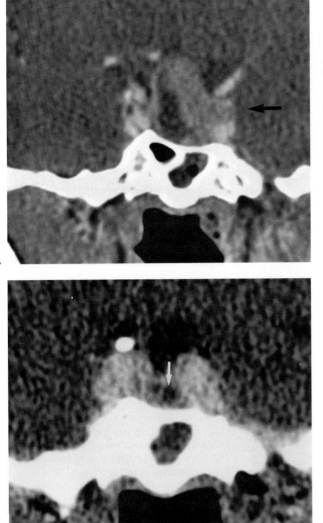

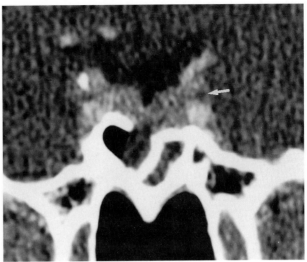

FIG. IIB-6. Postsurgical residual prolactinoma in a 29-year-old woman with hyperprolactinemia. **A:** Coronal contrast-enhanced CT shows a mixed enhancing and nonenhancing macroadenoma. There is a suggestion of extension into the left cavernous sinus (*arrow*). **B,C:** Postoperative enhanced CT was performed because of a persistently elevated serum prolactin level. **B:** Relatively nonenhancing residual tumor is seen in left cavernous sinus (*arrow*). **C:** Note low-attenuation postsurgical packing in the tumor bed (*arrow*).

patients and was difficult to delineate from the surrounding pituitary gland because of the relative similarity in signal intensities. In the remaining two patients, the gelatin foam appeared inhomogeneously hyperintense, possibly representing methemoglobin formation. After i.v. gadolinium contrast agent administration, the gelatin foam implant was readily differentiated from surrounding structures. The central portion of the gelatin foam implant did not enhance in any of the seven patients. In six of the seven patients, a thin peripheral rim of enhancement was noted surrounding the implant material. This rim of enhancement appeared hyperintense compared to the surrounding pituitary gland and helped determine the margins of the implant material. The authors suggested that the enhancing rim may represent granulation tissue. On follow-up MR, the gelatin foam implant decreased significantly in size or disappeared in almost all patients.

Dina et al. (30) described the MR appearance of Gelfoam packing in eight patients after transsphenoidal resec-

tion. Early and late postoperative MR scans were performed at less than 8 days and more than 4 months following surgery in all patients. On the early T_1-weighted spin-echo images, the surgical cavities packed with Gelfoam were peripherally isointense to the pituitary gland and displayed a central irregular area of decreased signal intensity. The authors suggest that this central area of decreased signal intensity may represent small air bubbles within the Gelfoam. Early T_2-weighted images also demonstrated decreased signal intensity within the surgical cavity. The late postoperative MR scans demonstrated complete resorption of the Gelfoam in five patients and a marked decrease in size in the remaining three patients.

Other types of postsurgical packing material are used less commonly, and their appearance on MR and CT is less well known. Because of the range of different packing materials in use, their variable appearance on MR and CT, and their change in appearance over time, it is easy to understand why postsurgical changes may be confused

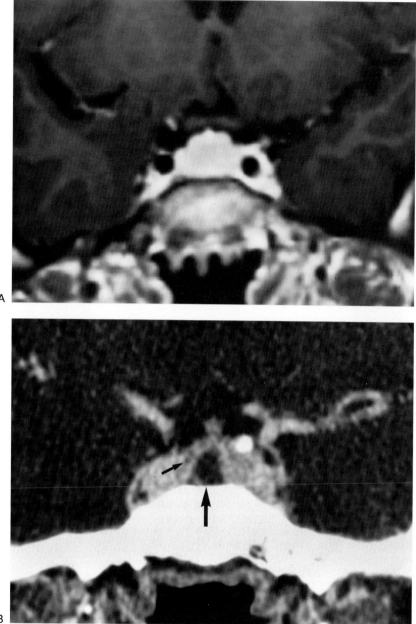

FIG. IIB-7. Early postsurgical appearance of the pituitary in a 23-year-old woman with an elevated serum prolactin level. **A:** Preoperative coronal T$_1$-weighted (TR = 500 msec, TE = 20 msec) gadolinium-enhanced MR image demonstrates diffuse enlargement of the pituitary gland, but no discreet pituitary adenoma is identified. Despite the MR finding, a prolactinoma was identified at the time of surgery and was resected via the transsphenoidal approach. **B:** Coronal contrast-enhanced CT performed 8 days postsurgery for persistent postoperative hyponatremia and SIADH. A well-defined area of decreased attenuation is present at the resection site consistent with Gelfoam packing (*large arrow*). There is a faint peripheral enhancing rim at the margins of the postsurgical packing (*small arrow*). The postoperative pituitary mass has changed little in size compared to the preoperative study.

with residual or recurrent tumor. For this reason, it is important for the radiologist to be familiar with the imaging appearance of surgical packing materials in use at his or her institution.

In addition to surgical packing material, the postoperative tumor bed may contain areas of hemorrhage (Fig. IIB-10). Early studies performed before the advent of CT or in the early CT era estimate the incidence of hemorrhage at between 0.5% and 2.5% (24,25,35,36). Later CT studies describe a higher incidence of hemorrhage (12,32). Kaplan et al. (12) noted hemorrhage in the postoperative tumor bed in 23 of 40 cases of macroadenoma but in only one of seven cases of microadenoma on CT scans performed within 21 days following surgery (12). Dolinkas and Simeone (32) detected postoperative

hemorrhage in 10 of 50 patients on CT scans performed within 1 week following transsphenoidal surgery. In six of these 10 patients, the hemorrhage was confined to the tumor bed. The authors observed that patients became symptomatic only if the bleeding involved structures outside the tumor bed (e.g., subarachnoid or intraventricular hemorrhage).

Air may be a normal finding within the postoperative tumor bed in the early period following transsphenoidal surgery (Fig. IIB-10). Kaplan et al. (12) observed air within the tumor bed or subarachnoid space on 22 of 40 postoperative CT scans. In almost all cases the air was resorbed within 21 days. In one case, a sudden increase in intracranial air accompanied massive CSF rhinorrhea, indicating the development of a CSF fistula.

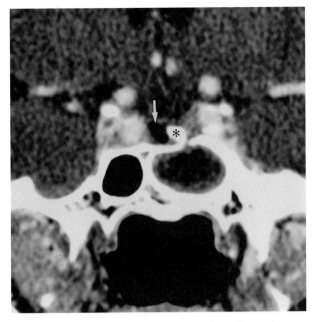

FIG. IIB-8. Postsurgical alterations of the sella turcica seen by CT of a 46-year-old man 6 months following transsphenoidal resection of a pituitary macroadenoma. Coronal contrast-enhanced CT shows postsurgical fat packing (*small arrow*) and calcification (*asterisk*) in the sellar floor.

Perhaps the most important finding on early postoperative CT and MR scans is the lack of change in size of the pituitary mass when compared to the preoperative scan (Figs. IIB-7 and IIB-10). Dina et al. (30) performed postoperative MR on 10 patients within 2 to 8 days following transsphenoidal resection. In two patients, the pituitary mass was unchanged in size; in five patients, it was slightly smaller; and in three patients, the pituitary mass actually increased in size. The lack of change in size of the pituitary mass in the immediate postoperative period has been ascribed to surgical packing in the tumor bed, postoperative hemorrhage, as well as adhesions between the diaphragma sella or tumor and brain tissue (theoretically preventing the outer margins of the tumor from collapsing inward).

Teng et al. (33) described the appearance of the pituitary mass on early postoperative CT as a central area of decreased attenuation with a thin peripheral enhancing rim (Fig. IIB-7). The authors attributed the central area of decreased attenuation to postsurgical packing, hemorrhage, and fluid. The peripheral enhancing rim has been described as a tumor capsule, but whether this tissue represents residual tumor or normal pituitary gland has not been determined. Dina et al. (30) observed a similar peripherally enhancing rim on i.v. gadolinium enhanced MR scans in three of 10 patients in the immediate postoperative period.

Although the dimensions of the pituitary mass may be unchanged in the immediate postoperative period, later postoperative CT and MR scans usually demonstrate sig-

nificant shrinkage of the pituitary mass (Fig. IIB-10). In a serial MR study of 10 patients, Dina et al. (30) observed a progressive decrease in height of the pituitary mass ranging from 21% to 75% (average of 54%) within 4 to 9 months following transsphenoidal surgery (30).

In light of this normal progressive involution in size of postoperative pituitary mass, several authors have recommended that baseline postoperative CT and MR scans be delayed for up to 4 to 6 months following surgery (31,33). Ciric et al. (34) suggest that the rate of tumor recurrence following transsphenoidal hypophysectomy is approximately 12% and that most recurrences occur between 4 and 8 years following surgery (Fig. IIB-11). This slow rate of growth of pituitary adenomas would add support to the recommendation that baseline CT or MR be delayed for up to 4 to 6 months after surgery.

The usual reason baseline postoperative CT or MR scans are performed in cases of macroadenoma is to determine the success of surgery and to assess the potential need for radiotherapy. Functioning microadenomas generally do not require a postoperative baseline CT or MR because residual or recurrent tumor can be detected biochemically.

On late postoperative MR and CT studies following transsphenoidal resection of a pituitary macroadenoma, the remaining normal pituitary gland demonstrates some degree of deformity. The gland is often eccentrically located within the sella, and the deformed shape of the gland has been described as club- or sickle-shaped (37). Herniation of the optic chiasm into a partially empty sella may also occur following resection of a macroadenoma (12,30) (Fig. IIB-12). Kaufman et al. (38) have observed a lack of correlation between the degree of optic chiasm herniation and the severity of visual symptoms, although some effect on vision may be attributable to this phenomenon.

The mortality and morbidity rates following transsphenoidal surgery are quite low (23,24,34,39–41). Despite the widespread acceptance of this procedure, serious and potentially life-threatening complications may arise. A detailed discussion of all the potential postoperative complications is beyond the scope of this chapter. However, Reddy et al. (41) have summarized the reported complications of transsphenoidal surgery that have appeared in the medical literature (41). Some of the important complications that rely on imaging studies for diagnosis are reviewed.

The transsphenoidal approach may traumatize the nasal cavity and paranasal sinuses, resulting in complications. Transient maxillary or ethmoid sinusitis may be seen, but this usually resolves within 2 months of surgery (32). Within the sphenoid sinus, postsurgical packing material, mucous membrane thickening, and other inflammatory changes are a common finding and may persist indefinitely (30–32) (Fig. IIB-13). These postsurgical changes in the sphenoid sinus are

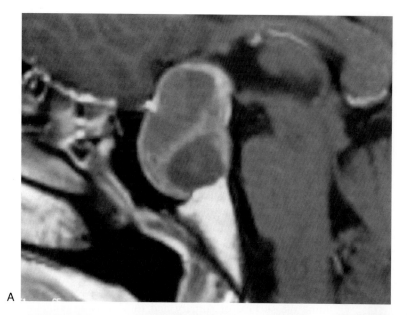

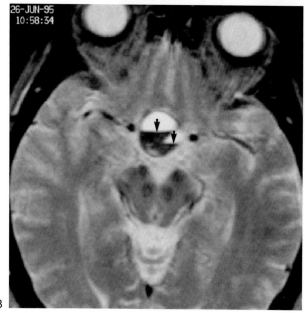

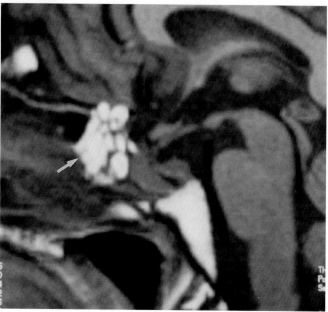

FIG. IIB-9. Postsurgical alterations of the sella turcica seen by MR of a 53-year-old man who presented with seizures and a visual field defect. (**A**) Preoperative sagittal gadolinium-enhanced T$_1$-weighted (TR = 500 msec, TE = 20 msec) MR and (**B**) axial T$_2$-weighted (TR = 2000 msec, TE = 90 msec) MR demonstrate a macroadenoma with intratumoral hemorrhage and layering of blood products (*arrows*). **C:** Five months post-surgery, sagittal unenhanced T$_1$-weighted (TR = 500 msec, TE = 20 msec) MR image demonstrates marked reduction in tumor size. Note hyperintense fat packing in sphenoid sinus and sellar floor (*arrow*).

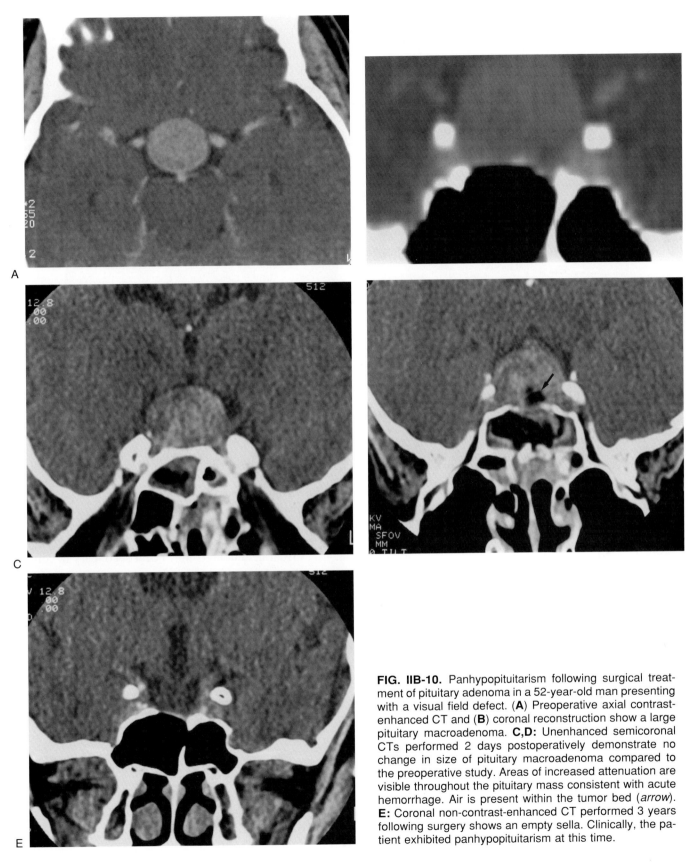

FIG. IIB-10. Panhypopituitarism following surgical treatment of pituitary adenoma in a 52-year-old man presenting with a visual field defect. (**A**) Preoperative axial contrast-enhanced CT and (**B**) coronal reconstruction show a large pituitary macroadenoma. **C,D:** Unenhanced semicoronal CTs performed 2 days postoperatively demonstrate no change in size of pituitary macroadenoma compared to the preoperative study. Areas of increased attenuation are visible throughout the pituitary mass consistent with acute hemorrhage. Air is present within the tumor bed (*arrow*). **E:** Coronal non-contrast-enhanced CT performed 3 years following surgery shows an empty sella. Clinically, the patient exhibited panhypopituitarism at this time.

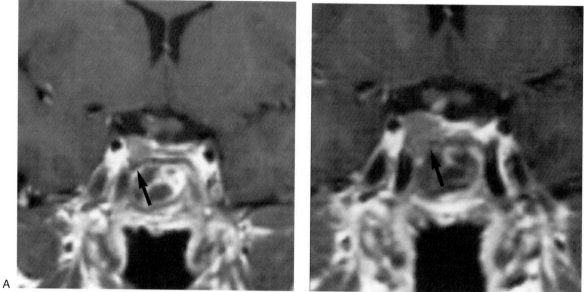

FIG. IIB-11. Recurrent postoperative pituitary adenoma in a 36-year-old woman with Cushing's disease who had persistently elevated serum cortisol levels despite previous treatment with bilateral adrenalectomy and total hypophysectomy. **A:** Postoperative coronal T_1-weighted (TR = 500 msec, TE = 20 msec) gadolinium-enhanced MR image shows small right-sided microadenoma (*arrow*). **B:** T_1-weighted (TR = 500 msec, TE = 20 msec) MR performed 2 years later reveals interval growth of the adenoma (*arrow*).

usually asymptomatic, but symptomatic chronic sinusitis may develop (36). Sphenoid sinus mucocele is a rare complication (36). Following transsphenoidal surgery, nasal complications include fractures of the medial wall of the maxillary sinus and nasal septal perforations, which may result in saddle nose deformity (36,40). Mucosal adhesions between the nasal

septum and lateral nasal wall may occur and impair ventilation (42).

Important intracranial complications include hemorrhage (intracerebral, subarachnoid, intraventricular), hydrocephalus, meningitis, thalamic infarction, pneumocephalus, and CSF fistula (12,24,34,40,41,43–46). Visual field deficits may occur secondary to com-

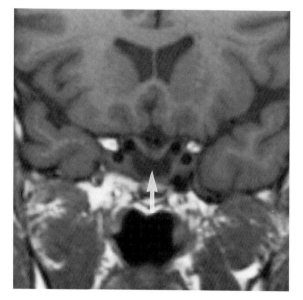

FIG. IIB-12. Asymptomatic postsurgical optic chiasm sellar herniation. Coronal T_1-weighted (TR = 500 msec, TE = 20 msec) MR image following resection of a macroadenoma shows herniation of optic chiasm into the partially empty sella (*arrow*). The patient was asymptomatic at this time.

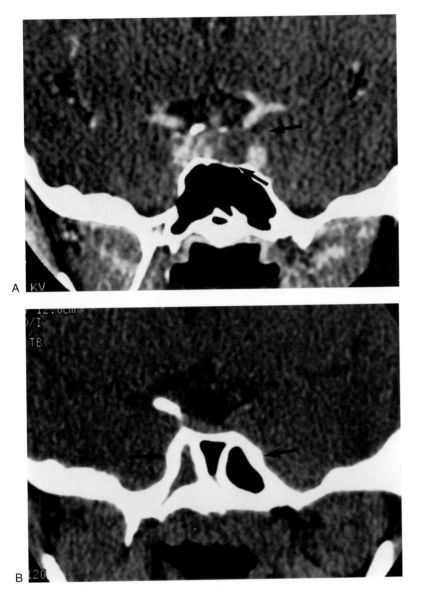

FIG. IIB-13. Postoperative changes in the sphenoid sinus in a 31-year-old woman with an elevated serum prolactin level. **A:** Preoperative coronal contrast-enhanced CT reveals a low-attenuation pituitary adenoma (*arrow*). **B:** Postoperative coronal unenhanced CT performed 16 months following transsphenoidal resection of the pituitary adenoma. Note the diffuse symmetric thickening of the bony walls and septum of the sphenoid sinus (*arrows*) compared to the preoperative scan. Inflammatory soft tissue is also present within the sphenoid sinus. The findings are consistent with chronic sphenoid sinusitis. The patient was asymptomatic.

pression or injury of the optic nerves or chiasm (40,47) (Fig. IIB-14). If the surgical dissection extends laterally into the cavernous sinus, then cranial nerve (3, 4, 5, or 6) palsy may ensue (34,43,46). A rare and dreaded complication of transsphenoidal surgery is inadvertant injury to the internal carotid artery within the cavernous sinus. This may result in life-threatening hemorrhage, false aneurysm formation, or arterial occlusion (43,46,48–50) (Fig. IIB-15).

Despite the low incidence of postoperative complications following transsphenoidal surgery, a variety of additional complications have been described in the medical literature. Awareness of potential complications combined with the knowledge of the normal appearance of the postoperative pituitary enables the radiologist to provide accurate interpretation of postoperative CT and MR scans.

RADIOTHERAPY

Although radiotherapy has been used with success as a primary treatment modality for pituitary macroadenomas (51,52), it is most frequently used for large pituitary macroadenomas after incomplete resection or persistently endocrinologically active pituitary adenomas following surgery. Radiotherapy can be performed in the immediate postoperative period or as late therapy following recurrence.

Because of the high recurrence rate of pituitary macroadenomas after surgery, adjuvant radiotherapy is frequently used in the immediate postoperative period (53). The overall results are excellent, with progression-free and overall survival rates of 62% to 89.4% and 81.5% to 90%, respectively (53–56). Patients are generally considered progression-free or disease-free if there is stabilization or normalization of hormone levels or lesion size on imaging studies. Of the endocrine-active tumors, prolactinomas are the most responsive (57). Growth-hormone-secreting tumors are more resistant. ACTH-secreting tumors and Nelson's syndrome typically have a variable response (58).

Radiation fields are generally formed by rotational arcs or parallel opposed lateral fields. Field size is generally within a 1-cm radius of the preoperative tumor. The median field size is approximately 5 to 5.5 cm. The fields generally include the perisellar optic pathways and the medial temporal lobes.

Dose fractionation is usually held under 225 cGy per day, as there is a reported increase in visual problems following high-dose fractionation (59). Response to therapy is clearly dose related. Doses of 4500 to 5000 cGy (60) are recommended to decrease the incidence of recurrence.

When the postradiotherapy pituitary gland is imaged, it is important to recognize that considerable residual soft tissue mass may persist in spite of normalization of hor-

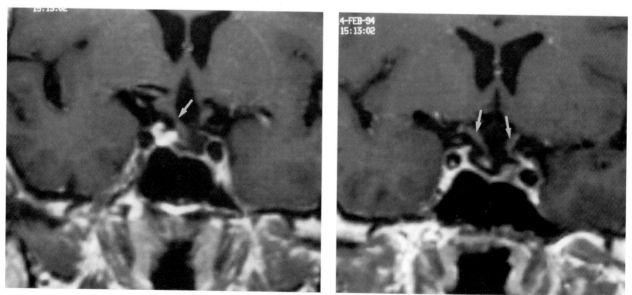

FIG. IIB-14. Visual deterioration from combined therapy of pituitary adenoma in a 54-year-old woman who presented 17 years earlier with a nonfunctioning macroadenoma and was treated with surgery and radiotherapy at that time. The patient now presents with progressive visual deterioration, and, therefore, MR was performed. **A,B:** Coronal T_1-weighted (TR = 500 msec, TE = 20 msec) gadolinium-enhanced MR demonstrates disruption and deformity of the optic chiasm (*arrows*), related to previous tumor compression and/or surgery. The patient's progressive visual impairment was attributed in part to radiation injury of the optic nerves and chiasm. Optic chiasm tethering may also have contributed to the visual deterioration.

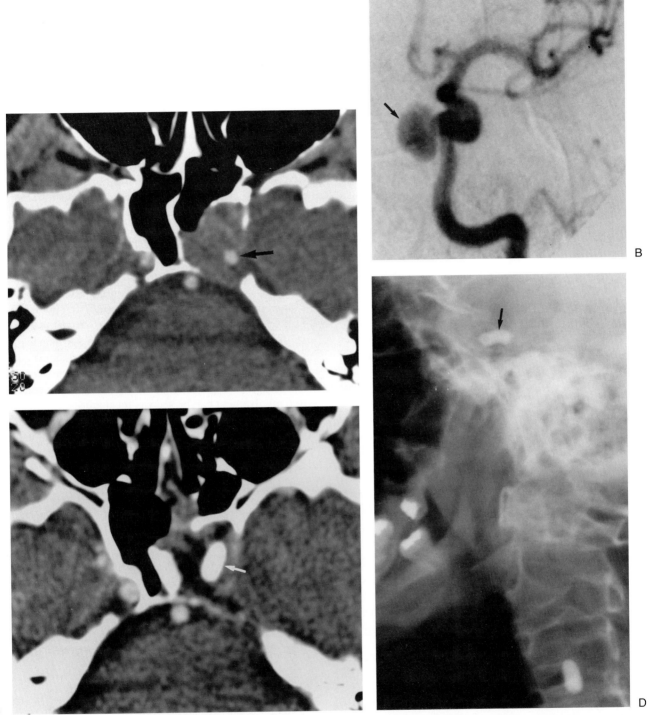

FIG. IIB-15. Postsurgical pseudoaneurysm formation following transsphenoid resection of pituitary adenoma in a 58-year-old man with hyperprolactinemia. **A:** Axial contrast-enhanced CT shows a pituitary macroadenoma with invasion of left cavernous sinus and possible encasement of left internal carotid artery (*arrow*). Patient underwent transsphenoidal resection. Intraoperatively, the carotid artery was inadvertently injured, resulting in massive life-threatening epistaxis. **B:** Angiogram shows a false aneurysm (*arrow*) arising from the internal carotid artery and extending into the sphenoid sinus. Following successful balloon test occlusion of the left internal carotid artery, the aneurysm was trapped with permanent balloon occlusion of the carotid artery (**C,D**) (*arrows*).

mone secretion and stabilization of tumor growth. There is frequently a delay of up to years in the endocrine and volume-reduction response to radiotherapy. Although the response may result in an "empty sella" appearance in some patients, the majority will have residual soft tissue after therapy. It is important to have a preradiotherapy baseline as well as follow-up examinations for assessment of tumor growth. Imaging follow-up is particularly important in nonsecretory adenomas and in prolactinomas treated with bromocriptine, when hormone levels are not reliable in assessing response to therapy.

Recent improvements in CT and MR imaging now enable accurate detection of tumor recurrence. This allows the option of radiotherapy being performed as so-called salvage therapy for recurrences rather than as routine postoperative treatment. Salvage radiotherapy has been shown to be effective in the control of recurrent tumors (53,55).

Complications of radiotherapy include hypopituitarism, which has been reported to occur in as many as 71% of individuals treated with radiation (61,62). The onset of hypopituitarism usually occurs within 3 to 4 years following radiotherapy but may be delayed in onset, supporting the concept of careful long-term follow-up of patients.

Delayed adverse effects of radiation therapy include cerebrovascular accidents, brain necrosis, optic atrophy, and secondary tumors (63) (Fig. IIB-16). For example, radiotherapy for pituitary adenomas has been implicated in an increased incidence of cerebrovascular accidents

(CVA) (64), although the larger series do not demonstrate a statistically significant increase (64). These infarctions typically involve the basal ganglia in the distribution of the lentriculostriate arteries and are well demonstrated by CT and MR. They frequently occur many years following radiation therapy. Other vascular complications included the development of cavernous carotid aneurysms (65,66) and Moya-Moya-like vascular changes (67).

Visual problems secondary to optic nerve and chiasm radiation effects have been shown to be dose related (59,68). Subjective cognitive and memory dysfunctions have been reported, presumably related to the inclusion of the medial temporal lobes and hypothalamus in the radiation field. Subjective complaints of cognitive memory impairment have been reported in as many as 11% of patients (53). Cognitive and memory dysfunction is also recognized preoperatively in patients with pituitary tumors (69).

Radiation necrosis of neural tissue can occur, although it is rare in the doses used for pituitary microadenomas. Frank radiation necrosis of the medial temporal lobes usually occurs only at higher doses (i.e., greater than 5500 cGy) (55,70,71) (Fig. IIB-17). Magnetic resonance imaging demonstrates high signal intensity on the intermediate and T_2-weighted images in the periventricular white matter adjacent to the temporal horns. Brainstem and pontine involvement can be seen as focal areas of high signal intensity on the intermediate and T_2-weighted sequences. Areas of radiation necrosis may also demonstrate en-

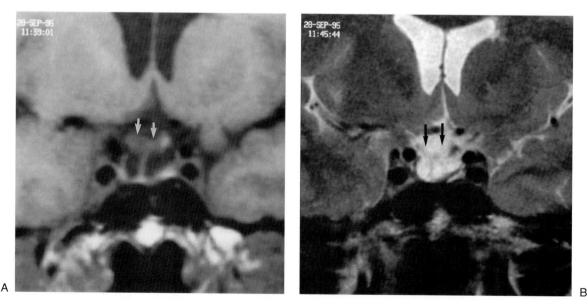

FIG. IIB-16. Radiation injury to the optic chiasm following radiotherapy for pituitary adenoma in a 48-year-old man treated 14 years earlier with surgery and radiotherapy for an FSH-producing macroadenoma who now presents with a worsening visual field defect. (**A**) T_1-weighted (TR = 500 msec, TE = 20 msec) and corresponding (**B**) coronal fast spin-echo T_2-weighted (TR = 4000 msec, TE = 90 msec) MR images demonstrate low signal intensity within the optic chiasm on the T_1-weighted acquisitions (*arrows*) and high signal intensity within the optic chiasm (isotense with CSF) on the T_2-weighted images (*arrows*), consistent with radiation injury.

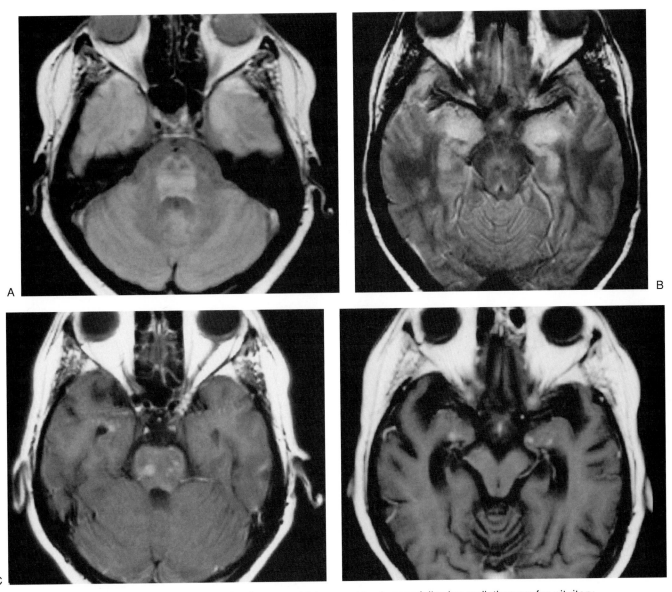

FIG. IIB-17. Radiation necrosis of temporal lobes and brainstem following radiotherapy for pituitary adenoma in a 39-year-old woman 6 years following radiotherapy for hypothalamic glioma. (**A**) Axial proton-density-weighted (TR = 2000 msec, TE = 40 msec), (**B**) T$_2$-weighted (TR = 2000 msec, TE = 90 msec), and (**C,D**) gadolinium-enhanced T$_1$-weighted (TR = 500 msec, TE = 20 msec) MR images demonstrate areas of increased signal intensity and enhancement in pons and medial temporal lobes bilaterally, consistent with radiation necrosis.

hancement on T$_1$-weighted images following i.v. gadolinium contrast agent administration. Medial temporal lobe atrophy occurs on a delayed basis.

Modern transsphenoidal surgical techniques make radiotherapy infrequently required for microadenomas. In our center, radiotherapy is generally reserved for cases of incompletely resected macroadenoma. Imaging is performed in conjunction with clinical and serologic assessment every 6 months to 1 year following surgery. If growth is demonstrated, then radiotherapy is performed. Radiotherapy for recurrent macroadenomas generally yields excellent results with series indicating overall 10-year survivals matching the expected (56).

CONCLUSIONS

Magnetic resonance has become the imaging examination of choice in the evaluation of pituitary adenomas. Computed tomography may also provide valuable information and remains in widespread use. Pituitary adenomas are usually treated medically, surgically, with radiotherapy, or with combination therapy. Following treatment, the normal anatomy of the pituitary gland and surrounding structures is frequently altered. The changes in the posttherapeutic pituitary may mimic residual or recurrent disease, making interpretation of posttreatment MR and CT difficult.

In order to provide accurate interpretation of posttherapeutic MR and CT, the radiologist must have access to the pretreatment examinations for comparison. Correlation with serum hormone levels is essential in order to determine the significance of the imaging findings. In addition, the radiologist must be familiar with the normal appearance of the pituitary following treatment as well as the potential complications that may arise.

Finally, despite the best efforts, it may be impossible to determine whether residual or recurrent tumor is present on a single examination. Following resection of a macroadenoma, the pituitary mass may continue to involute for up to 4 to 6 months postsurgery. Changes in the pituitary may continue for several years following radiotherapy or bromocriptine therapy. In light of these expected posttherapeutic changes, long-term follow-up may be needed to determine the ultimate success or failure of treatment.

REFERENCES

1. Mikhael MA, Ciric IS: MR imaging of pituitary tumors before and after surgical and/or medical treatment. *J Comput Assist Tomogr* 1988;12(3):441–445.
2. Peck WW, Dillon WP, Norman D, Newton TH, Wilson CB: High-resolution MR imaging of microadenomas at 1.5 T: experience with Cushing's disease. *Am J Neuroradiol* 1988;9(6):1085–1091.
3. Kulkarni MV, Francis Lee K, McArdle CB, Yeakley JW, Haar FL: 1.5 T MR imaging of pituitary microadenomas: technical considerations and CT correlation. *Am J Neuroradiol* 1988;9(1):5–11.
4. Lundin P, Bergstrom K, Thuomas KA, Lundberg PO, Muhr C: Comparison of MR imaging and CT in pituitary macroadenomas. *Acta Radiol* 1991;32(3):189–196.
5. Finelli DA, Kaufman B: Varied microcirculation of pituitary adenomas at rapid, dynamic, contrast-enhanced MR imaging. *Radiology* 1993;189(1):205–210.
6. Bonneville JF, Cattin F, Mouss-Bacha K, Portha C: Dynamic computed tomography of the pituitary gland: the "tuft sign." *Radiology* 1983;149:145–148.
7. Tien RD: Sequence of enhancement of various portions of the pituitary gland on gadolinium-enhanced MR images: correlation with regional blood supply. *Am J Roentgenol* 1992;158:651–654.
8. Bonneville JF, Cattin F, Gorczyca W, Hardy J: Pituitary adenomas: early enhancement with dynamic CT—implications in arterial blood supply and potential importance. *Radiology* 1993;187:1–5.
9. Teramoto A, Hirakawa K, Sanno N, Osamura Y: Incidental pituitary lesions in 1,000 unselected autopsy specimens. *Radiology* 1994;193(1):161–164.
10. Chong BW, Kucharczyk W, Singer W, George S: Pituitary gland MR: a comparative study of healthy volunteers and patients with microadenomas. *Am J Neuroradiol* 1994;15:675–679.
11. Hall WA, Luciano MG, Doppman JL: Pituitary magnetic resonance imaging in normal human volunteers: occult adenomas in the general population. *Ann Intern Med* 1994;120:817–820.
12. Kaplan HC, Baker HL, Houser OW, Laws ER, Abboud CF, Scheithauer BW: CT of the sella turcica after transsphenoidal resection of pituitary adenomas. *Am J Neuroradiol* 1985;6(5):723–731.
13. Scotti G, Scialfa G, Pieralli S, Chiodini PG, Spelta B, Dallabonzana D: Macroprolactinomas: CT evaluation of reduction of tumor size after medical treatment. *Neuroradiology* 1982;23:123–126.
14. Lundin P, Bergstrom K, Nyman R, Lundberg PO, Muhr C: Macroprolactinomas: serial MR imaging in long-term bromocriptine therapy. *Am J Neuroradiol* 1992;13:1279–1291.
15. Bassetti M, Spada A, Pezzo G, Giannattasio G: Bromocriptine treatment reduces the cell size in human macroprolactinomas: a morphometric study. *J Clin Endocrinol Metab* 1984;58:268–273.
16. Gen M, Uozumi T, Ohta M, Ito A, Kajiwara H, Mori S: Necrotic changes in prolactinomas after long term administration of bromocriptine. *J Clin Endocrinol Metab* 1984;59:463–470.
17. Esiri MM, Bevan JS, Burke CW, Adams CBT: Effect of bromocriptine treatment on the fibrous tissue content of prolactin-secreting and nonfunctioning macroadenomas of the pituitary gland. *J Clin Endocrinol Metab* 1986;63:383–388.
18. Weingarten K, Zimmerman RD, Deo-Narine V, Markisz J, Cahill PT, Deck MDF: MR imaging of acute intracranial hemorrhage: findings on sequential spin-echo and gradient-echo images in a dog model. *Am J Neuroradiol* 1991;12:457–467.
19. Ostrov SG, Quencer RM, Hoffman JC, Davis PC, Hasso AN, David NJ: Hemorrhage within pituitary adenomas: how often associated with pituitary apoplexy syndrome? *Am J Neuroradiol* 1989;10:503–510.
20. Dooms GC, Uske A, Brant-Zawadzki M, et al: Spin-echo MR imaging of intracranial hemorrhage. *Neuroradiology* 1986;28:132–138.
21. Yousem DM, Arrington JA, Zinreich SJ, Ashok JK, Bryan NR: Pituitary adenomas: possible role of bromocriptine in intratumoral hemorrhage. *Radiology* 1989;170:239–243.
22. Wolpert SM: The radiology of pituitary adenomas. *Endocrinol Metab Clin* 1987;16:553–584.
23. Hardy J: Transsphenoidal hypophysectomy. *J Neurosurg* 1971;34:582–594.
24. Wilson CB, Dempsey LC: Transsphenoidal microsurgical removal of 250 pituitary adenomas. *J Neurosurg* 1978;48:13–22.
25. Kenan PD: The rhinologist and the management of pituitary disease. *Laryngoscope* 1979;89(Suppl 14):1–26.
26. Zervas NT, Martin JB: Current concepts in cancer: management of hormone secreting pituitary adenomas. *N Engl J Med* 1980;320:210–214.
27. Laws ER, Kern EB: Special circumstances in operative management. In: Laws ER, Randall RV, Abboud CS, eds. *Management of Pituitary Adenomas and Related Lesions with Emphasis on Transsphenoidal Microsurgery*. New York: Appleton-Centry Crofts, 1982:271–276.
28. Post KD: General considerations in the surgical management of pituitary tumors. In: Post KD, Jackson IMD, Reichlin S, eds. *The Pituitary Adenoma*. New York: Plenum Press, 1980:341–363.
29. Spaziante R, de Divitilis E, Cappabianca P: Reconstruction of the pituitary fossa in transsphenoidal surgery: an experience of 140 cases. *Neurosurgery* 1986;17(3):453–458.
30. Dina TS, Feaster SH, Laws ER, Davis PO: MR of the pituitary gland postsurgery: serial MR studies following transsphenoidal resection. *Am J Neuroradiol* 1993;14:763–769.
31. Steiner E, Knosp E, Herold CJ, Kramer J, Stiglbauer R, Staniszewski K, Imhof H: Pituitary adenoma: findings of postoperative MR imaging. *Radiology* 1992;185:521–527.
32. Dolinkas CA, Simeone FA: Transsphenoidal hypophysectomy: post-surgical CT findings. *Am J Neuroradiol* 1985;6:45–50.
33. Teng MMH, Huang C, Chang T: The pituitary mass after transsphenoidal hypophysectomy. *Am J Neuroradiol* 1988;9:23–26.
34. Ciric I, Mikhael M, Stafford T, Lawson L, Garces R: Transsphenoidal microsurgery of pituitary macroadenomas with long-term follow-up results. *Neurosurgery* 1983;59:395–401.
35. Kern EB, Pearson BW, McDonald TJ, Laws ER: The transseptal approach to lesions of the pituitary and parasellar regions. *Laryngoscope* 1979;89(Suppl 15):1–34.
36. Laws ER, Kern EB: Complications of transsphenoidal surgery. *Clin Neurosurg* 1975;22:401–405.
37. Steiner E, Math G, Knosp E, Mostbeck G, Kramer J, Herold CJ: MR appearance of the pituitary gland before and after resection of pituitary macroadenomas. *Clin Radiol* 1994;49:524–530.
38. Kaufman B, Tomsak RL, Kaufman BA, et al: Herniation of the suprasellar visual system and third ventricle into empty sella: morphologic and clinical consierations. *Am J Neuroradiol* 1989;10:65–76.
39. Baskin DS, Boggan JE, Wilson CB: Transsphenoidal microsurgical removal of growth hormone secreting pituitary adenomas—a review of 137 cases. *J Neurosurg* 1982;56:634–641.
40. Kennedy DW, Cohn S, Papel ID, et al: Transsphenoidal approach to the sella: the John Hopkins experience. *Laryngoscope* 1984;94:1066–1074.

41. Reddy K, Fewer D, West M: Complications of the transsphenoidal approach to sellar lesions. *Can J Neurol Sci* 1991;18(4):463–466.

42. Karduck A, Bock WJ: Rhinological findings following transsphenoidal surgery of the pituitary gland. *Acta Otolaryngol (Stockh)* 1978;85:449–452.

43. Laws ER, Trautmann JC, Hollenhurst RW Jr: Transsphenoidal decompression of the optic nerve and chiasm—visual results in 62 patients. *J Neurosurg* 1977;46:717–722.

44. Gransden WR, Wickstead M, Eykyn S: Meningitis after transsphenoidal excision of pituitary tumors. *J Laryngol Otol* 1988;102:33–36.

45. Shields CB, Valdes-Rodriquez AG: Tension pneumocephalus after transsphenoidal hypophysectomy—case report. *Neurosurgery* 1982;11(5):687–689.

46. Zervas NT: Surgical results in pituitary adenomas: results of an international survey. In: Black PMcL, Zervas NT, Ridgway EC Jr, Martin JB, eds. *Secretory Tumors of the Pituitary Gland.* New York: Raven Press, 1984:377–385.

47. Barrow DL, Tindall GT: Loss of vision after transphenoidal surgery. *Neurosurgery* 1990;27(1):60–68.

48. Carbezudo JM, Carrillo R, Vaguero J, et al: Intracavernous aneurysm of the carotid artery following transsphenoidal surgery—case report. *J Neurosurg* 1981;54:118–121.

49. Paullus WS Jr, Norwood CW, Morgan HW: False aneurysm of the cavernous carotid artery and progressive external ophthalmoplegia after transsphenoidal hypophysectomy—case report. *J Neurosurg* 1979;59:707–709.

50. Reddy K, Lesiuk H, West M, et al: False aneurysm of the cavernous carotid artery: a complication of transsphenoidal surgery. *Surg Neurol* 1990;33:142–145.

51. Rush SC, Newall J: Pituitary adenoma: the efficacy of radiotherapy as the sole treatment. *Int J Radiat Oncol Biol Phys* 1989;17(1):165–169.

52. Grigsby PW, Stokes S, Marks JE, Simpson JR: Prognostic factors and results of radiotherapy alone in the management of pituitary adenomas. *Int J Radiat Oncol Biol Phys* 1988;15(5):1103–1110.

53. Clark SD, Woo SY, Butler EB, Dennis WS, Lu H, et al: Treatment of secretory adenoma with radiation therapy. *Radiology* 1993;188(3):759–763.

54. Fisher BJ, Gaspar LE, Noone B: Giant pituitary adenomas: role of radiotherapy. *Int J Radiat Oncol Biol Phys* 1993;25(4):677–681.

55. Kovalic JJ, Grigsby PW, Fineberg BB: Recurrent pituitary adenomas after surgical resection: the role of radiation therapy. *Radiology* 1990;177(1):273–275.

56. Grigsby PW, Simpson JR, Emami BN, Fineberg BB, Schwartz HG: Prognostic factors and results of surgery and postoperative irradiation in the management of pituitary adenomas. *Int J Radiat Oncol Biol Phys* 1989;16:(6)1411–1417.

57. Barkan AL: Acromegaly: diagnosis and therapy. *Endocrinol Metab Clin North Am* 1989;18:277–310.

58. Jenkins PJ, Trainer PJ, Plowman PN, Shand WS, Grossman AB, et al: The long-term outcome after adrenalectomy and prophylactic pituitary radiotherapy in adrenocorticotropin-dependent Cushing's syndrome. *J Clin Endocrinol Metab* 1995;80(1):165–171.

59. Harris JR, Levene MB: Visual complications following irradiation for pituitary adenomas and craniopharyngiomas. *Radiology* 1976;120:167–171.

60. McCollough WM, Marcus RB, Rhoton AL, Ballinger WE, Million RR: Long-term follow-up of radiotherapy for pituitary adenoma: the absence of late recurrence after >4500 cGy. *Int J Radiat Oncol Biol Phys* 1991;21:607–614.

61. Halberg FE, Sheline GE: Radiotherapy of pituitary tumors. *Endocrinol Metab Clin* 1987;16:667–681.

62. Zaugg M, Adaman O, Pescia R, Landolt AM: External irradiation of macroinvasive pituitary adenomas with telecobalt: a retrospective study with long-term follow-up in patients irradiated with doses mostly of between 40–45 Gy. *Int J Radiat Oncol Biol Phys* 1995;32(3):671–680.

63. Fisher BJ, Gaspar LE, Noone B: Radiation therapy of pituitary adenoma: delayed sequelae. *Radiology* 1993;187:843–846.

64. Bowen J, Paulsen CA: Stroke after pituitary irradiation. *Stroke* 1992;23:908–911.

65. McConachie NS, Jacobson I: Bilateral aneurysms of the cavernous internal carotid arteries following yttrium-90 implantation. *Neuroradiology* 1994;36(8):611–613.

66. Sutton LN: Vascular complications of surgery for craniopharyngioma and hypothalamic glioma. *Pediatr Neurosurg* 1994;21(Suppl 1):124–128.

67. Bitzer M, Topka H: Progressive cerebral occlusive disease after radiation therapy. *Stroke* 1995;26(1):131–136.

68. Croisile B, Piperno D, Bascoulergue Y, Romestaing P, Trillet M, et al: Chiasmal radionecrosis after irradiation of the sella turcica using a conventional dosage. Contribution of magnetic resonance imaging. *Rev Neurol (Paris)* 1990;146(1):57–60.

69. Grattan-Smith PJ, Morris JG, Shores EA, Batchelor J, Sparks RS: Neuropsychological abnormalities in patients with pituitary tumors. *Acta Neurol Scand* 1992;86(6):626–631.

70. Kleinschmidt-DeMasters BK: Necrotizing brainstem leukoencephalopathy six weeks following radiotherapy. *Clin Neuropathol* 1995;14(2):63–68.

71. Bederson JB, Harsh GR 4th, Walker JA, Wilson CB: Radiation-induced bilateral cystic temporal lobe necrosis: reversal of memory deficit after fenestration and internal shunting. Case report. *J Neurosurg* 1990;72(3):503–505.

Posttherapeutic Neurodiagnostic Imaging,
edited by J.R. Jinkins,
Lippincott-Raven Publishers, New York © 1997.

CHAPTER IIC

The Posttherapeutic Temporal Bone

Suresh K. Mukherji and Mauricio Castillo

Interpretation of the postoperative temporal bone is a challenging area for radiologists and requires a basic understanding of its normal and pathologic anatomy. Distortion of normal anatomy from previous surgery further increases the difficulty of interpreting images of this region. Knowledge of the various surgical procedures significantly aids in the understanding and interpretation of images of the postoperative temporal bone. Knowledge of the various procedures also helps to determine the specific type and extent of prior surgery in patients whose surgical records are incomplete or unavailable. Computed tomography (CT) is ideal for the evaluation of the postsurgical external and middle ear, and magnetic resonance (MR) is the imaging method of choice for the evaluation of the postsurgical internal auditory canal. Plain radiographs are helpful in the evaluation of cochlear implants. This chapter describes the imaging features of the most common surgical procedures employed for treatment of temporal bone disease as well as the changes resulting from irradiation and chemotherapy.

IMAGING PROTOCOL

Computed tomography is preferred for imaging patients who have undergone mastoidectomies for otomastoid disease and/or ossicular reconstructions. The CT is superior to MR for evaluation of underlying bony anatomy including the status of the sigmoid plate, tegmen tympani, and the bone covering of the facial nerve. The CT also provides optimal visualization of the ossicles and permits evaluation of the inner ear for presence of congenital abnormalities, obliterative labyrinthitis, and otosclerosis. Magnetic resonance is superior to CT for visualizing the cranial nerves and is the preferred modality for evaluating the intracanalicular portions of the facial and vestibuloco-

chlear nerves for recurrent or residual facial or vestibular schwannoma.

The CT of the temporal bone includes axial and coronal noncontrast contiguous 1.0-mm-thick sections performed parallel to the infraorbital–meatal line. Image acquisition starts superior to the arcuate eminence of the temporal bone and extends to the floor of the external auditory canal. Coronal images are obtained perpendicular to the infraorbital–meatal line from the posterior aspect of the mandibular condyle to the posterior semicircular canal. Coronal images should be acquired only directly. If direct coronal images are not possible, helical CT with a slice thickness of 1 mm (pitch = 1) results in adequate coronal reconstructions. If there are signs of infection, intravenous contrast administration is indicated. The CT should be performed with high-mAs technique and reconstructed using the high-resolution bone algorithm. Optimal visualization of middle- and inner-ear anatomy is obtained by targeting and reconstructing each side separately using a small field of view (9 to 10 cm).

The MR image is obtained using 3-mm-thick T_1-weighted images (TR = 650 msec, TE = 15 msec) through the internal auditory canals. Images should have a minimal interslice gap (10% or less), and two to four signal averages are required to obtain an adequate signal-to-noise ratio. Precontrast images are obtained only in the axial projection. These images serve to screen for the presence of blood or fat within the surgical bed. Postcontrast images should be performed in both axial and coronal projections. The study is complemented by axial T_2-weighted images (TR = 3500 to 4000 msec, TE = 19/90 msec) throughout the brain to assess the integrity of auditory pathways. Comparison with prior studies, including a preoperative one, is extremely helpful.

SURGICAL PROCEDURES

Mastoidectomy

There are several mastoidectomies and their nomenclature varies with each type of approach and the structures re-

S. K. Mukherji, M. Castillo: Departments of Radiology and Surgery, and Department of Radiology, University of North Carolina School of Medicine, Chapel Hill, North Carolina 27599.

moved. This nomenclature also varies among institutions. Mastoidectomies are classified as "canal-wall-up" (closed-cavity) and "canal-wall-down" (open-cavity) procedures (1). The term "simple mastoidectomy" (cortical mastoidectomy) refers to a procedure that respects the epitympanum. The canal-wall-up mastoidectomy (CWUM) is a variation of the simple mastoidectomy. The CWUM extends to the epitympanum and allows direct inspection of the ossicles and preservation of the posterior bony wall of the external auditory canal (Fig. IIC-1). This procedure includes exenteration of mastoid air cells and overlying cortex and removal of Körner's septum, which allows the surgically created cavity ("mastoid bowl") to communicate with the antrum and epitympanum. The posterior wall of the external auditory canal (EAC) is preserved. A CWUM is similar to a simple (cortical) mastoidectomy; however, the latter does not enter the antrum or epitympanum and does not allow direct visualization of the ossicles. A CWUM is the treatment of choice for coalescent mastoiditis. This procedure may also be performed for resection of cholesteatoma in adults, but it carries a relatively high rate of recurrence (25% to 35%). Similar surgical approaches may be utilized for cochlear implantation and endolymphatic duct surgeries (2,3).

The most commonly performed mastoidectomy is the canal-wall-down mastoidectomy (CWDM), which may be classified as modified radical or radical (1). The specific type of procedure performed is based on a combination of institutional preference and extent of disease. Extensive disease requires a radical mastoidectomy. The posterosuperior wall of the external auditory canal is removed, allowing it to communicate with the mastoid cavity ("canal wall down") (Fig. IIC-2). Next, for disease limited to the epitympanum, access is obtained by resecting the scutum, thereby allowing limited exposure of the middle ear. This does not require manipulation of the ossicles. If disease involves the ossicles, access to the middle ear cavity can be improved by separating the tympanic membrane from its annulus and skeletonizing the descending facial canal. If the ossicles are eroded by the underlying disease, a surgical reconstruction may be performed to preserve ossicular continuity. This procedure is referred to as a "modified radical mastoidectomy." For extensive disease encompassing the middle ear cavity, the previously mentioned procedure may be extended to include complete removal of the tympanic membrane, malleus, and incus while attempting to preserve the superstructure of the stapes. The descending facial canal is skeletonized, and the mucosa of the middle ear cavity and the eustachian tube is stripped. The eustachian tube orifice may then be occluded using a plug composed of fascia and/or fat (2,3). The latter procedure is known as a radical mastoidectomy and middle ear obliteration (2,3). A CWDM is performed for resection of middle ear cholesteatomas. Because this procedure allows exposure of the middle cavity, the recurrence rate of cholesteatoma is lower than that of a CWUM.

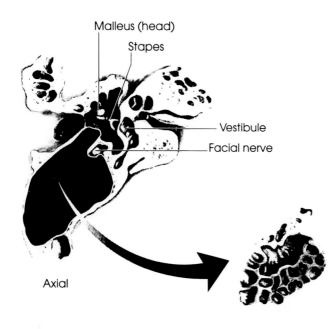

Canal Wall Up Mastoidectomy

FIG. IIC-1. Diagram showing resection of mastoid air cells and preservation of posterior wall of external auditory canal. (Drawing courtesy of Neill Biomedical Art, Gainesville, FL. From ref. 1, with permission.)

Ossicular Reconstruction

These reconstructions are performed in patients with otosclerosis or in patients whose ossicles are eroded or disrupted by either cholesteatoma or trauma. A procedure commonly performed in patients with otosclerosis is a stapedectomy. This procedure entails placement of a stapes prosthesis extending from the oval window to the incus (Fig. IIC-3). Initially, the tympanic membrane is lifted off the annulus posteriorly (tympanomeatal flap) along with a small amount of bone. The stapes suprastructure is resected, and a small hole is drilled into its footplate. One end of the prosthesis is placed into this opening, and the opposite end is attached to the incus. The prosthesis may be composed of Teflon, Silastic, or stainless steel (4).

An incus interposition procedure attempts to preserve ossicular continuity by altering the configuration and position of the native incus. This modification allows an abnormal incus to transmit vibrations from malleus to stapes (Fig. IIC-4). The incus is completely disarticulated, and a depression is drilled on the undersurface of its body in order to allow it to articulate between the head of the stapes and the manubrium of the malleus. This procedure is commonly used in patients who have ossicular destruc-

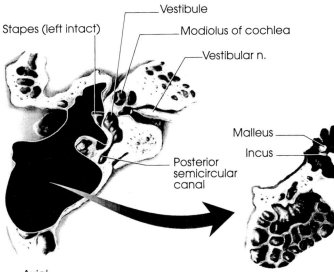

Stapes (left intact) — Vestibule

Vestibule

Modiolus of cochlea

Vestibular n.

Malleus

Incus

Posterior
semicircular
canal

Axial

Canal Wall Down
Radical Mastoidectomy

A

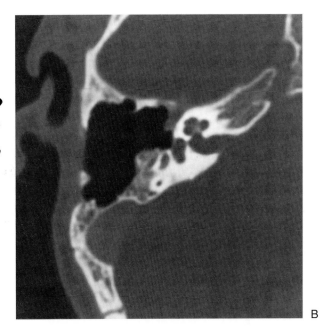

B

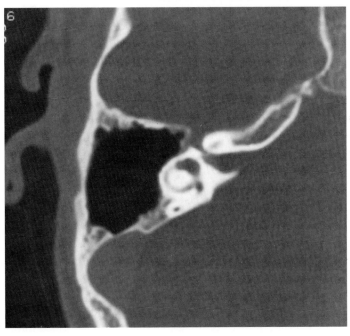

C

FIG. IIC-2. A: Diagram shows removal of mastoid and posterior wall of the external auditory canal but preservation of stapes (radical modified) (Drawing courtesy of Neill Biomedical Art, Gainesville, FL. From ref. 1, with permission.) **B:** Axial CT shows canal-wall-down mastoidectomy and, in addition, complete ossicular resection. **C:** Axial CT showing superior extent of this mastoidectomy.

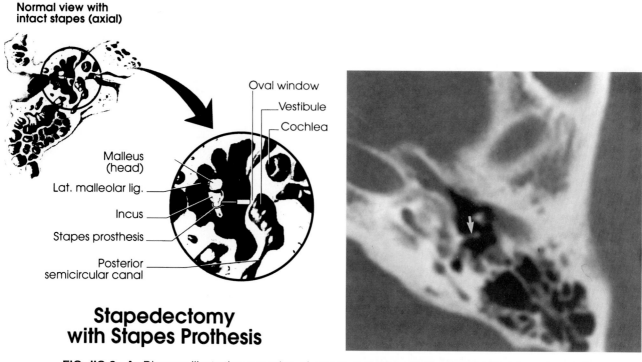

Normal view with intact stapes (axial)

Oval window
Vestibule
Cochlea

Malleus (head)
Lat. malleolar lig.
Incus
Stapes prosthesis
Posterior semicircular canal

Stapedectomy with Stapes Prothesis

A

B

FIG. IIC-3. A: Diagram illustrating resection of stapes and wire prosthesis extending from the oval window to the long process of the incus. (Drawing courtesy of Neill Biomedical Art, Gainesville, FL. From ref. 1, with permission.) **B:** Axial CT shows wire prosthesis (*arrow*) replacing stapes.

tion or displacement as a result of chronic otitis, cholesteatoma, or trauma (5).

A prosthesis may also extend directly from the tympanic membrane to the stapes or directly to the oval window. Synthetic ossicular prosthetics are constructed from hydroxyapatite, polytetrafluoroethylene–vitreous carbon (Proplast), and high-density polyethylene sponge (Plastipore) (5). The most common middle ear prosthesis is a partial ossicular (replacement) prosthesis (POP or PORP) (Fig. IIC-5A). This prosthesis rests on the capitulum of the stapes and attaches to the underside of the tympanic membrane in order to preserve conductive hearing. The other major type of prosthesis is the total ossicular (replacement) prosthesis (TOP or TORP) (Figs. IIC-5 A& B). In this procedure, a prosthesis extends from the undersurface of the tympanic membrane to the footplate of the stapes. Portions of the stapes (head, crura) are resected, and the footplate of the stapes and its attachment to the oval window are preserved. The incus and malleus may be preserved or resected, depending on their condition. Synthetic prostheses are most commonly used in patients with ossicular destruction or disruption caused by cholesteatoma and chronic otitis media (6). They are also used in patients with congenital ossicular malformations.

Tympanoplasty

Tympanoplasties comprise several reconstructive procedures that attempt to preserve sound conduction. There

are five types of tympanoplasties, which vary from isolated repairs of the tympanic membrane to extensive procedures. The exact procedure performed depends on the status of the ossicles.

Type I tympanoplasty consists of repairing the tympanic membrane without altering the underlying ossicles (7). This procedure is also known as a myringoplasty.

Type II tympanoplasty preserves the articulation between the stapes and incus (7). This procedure is most commonly performed when there is erosion of the lenticular process or the head of the stapes, or both. The continuity of the ossicular chain is preserved by placing a bone strut between the capitulum of the stapes and the long process of the incus. Both type I and type II tympanoplasties are done without need for a mastoidectomy (7).

Type III is one of the most commonly performed forms of tympanoplasty (7). Commonly, type III tympanoplasty consists of placing the tympanic membrane or a graft directly on the capitulum of an intact stapes. This procedure, also known as a ''stapes-columella,'' is typically done following a radical mastoidectomy in which the incus and malleus have been eroded but the stapes is intact. This procedure, when performed in an otherwise normal ear, results in only a 30 dB conductive hearing loss. Two other procedures of type III tympanoplasties exist. The ''minor-columella'' procedure consists of placement of a strut between the tympanic membrane and an intact stapes. If a synthetic material is used, this procedure is similar to a PORP. The ''major-columella'' procedure con-

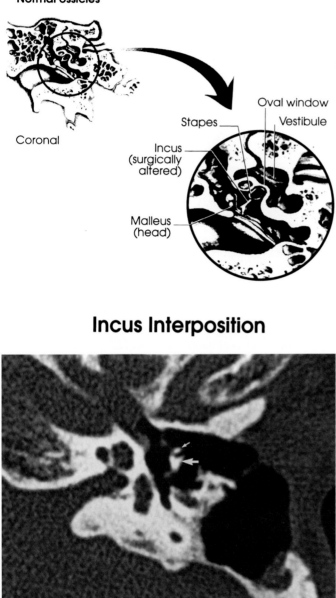

A

Incus Interposition

B

C

FIG. IIC-4. A: Diagram shows surgically rotated incus placed between the superstructure of the stapes and the neck of the malleus. (Drawing courtesy of Neill Biomedical Art, Gainesville, FL. From ref. 1, with permission.) **B:** Axial CT showing rotated incus (*arrow*) after interposition. Note mastoidectomy defect. **C:** Axial CT in a different patient shows incus (*larger arrow*) interposed between the stapes and the malleus (*smaller arrow*). Note mastoidectomy defect.

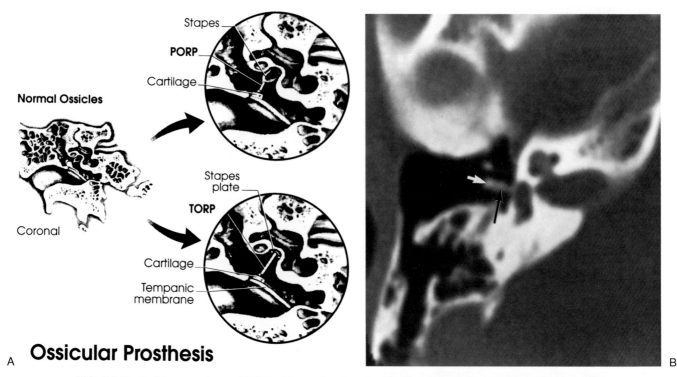

Ossicular Prosthesis

A

B

FIG. IIC-5. A: Diagram shows PORP with prosthesis extending from the superstructure of the stapes to the tympanic membrane and TORP with prosthesis between the footplate of the stapes and the tympanic membrane. (Drawing courtesy of Neill Biomedical Art, Gainesville, FL. From ref. 1, with permission.) **B:** Axial CT after TORP shows wire prosthesis (*long black arrow*) extending from oval window to tympanic membrane (*white shorter arrow*). (From Mukherji et al., ref. 1, with permission.)

sists of placing a prosthesis that extends from the tympanic membrane to the stapes footplate. This procedure is performed when the capitulum and the crura and the footplate are eroded and is similar to a TORP (7).

Type IV tympanoplasty is performed when the head and the crura of the stapes are eroded (7). In this procedure, the stapes footplate is exteriorized and directly exposed to sound. A thin skin graft is placed directly over the oval window to prevent fibrous obliteration. The tympanic membrane or a graft is placed over the cochlear promontory and serves to protect the round window and eustachian tube orifice (7).

Type V tympanoplasty is performed following types III or IV tympanoplasties in patients who have persistent hearing loss with an aerated round window (7). This procedure consists of removal of the stapes footplate and subsequent packing of the oval window with fat and placement of an overlying graft. Fenestration of the lateral semicircular canal is performed in order to bypass the nonfunctional oval window (8).

Tympanotomy Tubes

These tubes are inserted with the goal of providing drainage for ventilation and equalization of pressure in the middle ear. The tubes are made up of plastics (which may be somewhat radiopaque) or metal. Their shape may be straight or bobbin-like. The latter shape conveys a greater stability and lessens the possibility of dislodgement. On CT, bobbin tubes should not be confused with foreign objects. Their midportion should normally be parallel to the course of the tympanic membrane. Identification of these tubes may be difficult if they are surrounded by fluid or become dislodged (Fig. IIC-6).

Cochlear Implants

Postoperative imaging in patients who have undergone cochlear implantation is performed because of the possibility that the electrode may be malpositioned. A malpositioned electrode may lie in the middle ear cavity, internal auditory canal, or cochlear aqueduct (1). The electrode should not touch the facial nerve. The electrode usually has small radiopaque markers identifying the position of each channel. The number of channels that are required to lie inside the cochlea for proper functioning varies with the type of unit utilized. At our institution, multichannel cochlear implants have 22 markers on their electrodes. Of these, 12 need to be inside the cochlea. Fewer than this number may result in suboptimal function and the inability of the patient to recognize all the intended frequencies. The initial 10 markers on these electrodes serve

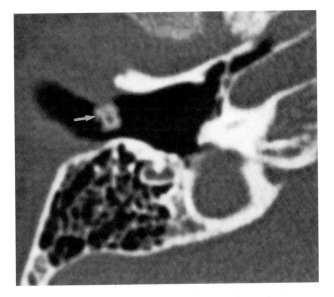

FIG. IIC-6. Dislodged pressure equalization tube. Axial CT shows pressure equalization tube (*arrow*) in external auditory canal. This appearance should not be confused with an osteochondroma.

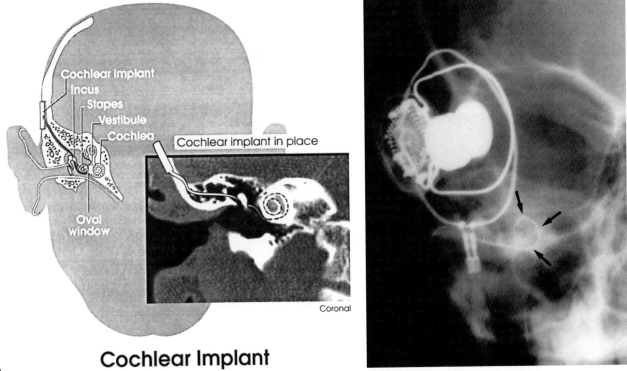

A

Cochlear Implant

B

FIG. IIC-7. A: Diagram shows position of implant. The electrode enters the cochlea via the round window and lies in the proximal 1.5 turns (Drawing courtesy of Neill Biomedical Art, Gainesville, FL. From ref. 1, with permission.) **B:** Frontal radiograph shows electrode (*arrows*) adequately positioned inside the cochlea.

as stiffeners. In our opinion, plain radiographs are a simple, inexpensive method to assess the position of an electrode (Fig. IIC-7). However, detailed examination of its course may require CT scanning.

Surgery for Vestibular Schwannoma

At our institution, surgery for acoustic schwannomas is performed via a lateral suboccipital approach. However, in some institutions, a middle cranial fossa approach is used (9). If a translabyrinthine approach has been used,

the normal structures of the inner ear are resected, and a soft tissue graft, which commonly contains fat, is placed in the surgical bed (1) (Fig. IIC-8).

Irrespective of the surgical approach, several changes occur in the internal auditory canal (IAC) after surgery. Commonly, there is atrophy of the ipsilateral cerebellar hemisphere secondary to retraction during surgery or to long-term compression by the mass. Because the dura is opened, dural enhancement in the posterior fossa is common and may persist for the remainder of the patient's life. In this type of surgery, the posterior wall of the IAC is exposed by burring the posterior petrous bone (10)

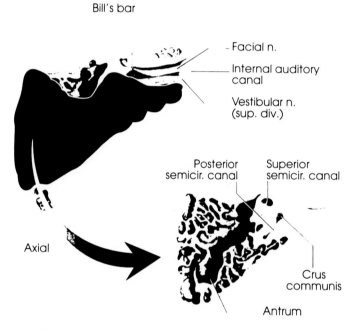

Bill's bar

- Facial n.
- Internal auditory canal
- Vestibular n. (sup. div.)

Posterior semicir. canal
Superior semicir. canal

Axial

Crus communis

Antrum

Translabyrinthine Approach

A

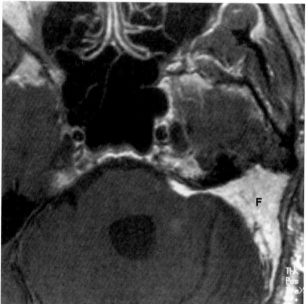

B

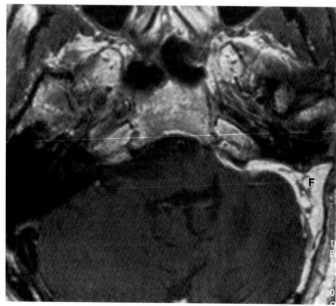

C

FIG. IIC-8. Translabyrinthine approach to the internal auditory canal. **A:** Diagram showing removal of mastoid and middle inner ear structures to approach the posterior aspect of the internal auditory canal. (Drawing courtesy of Neill Biomedical Art, Gainesville, FL. From ref. 1, with permission.) **B:** Postcontrast T_1-weighted MR image after translabyrinthine resection of acoustic schwannoma shows fat graft (F) in place and dural enhancement along the dorsal petrous bone tip. **C:** In the same patient, the left inner ear structures are missing and replaced by the fat graft (F).

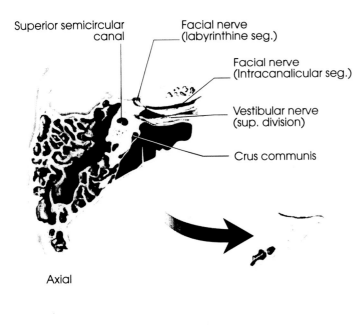

Superior semicircular canal

Facial nerve (labyrinthine seg.)

Facial nerve (Intracanalicular seg.)

Vestibular nerve (sup. division)

Crus communis

Axial

Retrosigmoid Approach

FIG. IIC-9. Retrosigmoid (suboccipital) approach to the internal auditory canal. The posterior wall of the internal auditory canal is resected with preservation of the middle ear structures. (Drawing courtesy of Neill Biomedical Art, Gainesville, FL. From ref. 1, with permission.)

(Fig. IIC-9). This may lead to abnormal communications between the IAC and the neighboring mastoid air cells. The communications are commonly sealed by placing a soft tissue graft, which may contain fat. Residual tumor may also be left in the fundus of the IAC. We commonly perform the initial postsurgery MRI study 6 months after surgery to allow some of the induced inflammatory changes to decrease.

We have noticed four different appearances of the postoperative IAC (11). In type I, the IAC appears empty but may have some nonenhancing soft tissue strands within it. These are probably related to distorted cranial nerves or nonenhancing scars. This appearance occurs in 20% to 30% of cases. Type II is the most common appearance (up to 50% of cases) and shows linear dural enhancement along the walls of the IAC (Fig. IIC-10A). This finding may remain unchanged indefinitely or decrease slightly over time. It reflects dural inflammation and fibrosis. In type III, there are globular areas of enhancement within the IAC or at the porus acousticus (Fig. IIC-10B). Although this appearance is likely to be secondary to inflammation and retraction of the meninges, it may mask early recurrent tumor or small amounts of residual tumor. Thus, these patients need careful follow-up. Type IV are those patients in whom a graft was placed. These grafts may be of high T_1 signal intensity. Therefore, they may enhance and mask residual or recurrent tumor (Figs. IIC-10C,D). These patients also require periodic and careful follow-up MRI studies. In our experience, there is no correlation between the postoperative appearance of the IAC and hearing or facial nerve function preservation.

Petrous Apex Surgery

This section addresses changes following resection of petrous apex cholesterol cysts. These masses may be exenterated or marsupialized (9). Regardless of the mode of treatment, the increased signal intensity that is seen preoperatively should disappear after surgery. Residual T_1 and T_2 brightness in the petrous apex indicates a residual cholesterol cyst. However, after marsupialization, this brightness may temporarily persist. Increased signal intensity more than 6 months after surgery is indicative of surgical failure. Continued growth of the lesion is a very reliable sign of surgical failure.

RADIATION THERAPY

The most common primary tumor of the petrous bone is a paraganglioma. Primary lesions, which arise from the external auditory canal, include squamous cell carcinoma, basal cell carcinoma, squamous cell papilloma, melanoma, and cerumen gland adenocarcinoma. Radiation therapy (RT) may be used as adjuvant therapy following surgery, as a primary modality of treatment, or in patients who are poor surgical candidates. Following RT, at least one-half of the patients develop a serous otitis media that is seen by imaging as opacification of the middle ear cavity by fluid or soft tissue. These patients also develop a reactive osteitis with opacification of mastoid air cells. Progressive erosion is not expected and, if present, is suggestive of tumor progression or osteoradionecrosis. Differentiation between these two entities is often difficult

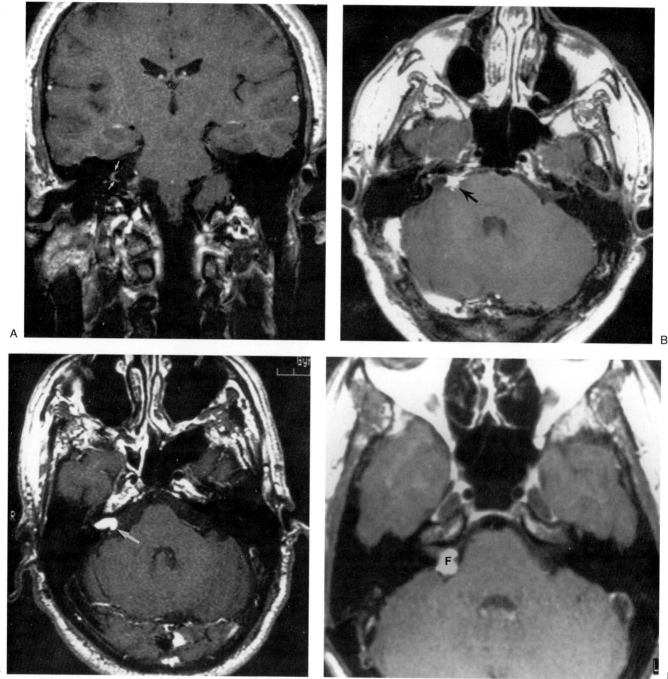

FIG. IIC-10. Changes after suboccipital resection of acoustic schwannoma. **A:** Coronal postcontrast T₁-weighted MR image shows dural enhancement (*arrows*) in the fundus of the right internal auditory canal. **B:** Axial postcontrast T₁-weighted MR image shows nodular dural enhancement (*arrow*) in the porus acousticus and linear enhancement along the walls of the internal auditory canal. **C:** Postcontrast T₁-weighted MR image shows fat graft (*arrow*) that could easily be mistaken for recurrent or residual tumor. **D:** Axial postcontrast T₁-weighted MR image shows fat graft (F) mostly in the cerebellopontine angle cistern.

by imaging alone and may require biopsy. Radiation-induced sarcomas arising from the temporal bone are rare but have been described (10) (Fig. IIC-11). Following chemotherapy or RT, tumors that previously eroded the temporal bone become smaller and show reossification of the destroyed portions of the temporal bones (Fig. IIC-12). Continued growth and bone erosion are signs of tumor progression and treatment failure.

The post-RT appearance of paragangliomas has been described in the literature (12). Successfully treated para-

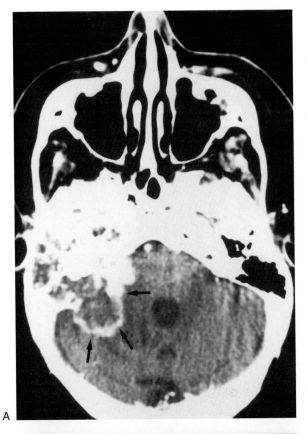

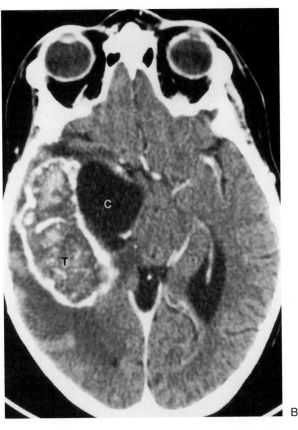

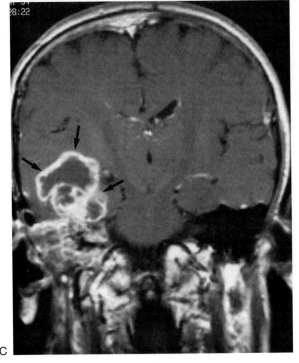

FIG. IIC-11. Postirradiation squamous cell carcinoma of the middle ear. **A:** Axial postcontrast CT in a patient who underwent radiation therapy for cerebellar medulloblastoma. There is a large mass (*arrows*) destroying the petrous bone and protruding into the posterior fossa. **B:** In the same patient, the tumor (T) invades the right temporal bone. Note tumor cyst (C) and mass effect. There is edema in the white matter of the right occipital lobe. **C:** Coronal postcontrast T$_1$-weighted MR image through the posterior aspect of the tumor (*arrows*) shows central necrosis.

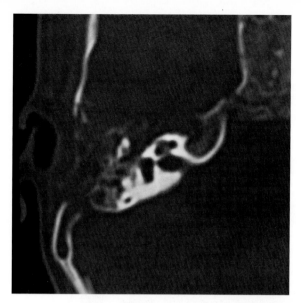

FIG. IIC-12. Treated rhabdomyosarcoma. Axial CT after completion of radiation and chemotherapy shows early remineralization of the petrous bone in patient with middle ear rhabdomyosarcoma.

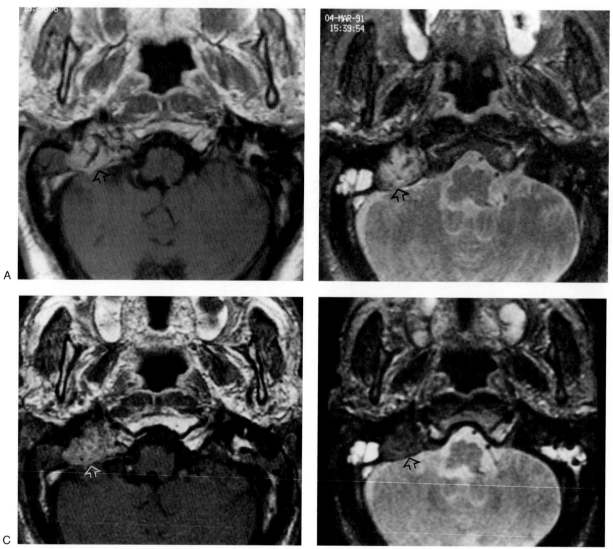

FIG. IIC-13. Treatment-induced changes in paraganglioma. **A:** Pretreatment axial postcontrast T_1-weighted MR image shows right glomus jugulare tumor (*arrow*) with internal flow voids secondary to large intratumoral vessels. **B:** Corresponding T_2-weighted image shows tumor (*arrow*) to be of increased signal intensity. Note bright secretions in right mastoid. **C:** Axial postcontrast T_1-weighted MR image after irradiation shows decreased size of flow voids and less enhancement. The tumor (*arrow*), however, remains unchanged in size. **D:** Corresponding T_2-weighted image shows markedly decreased signal intensity in tumor (*arrow*).

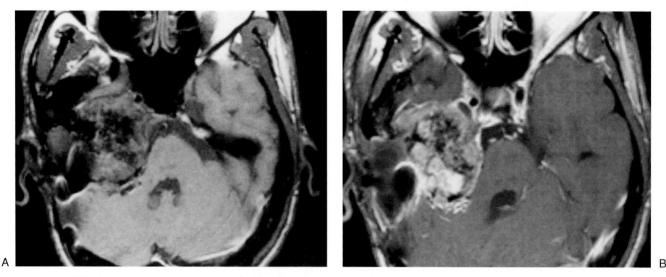

FIG. IIC-14. Failed treatment in paraganglioma. **A:** Axial precontrast T_1-weighted MR image in right glomus jugulare tumor that was previously irradiated and partially resected. Note large size of tumor with multiple central flow voids. **B:** After contrast administration, there is intense tumor enhancement.

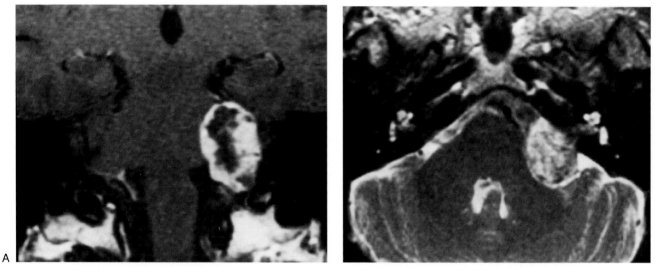

FIG. IIC-15. Acoustic schwannoma after stereotactic radiation therapy. **A:** Coronal postcontrast T_1-weighted MR image shows large left tumor with central necrosis and peripheral enhancement. **B:** Axial T_2-weighted MR image shows mostly hyperintense left-sided tumor.

gangliogliomas show as residual masses; therefore, the presence of a mass is not indicative of treatment failure. The MR signs that correlate with adequate treatment include reduction in size, decreased contrast enhancement, diminution in the number and size of flow voids related to the presence of intratumoral vessels, lack of progression of bone erosion, bone remineralization, and diminished T_2 signal intensity (Figs. IIC-13 and IIC-14).

The imaging characteristics of acoustic schwannoma after stereotactic radiosurgery are well known (13). In a series of 88 stereotactic radiosurgically treated patients who were followed with MR over a 3-year period, tumor size was unchanged in 73%, smaller in 23%, and increased in 4% (13). Tumor shrinkage was noted mostly during the year following RT. Most tumors showed decreased signal intensity and decreased enhancement in their central portion that was probably related to necrosis (Fig. IIC-15).

CONCLUSIONS

In summary, the imaging modality that should be used to evaluate the temporal bone depends on the clinical scenario. CT is the modality of choice for evaluating patients who have undergone prior mastoidectomy and present with symptoms of recurrent otomastoid disease. Plain films are the initial modality of choice for evaluating patients with cochlear implants. Patients who have undergone previous treatment for neoplasms involving the temporal bone or skull base should be evaluated with MR imaging.

REFERENCES

1. Mukherji SK, Mancuso AA, Kotzur IM, et al: CT of the temporal bone: findings after mastoidectomy, ossicular reconstruction, and cochlear implantation. *Am J Roentgenol* 1994;163:1467–1471.
2. Chole RA, Brodie HA: Surgery of the mastoid and petrosa. In Bailey BJ, ed. *Head and Neck Surgery,* vol 2. Philadelphia: JB Lippincott, 1993:1647–1665.
3. Nadol JB: Osseous approaches to the temporal bone. In: Nadol JB, Schuknecht HF, eds. *Surgery of the Ear and Temporal Bone.* New York: Raven Press, 1993:99–109.
4. Schuknecht HF: Otosclerosis surgery. In: Nadol JB, Schuknecht HF, eds. *Surgery of the Ear and Temporal Bone.* New York: Raven Press, 1993:223–244.
5. Montandon P: Ossiculoplasty and tympanoplasty combined with surgery for active chronic otitis media. In: Nadol JB, Schuknecht HF, eds. *Surgery of the Ear and Temporal Bone.* New York: Raven Press, 1993:245–254.
6. Arrigg FG: Ossicular reconstruction in chronic inactive otitis media. In: Nadol JB, Schuknecht HF, eds. *Surgery of the Ear and Temporal Bone.* New York: Raven Press, 1993:255–262.
7. Montandon P: Ossiculoplasty and tympanoplasty combined with surgery for active chronic otitis media. In: Nadol JB, Schuknecht HF, eds. *Surgery of the Ear and Temporal Bone.* New York: Raven Press, 1993:245–254.
8. Gacek R: Symposium on tympanoplasty. I. Results of modified type V tympanoplasty. *Laryngoscope* 1973;83:437–447.
9. Linskey ME, Lunsford LD, Flickinger JC: Neuroimaging of acoustic nerve sheath tumor after stereotaxic radiosurgery. *Am J Neuroradiol* 1991;12:1165–1175.
10. Million RR, Cassisi NJ, Mancuso AA, Stringer SP: Temporal bone. In: Million RR, Cassisi NJ, eds. *Management of Head and Neck Cancer: A Multidisciplinary Approach.* Philadelphia: JB Lippincott, 1994:751–764.
11. Smith M, Castillo M, Campbell J, Pillsbury H, Walters T: Baseline and follow-up MR imaging of the IAC after suboccipital resection of acoustic schwannoma: appearance and clinical correlations. *Neuroradiology* 1995;37:317–320.
12. Mukherji SK, Kasper ME, Tart RP, Mancuso AA: Irradiated paragangliomas of the head and neck: CT and MR appearance. *Am J Neuroradiol* 1994;15:357–363.
13. Mueller DP, Gantz BJ, Dolan KD: Gadolinium-enhanced MR of the postoperative internal auditory canal following acoustic neuroma resection via the middle fossa approach. *Am J Neuroradiol* 1992; 13:197–200.

Posttherapeutic Neurodiagnostic Imaging,
edited by J.R. Jinkins,
Lippincott-Raven Publishers, New York © 1997.

CHAPTER **IID**

The Posttherapeutic Paranasal Sinuses

Kent B. Remley

Surgical treatment of sinonasal disease is common, and postoperative imaging is often performed to assess the outcome of such therapy or to evaluate recurrent signs and symptoms. Operative therapy for benign chronic inflammatory disease has significantly increased as a result of the widespread popularity of functional endoscopic sinus surgery (FESS). Computed tomography (CT) has become an important part of the preoperative and postoperative evaluation of these patients (1–3). Although benign and malignant tumors of the sinonasal region are uncommon, both pretreatment and posttherapeutic imaging play an important role in patient management (4,5). Radiographic assessment is also occasionally necessary after surgical treatment of congenital sinonasal lesions, craniofacial malformations, and facial trauma.

Physicians who image or treat patients with disorders of the sinonasal region must be familiar with the radiographic appearance of this area after therapeutic intervention. The goal of this chapter is fourfold: (a) to acquaint the reader with the more commonly used surgical procedures for treatment of many benign and malignant diseases of the paranasal sinuses; (b) to review the "normal" or uncomplicated postoperative appearance of the sinonasal cavities following surgery for inflammatory and neoplastic disorders; (c) to demonstrate imaging findings associated with procedural complications, treatment failure, tumor recurrence, and postradiation change; and (d) to discuss changes involving the sinuses that may be associated with surgical approaches to the orbit, anterior cranial fossa, skull base, and sella.

Accordingly, the chapter is divided into four sections. The first section gives general principles in approaching the posttherapeutic paranasal sinus. The second section addresses the sinonasal cavities after intervention for inflammatory disease, with an emphasis on FESS. The third section deals with postoperative imaging after resection of benign and malignant sinonasal tumors. Imaging after

craniofacial resection is included in this section. The last section discusses postoperative changes affecting the sinuses after transsphenoidal approaches to the sella and procedures for orbital decompression, and changes involving the sinuses after radiation and chemotherapy.

GENERAL APPROACH TO THE POSTTHERAPEUTIC PATIENT

As is true with other areas of the head and neck, proper radiographic evaluation and interpretation of head and neck examinations require the radiologist to be knowledgeable of several key concepts. Invariably, patients are referred for pretherapeutic imaging, and the accompanying clinical history is frequently inadequate to allow a proper tailoring of the imaging study. Interpretation of head and neck imaging studies without adequate history may lead to misleading radiologic reporting at least and to unnecessary complications and poor patient management at the worst. Therefore, at a minimum, the medical imaging specialist needs to be cognizant of the preoperative clinical diagnosis, the operation or treatment performed, and the timing of the therapeutic measure relative to the imaging examination.

The normal paranasal sinus anatomy is frequently altered by the primary disease process and is further distorted by surgery. Knowing the preoperative diagnosis enables the radiologist to anticipate potential complications or disease recurrence and tailor the imaging study as needed. Some familiarity with the operative procedure performed is important in approaching the postoperative study. Bony and soft tissue defects are often created at the time of surgery. Furthermore, soft tissue flaps, bone struts and grafts, and various prosthetic materials may be used to repair these defects. Without proper knowledge of the surgical procedure, these soft tissue and bony changes may be falsely interpreted as pathologic. After surgery and radiation therapy, bony changes and soft tissue reaction take place. The extent of this reaction and the imaging appearance change over time. In the acute

K. B. Remley: Department of Radiology, University of Minnesota Medical School, Minneapolis, Minnesota 55455.

setting, edema, hemorrhage, and inflammatory changes can be difficult to differentiate from tumor or infection. With time, scar and granulation tissue mature, taking on a different appearance (6). As a result, the length of time separating the operation from the date of the imaging exam has important implications for image interpretation.

The question frequently arises as to whether CT or magnetic resonance (MR) is the optimal imaging technique for the paranasal sinuses. Pathologic changes are most easily detected when the current examination is compared to a posttherapeutic baseline or prior study using the same imaging modality. The choice of imaging modality depends on several factors, including the status or stability of the patient, modality availability, cost, and the patient's diagnosis. In general, inflammatory disease is most easily followed by CT because imaging in the coronal plane is preferred by surgeons performing FESS; contrast administration is usually not necessary. Although CT, or a combination of CT and MR, is often obtained for neoplastic disease preoperatively, the advantages of MR over CT make it the preferred modality in most cases for sequential follow-up after treatment. Differentiation between inflammatory tissue and tumor can be impossible with CT. With MR, on the other hand, sinonasal inflammatory tissue is usually low or low-intermediate signal intensity on T_1-weighted (T_1W) images and hyperintense on T_2-weighted (T_2W) acquisitions (7). When compared to inflammatory tissue, the vast majority of sinonasal neoplasms have lower signal intensity on T_2W images, making the distinction between tumor and inflammatory disease much less difficult. Although it is somewhat variable, scar tissue usually has a lower signal intensity than tumor on T_2W images (6). Unlike the preoperative patient, MR contrast agents are less useful in the postoperative setting. Both inflammatory and neoplastic tissue enhance, although inflamed mucosa enhances intensely, whereas tumor enhancement is more variable. However, scar and granulation tissue may also enhance, particularly early in the postoperative period (8). Thus, a definitive distinction is not always possible, and the radiologist should not hesitate to recommend biopsy when appropriate.

From the above comments, the importance of the post-therapeutic baseline or reference study for comparison becomes obvious, and this comparison is strongly encouraged, particularly in monitoring the higher-risk patient. In addition, the proper timing of this examination is crucial. Complete resolution of any postoperative tissue reaction is desired prior to obtaining the initial posttherapeutic study; however, in waiting too long, one runs the risk of reducing the detection of early recurrence. Furthermore, cost and patient convenience frequently play a part in the timing of this study. Therefore, it is recommended that the posttherapeutic baseline study be obtained approximately 6 to 12 weeks after treatment, erring toward the shorter waiting period in the higher-risk patient. Subsequently, follow-up imaging in patients with tumors should

be performed at 4- to 6-month intervals for the first 3 years and 6- to 12-month intervals for the following 2 or 3 years (4,9). Ultimately, the posttreatment imaging protocol should take into account patient reliability, histopathology of the primary tumor, and risk factors for recurrence or the appearance of a second primary neoplasm.

INFLAMMATORY DISEASE

The surgical management of chronic inflammatory sinonasal disease has evolved significantly over the past 10 to 15 years. The work of Messerklinger (10) and others (11,12) has demonstrated that most cases of chronic recurrent sinusitis are the result of interference with mucociliary clearance through the natural drainage pathways of the paranasal sinuses. Technological advances in instrumentation and endoscopes, coupled with advances in CT imaging, have led to the widespread acceptance of endoscopic (FESS) techniques as the primary method for treatment of chronic inflammatory disease. However, conventional surgical techniques are still occasionally performed in selected cases. In this section, traditional surgery methods and the associated postoperative imaging findings are reviewed, followed by a more in-depth discussion of FESS techniques. The appearance of the sinonasal region after FESS and indications for revision surgery are addressed. The section concludes with an overview of the potential complications associated with endoscopic techniques and useful adjunctive imaging techniques for evaluating those complications.

Conventional Surgical Techniques

Conventional surgical procedures for treatment of chronic inflammatory disease are used much less commonly today than they were prior to the development of endoscopic sinus surgery. Nevertheless, because of the prevalence of inflammatory sinus disease, postsurgical changes from these procedures are still frequently encountered on imaging examinations, and these techniques may be used in selected cases such as frontal sinus obliteration. This section covers the imaging appearances of the more common techniques used for the maxillary, ethmoid, and frontal sinuses, respectively.

Prior to the development of FESS, the Caldwell–Luc operation was considered the standard procedure for treatment of chronic maxillary sinusitis. This procedure may still be used for treatment of fungal sinusitis, massive polyposis, mucocele removal, or resection of uncomplicated dental origin cysts (13). The operation involves an incision in the upper gingivobuccal sulcus over the canine fossa. An opening is then created in the lower anterior wall of the maxillary sinus (Fig. IID-1). After inspection, all diseased tissue is removed, and the mucosa is stripped. The anterior bony defect is left to fill in with hematoma that eventually fibroses.

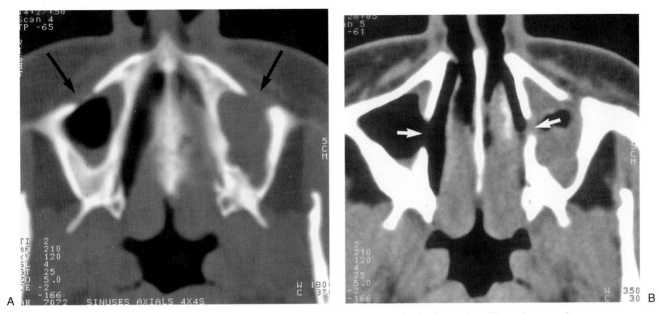

FIG. IID-1. Caldwell–Luc procedure. **A:** Axial CT image through the lower maxillary sinuses shows anterior wall defects (*arrows*) from bilateral Caldwell–Luc procedures. Prominent mucosal disease is present on the left, with mild mucoperiosteal thickening on the right. There is thickening of the sinus walls bilaterally. **B:** CT image cephalad to **A** shows bilateral nasoantral windows (*short arrows*). An intranasal antrostomy is usually performed in conjunction with the Caldwell–Luc procedure.

Infection and oroantral fistula represent early complications. The majority of patients will show radiographic improvement after the Caldwell–Luc procedure (14). However, bony changes can occur that can be directly attributed to the procedure. These changes include reactive fibroosseous proliferation (Fig. IID-2), with or without antral contraction and compartmentalization (Figs. IID-3 and IID-4). Although these reactive bony changes are occasionally quite pronounced, they should not be misinterpreted as postoperative osteomyelitis.

The intranasal antrostomy, or nasoantral window, involves creating an opening in the medial wall of the maxillary sinus under the inferior turbinate (Fig. IID-5). This procedure may be performed alone or in conjunction with the Caldwell–Luc procedure in order to provide ventilation of the maxillary sinus. If the opening into the nasal cavity is inadequate in size, the surgical defect can scar over. The intranasal antrostomy is infrequently performed alone at the present time for the initial treatment of chronic sinusitis. Because the mucus blanket within the sinus continues to be swept toward the natural ostium rather than the nasoantral window, the procedure fails to provide adequate drainage in many cases. However, in instances of primary ciliary dysfunction, the inferior nasal antrostomy becomes the operation of choice.

Conventional treatment of inflammatory frontal sinus disease consists of several options. Trephination of the

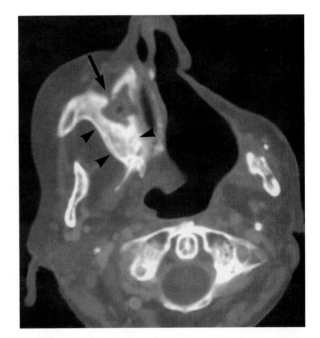

FIG. IID-2. Caldwell–Luc procedure with bony reaction. Axial CT image shows an anterior wall defect (*arrow*) with marked thickening of the medial and lateral antral walls (*arrowheads*) secondary to fibroosseous proliferation after a Caldwell–Luc procedure, producing antral contraction. A small inferior antrostomy is present medially. Postoperative changes following total maxillectomy are noted on the left.

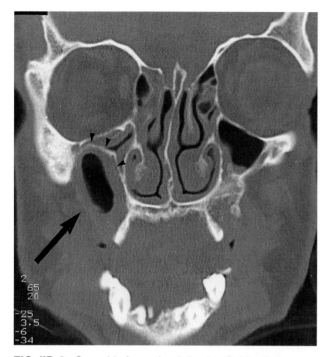

FIG. IID-3. Synechia formation following Caldwell–Luc procedure. Coronal CT image, obtained many years after a right Caldwell–Luc procedure, reveals a large defect of the maxillary sinus (*arrow*) with persistent mucoperiosteal thickening. Scar formation, a complication of the procedure, has resulted in compartmentalization of the antrum. In this case, the bridging scar tissue has calcified (*arrowheads*).

frontal sinus is performed for acute frontal sinusitis that is unresponsive to antibiotics. This procedure is essentially an incision and drainage procedure. A small incision is made in the superomedial aspect of the orbit, and the sinus is entered through the inferior edge of the supraorbital rim. The defect in the frontal sinus floor is usually less than 1 cm in size. The inflammatory secretions are evacuated, and the sinus mucosa is left intact. A drainage tube or cannula is usually left in place for 1 to 2 weeks and then removed to prevent foreign body reaction. Potential complications include penetration into the orbit below or drilling into the anterior cranial fossa through the posterior sinus wall above. Because the defect is small, it may not be readily visible on routine axial or coronal CT scans.

Options for treatment of chronic frontal sinusitis include mucosa-preserving and mucosa-eliminating procedures. The three nonobliterative procedures involving the frontal sinuses include the Lynch, Killian, and Reidel procedures. The Lynch procedure is primarily utilized as external ethmoidectomy; however, it also removes a large part of the medial floor of the frontal sinus, which allows entry into the sinus below and behind the orbital rim, in the region of the nasofrontal duct. The frontal sinus mucosa is then removed, and a drainage tube is placed from the sinus into the nasal cavity. The drain is typically left in place for 6 to 8 weeks.

For more extensive disease in moderate to large frontal sinuses, the Killian and Reidel procedures have been described (8). In both of these procedures, the mucosa of

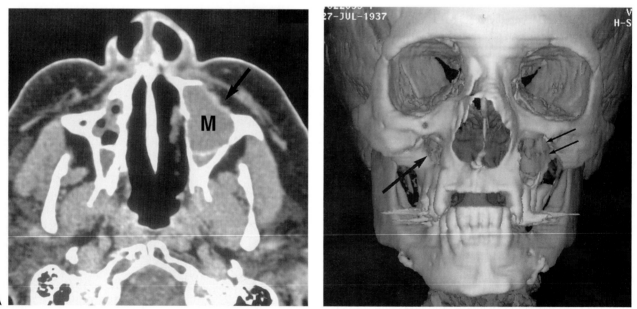

FIG. IID-4. Post-Caldwell–Luc complication. **A:** Axial CT scan shows typical post-Caldwell–Luc changes on the right and a large soft tissue mass (M) in the left antrum. There is expansion of the sinus and enlargement of the postoperative defect (*arrow*). **B:** Three-dimensional CT (shaded surface display) image shows the normal posttherapeutic changes on the right (*arrow*) and enlargement of the bony defect on the left (*double arrows*). Scar formation following the Caldwell–Luc procedure resulted in mucocele formation in the left antrum.

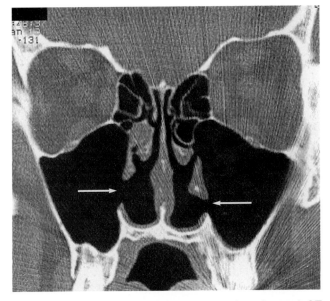

FIG. IID-5. Bilateral intranasal antrostomies. Coronal CT image through the maxillary sinuses demonstrates the normal posttherapeutic appearance of intranasal antrostomies (*white arrows*). This procedure may be performed alone or in combination with a Caldwell–Luc operation.

the sinus is entirely stripped. With the Killian procedure, a large bony defect is created within the frontal sinus, and a second defect is created below the orbital rim into the sinus floor. The rim is left intact, and the mucosa is stripped. The Reidel operation differs from the Killian procedure in that the orbital rim is also removed. This results in significant deformity, as the soft tissues over the upper brow and lower forehead collapse inward toward the posterior wall of the residual sinus. Because of the cosmetic defects from the Reidel and Killian procedures, they are rarely performed at the present time. However, they may be indicated for frontal sinusitis with osteomyelitis of the anterior table of the skull (13).

The osteoplastic flap procedure, an external mucosa-eliminating procedure, is the method of choice in most circumstances for surgical treatment of chronic frontal sinusitis (15). This procedure involves creating an anterior frontal bone flap through a bicoronal or brow incision. A posterior–anterior radiograph of the sinus or coronal CT scan can be used as an intraoperative template to define the borders of the bone flap. The flap is fractured along the inferior margin but remains attached by periosteum. The mucosa of the sinus is then stripped. There are several methods of managing the sinus cavity and frontal recess. Most commonly, the nasofrontal ducts are plugged with fascia, and the sinuses obliterated with nonvascularized fat tissue from the abdomen or thigh (Fig. IID-6). Alternatively, if the opposite frontal recess is patent and functional, the intersinus septum may be removed with drainage into the functional side.

Radiographic assessment in patients who have under-

gone osteoplastic frontal sinus flaps for inflammatory sinonasal disease can be frustrating. When patients present with recurrent symptoms, the differential diagnosis includes infection, with or without osteomyelitis, and mucocele formation. In the absence of osteomyelitis, CT is of limited use in differentiating infection from fibrotic tissue and/or early mucocele formation (Fig. IID-7) (16). Experience with MR has been somewhat limited to date. Theoretically, early mucocele formation should be readily differentiated from fibrosis and fat tissue with a combination of T_1W and T_2W images. Unfortunately, focal areas of T_2 hyperintensity within the sinus are often encountered (Fig. IID-8). In one study, the investigators found areas of T_2 hyperintensity and some degree of tissue enhancement in all patients, and the imaging findings showed poor correlation with patient symptoms (17). Therefore, unless there are obvious bony changes related to mucocele formation or osteomyelitis, MR presently appears to have limited utility in predicting the outcome in symptomatic patients who have undergone prior osteoplastic frontal sinus flap procedures.

Conventional ethmoidectomy can be accomplished through intranasal (internal), transmaxillary, or external approaches (18). Indications for ethmoidectomy include chronic refractory ethmoid sinusitis, recurrent sinonasal polyposis uncontrollable by local polypectomy, and exploration for CSF leak. The use of conventional ethmoidectomy for soft tissue tumors of the ethmoid region and transethmoid surgical approaches to the orbit for thyroid disease are discussed later in this chapter.

Internal or intranasal ethmoidectomy is best suited for limited ethmoid inflammatory disease or biopsy of soft

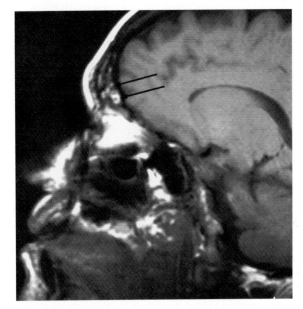

FIG. IID-6. Osteoplastic frontal sinus obliteration. Midline sagittal T_1W MR image shows high-signal-intensity material (fat) within the obliterated frontal sinuses (*arrows*) after an osteoplastic flap procedure.

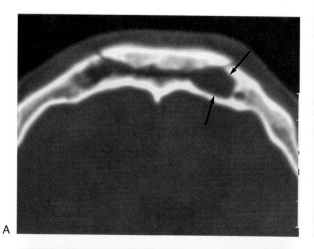

A

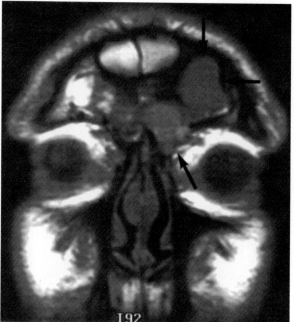

B

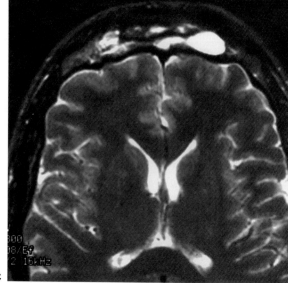

C

FIG. IID-7. Mucocele formation following osteoplastic flap. **A:** Axial CT image in this patient with recurrent headaches unresponsive to medical therapy demonstrates soft tissue within the obliterated frontal sinus. The bone flap is in a satisfactory position, and the margins of the flap are sharp. The internal bony contour on the left side (*arrows*) is smoother than that on the right. **B:** Coronal T$_1$W MR image through the obliterated frontal sinuses reveals high-signal-intensity fat on the right. Lower-signal-intensity soft tissue (*arrows*) has replaced the fat signal on the left. **C:** Axial T$_2$W MR image shows normal hypointense fat signal on the right. The central and left regions contain high-signal-intensity material. At surgery, a mucocele was discovered on the left. Small regions of hyperintensity can be seen, however, as a normal postoperative finding on T$_2$W images.

tissue masses but may be utilized for more extensive disease if the patient desires to avoid an external incision. After resection of the middle turbinate, the ethmoid sinuses are entered through the ethmoidal bulla. The air cells posterior to the ethmoid bulla are opened and resected, followed by resection of the anterior air cells. Intranasal ethmoidectomy can also be used for treatment of sinonasal polyposis. However, the procedure can be difficult and dangerous in these patients because of bleeding that compromises visualization of the anatomy (19). Inadvertent entry into the orbit through the lamina papyracea can occur, leading to serious consequences (20).

External ethmoidectomy is performed through a vertical incision between the medial canthus and the dorsum of the nose (Lynch incision). The periosteum is elevated, and the lamina papyracea is directly inspected. The frontoethmoid suture (at the level of the anterior and posterior ethmoidal artery canals) identifies the level of the cribriform plate and the rostral border of the posterior ethmoid air cells. The anterior air cells are initially entered via the lamina, and exploration is carried posteriorly as indicated. Through this approach, the supraorbital air cells, frontal sinus, sphenoid sinus, and orbit can all be accessed. An external approach for ethmoidectomy is indicated if the anterior lamina papyracea is absent. The transmaxillary ethmoidectomy is done through a Caldwell–Luc approach and is performed if there is coexistent maxillary sinus disease or the other approaches are contraindicated (Fig. IID-9). The upper maxillary sinus wall is resected, giving the surgeon access to the ethmoid complex.

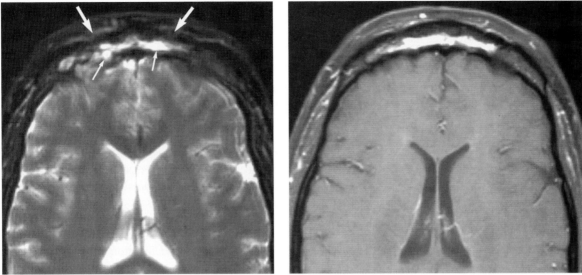

A   B

FIG. IID-8. Presumed infection after osteoplastic flap procedure. **A:** Axial T$_2$W MR image in a patient with headaches and mild upper facial swelling shows multiple small areas of increased signal intensity (*small arrows*) within the fat tissue of the obliterated frontal sinuses. The flap margins are difficult to identify, but there is no elevation of the flap (*large arrows*). **B:** Contrast-enhanced T$_1$W image with fat suppression shows enhancement within the obliterated frontal sinuses without enhancement of surrounding bone or dura, consistent with low-grade or early infection of the fat. Nevertheless, caution should be used when interpreting MR studies of these patients, as small areas of enhancement can be seen normally.

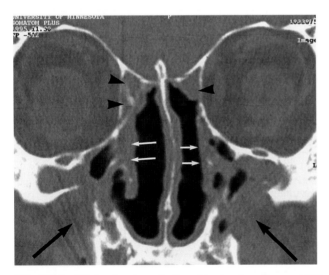

FIG. IID-9. Bilateral external ethmoidectomies. Coronal CT image demonstrates the postoperative changes of bilateral ethmoidectomies. Both superior and middle turbinates and the left inferior turbinate have been resected. The ethmoidectomies in this patient were performed using Caldwell–Luc approaches (*arrows*). Scarring from the operation (*small arrows*) has resulted in bilateral maxillary sinus inflammatory disease. Residual ethmoid inflammatory disease or postoperative scarring is also noted (*arrowheads*).

The sphenoid sinuses can be accessed by several different conventional operations, including the transnasal, transethmoid, and transseptal routes. The first two approaches are discussed below. The transseptal approach, utilized in transsphenoidal hypophysectomy, is covered later in this chapter. The choice of approach depends on the suspected pathology, the experience of the surgeon, and the presence or absence of coexistent ethmoid disease. In the absence of ethmoid disease, the transnasal route is preferable; however, the presence of ethmoid disease usually necessitates the transethmoidal approach. The transethmoidal approach may be intranasal, transantral (Caldwell–Luc), or through an external ethmoidectomy. Once the sphenoid sinus is reached, a sphenoid sinusotomy is performed in which the anterior wall of the sinus is removed. The sinuses then drain directly into the nasopharynx. The choice of procedure will dictate the expected postoperative appearance. When the transnasal route is used, adequate exposure necessitates removal of the posterior aspects of the middle and superior turbinates, sometimes accompanied by resection of the posterior ethmoid air cells. Transantral and external ethmoidectomy approaches require more extensive ethmoid resection. A sphenoid sinusotomy may be difficult to appreciate on conventional coronal sinus CT because the bony defect is in the plane of the scan slice. It is important to remember that the bony wall of the sphenoid sinus overlying the internal carotid artery may be extremely thin or dehiscent (21). Therefore, a soft tissue mass in the postoperative sphenoid sinus near the carotid artery, when associated with bony dehiscence of the sinus wall, should be evaluated further with contrast-enhanced CT or MR to exclude a postoperative carotid artery pseudoaneurysm prior to biopsy.

Functional Endoscopic Sinus Surgery

The popularity of FESS has increased dramatically over the past decade, and coronally oriented CT scanning has become an integral part of the preoperative work-up (1,22,23). FESS should be considered in the category of limited sinus surgery, the purpose of which is to restore normal sinus mucociliary clearance (11). The techniques utilized with FESS allow the surgeon to tailor the procedure, treating the area of disease and reestablishing drainage and ventilation while preserving normal, healthy mucosa. Hence, the postoperative imaging appearance of patients undergoing FESS will vary, depending on the preoperative extent of disease and aggressiveness of the surgeon. This section covers the postoperative imaging appearance(s) of FESS techniques when surgery is successful, as well as the radiographic appearances of postoperative complications. Although surgical complications

with FESS are becoming less common as surgeons gain greater experience, it is important for the radiologist to be knowledgeable of these potential complications so that appropriate recognition takes place on CT and/or MR imaging studies and further imaging, if necessary, is optimized. Radiographic assessment of the patient with recurrent inflammatory disease after FESS is discussed in the next section on Radiographic Evaluation after FESS.

There are two general approaches to endoscopic sinus surgery in use, the Messerklinger technique and the Wigand technique (13,23). The Messerklinger technique, the most widely utilized approach in the United States, is an anterior-to-posterior dissection based on the central theme that the anterior ethmoids and ostiomeatal complex (OMC) plays a critical role in the pathogenesis of most chronic sinonasal inflammatory disease (10). Therefore, this approach involves resection of the medial aspect of the anterior ethmoid complex from the fovea ethmoidalis superiorly to the anterior attachment of the uncinate process, behind the nasolacrimal duct.

In an attempt to standardize the FESS approach based on the extent of sinonasal inflammatory disease, Panje and Anand (25) created a classification scheme linking the preoperative extent of disease with CT imaging and clinical history with the appropriate FESS technique. This classification system, in modified form, is listed in Table IID-1. On further review of this system, it is obvious that

TABLE IID-1. *FESS: The Anand and Panje classification*

Type	Procedure	Indications
Type I	Uncinatectomy ± agger nasi cell exenteration	Isolated OMC thickening of mucous membrane Infundibular disease Patent maxillary sinus ostia without sinus membrane thickening or cysts Unsuccessful prior inferior nasal antrostomy or antrotomy with irrigation Prior septoplasty or adenoidectomy with continued paranasal sinus symptoms
Type II	Uncinatectomy Bulla ethmoidectomy Removal of sinus lateralis mucous membrane Exposure of frontal recess or frontal sinus	OMC thickening of mucous membrane Evidence of anterior ethmoid opacification, including obstruction of infundibulum Limited frontal recess disease Unsuccessful prior inferior nasal antrostomy or antrotomy with irrigation Prior septoplasty or adenoidectomy with continued paranasal sinus symptoms

Type III	Type II procedure
	Maxillary sinus antrostomy through the natural sinus ostium
		Same as type II with the following:
		  Maxillary sinusitis as evidenced by membrane thickening or sinus opacification
		  Stenotic or edematous maxillary sinus ostium

Type IV	Type III procedure Complete posterior ethmoidectomy	Total ethmoid involvement Nasal polyposis with extensive ethmoidal and maxillary sinus disease Prior type 1 or type II FESS without response or with progression of sinus disease

Type V	Type IV procedure
	Sphenoidectomy
	Stripping of mucous membrane
		Same as type IV with the following:
		  Evidence of sphenoid sinusitis
		  Pansinusitis and rhinitis

Anand–Panje (AP) type I surgery is the most limited dissection within the Messerklinger approach and that progression from AP type I to type II simply represents the next step of the surgical dissection. Modifications of this routine, as well as the point at which the surgeon stops, are determined by the preoperative indications and surgical findings. A brief synopsis of the FESS procedure is presented here, and the reader is referred to several references for a more complete description (24–26).

The Messerklinger approach to FESS may be performed under either local or general endotracheal anesthesia, both of which have their advantages and disadvantages. In either case, topical anesthetic agents are used for maximal mucosal vasoconstriction. A 4-mm straight-forward viewing (0°) endoscope is preferred for most portions of the operation. The procedure begins by opening the ethmoid infundibulum and removing the entire uncinate process. Once the uncinectomy is completed, the ethmoidal bulla and the anterior ethmoid air cells are then opened and removed until the basal or ground lamella is identified. The frontal recess is subsequently exposed and cleared of disease (AP type II), and the natural maxillary sinus ostium is enlarged (AP type III) as needed. A diameter of 7 to 10 mm is usually adequate, and further enlargement runs the risk of damage to the orbital floor or nasal lacrimal duct. For more extensive inflammatory disease and in advanced cases of sinonasal polyposis, the posterior ethmoid air cells are exenterated, and a sphenoidectomy is performed (AP types IV and V, respectively). Although middle turbinectomy is performed as a routine part of FESS by some surgeons, most feel it is usually not necessary, and it increases the risk of postoperative adhesions (13). However, partial turbinectomy is routinely done in cases where concha bullosa is present.

The Wigand technique, less commonly used in the United States, involves a posterior-to-anterior dissection and is usually performed under general anesthesia (23). The operation begins with an anterior sphenoidotomy. The posterior ethmoid sinus septations are then systematically taken down, following the skull base from posterior to anterior. The natural ostium of the maxillary sinus and the nasofrontal recess are enlarged. Thus, at the conclusion of the procedure, a complete ethmoidectomy has been performed, and all sinuses are opened into the ipsilateral nasal cavity. Because the Wigand procedure is more extensive than the Messerklinger operation, it is usually reserved for more severe disease such as extensive sinonasal polyposis.

Endoscopic techniques can also be used to treat other processes that involve the sinuses, orbits, and skull base. The use of endoscopy for the treatment of thyroid ophthalmopathy and endoscopic approaches to the sella are discussed later in this chapter in the section on Miscellaneous Changes, Radiation Therapy, and Chemotherapy. Endoscopic surgery has been advocated for the initial treatment of frontal and ethmoid mucoceles (27). Although CSF rhinorrhea is a known complication of FESS, endoscopic techniques can also be utilized to close defects of the anterior skull base, thus avoiding the morbidity associated with a formal craniotomy. Other indications include resection of benign soft tissue masses, osteomas, and treatment of nasolacrimal duct obstruction.

Radiographic Evaluation after FESS

The majority of patients who undergo FESS have satisfactory resolution of their preoperative symptoms, and postoperative imaging is not necessary. However, recurrent symptoms or inflammatory disease occur in 7% to 18% of patients after FESS (28,29). Clinical evaluation and plain film imaging are often inadequate for determining the reason for failure or recurrent symptoms. Residual or recurrent disease of the OMC is a major reason for surgical failure. Computed tomography is valuable in evaluating the postoperative sinonasal region (30), not only to detect recurrent disease but to accurately visualize the extent of surgery, because operative reports frequently overestimate the extent of dissection. In a manner similar to the evaluation of the preoperative patient, the coronal projection is preferred. Additionally, it may be necessary to obtain images in the axial plane in some cases. A systematic method of evaluation with emphasis on anatomic structure is stressed, concentrating on the same areas that are emphasized on the preoperative study (Table IID-2). As with any postoperative imaging study, comparison with the preoperative study is helpful to identify the pattern of inflammatory disease and the preoperative integrity of the bony structures. This approach to the analysis of the imaging study will help determine the type and extent of surgery as well as recognize complications and/or recurrent disease.

In order to evaluate the postoperative patient adequately, familiarity with the expected postsurgical imaging appearance is necessary. With the Messerklinger approach to FESS, the idea is to limit surgical dissection to only those areas that are diseased, with the focus begin-

TABLE IID-2. *Structural landmarks for sinus CT interpretation*

Frontal sinus
Frontal recess and nasofrontal duct
Agger nasi cell and anterior ethmoid sinus
Ethmoid bulla
Ethmoid roof
Uncinate process and ethmoid infundibulum
Middle meatus
Maxillary sinus and natural ostium
Basal (ground) lamella
Sinus lateralis
Posterior ethmoid sinus (Onodi cell)
Sphenoid sinus (intersinus septum and optic canal)
Nasal septum and nasal turbinates

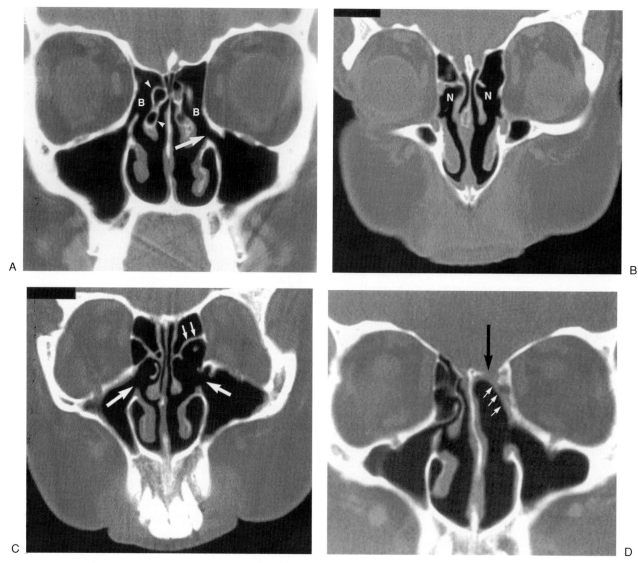

FIG. IID-10. Imaging evaluation after FESS. **A:** Coronal CT scan after FESS shows Anand and Panje type 2 changes (see Table IID-1) on the left consisting of uncinectomy (*arrow*) and ethmoid bullectomy (B). Ethmoid bullectomy (B) has also been performed on the right, but the uncinate process has been left intact. A septated right concha bullosa (*arrowheads*) is present in addition. **B,C:** Coronal CT images from a different patient show type 3 changes. The agger nasi cells have been opened in conjunction with exposure of the nasofrontal recesses (N). More posteriorly, uncinectomies have been performed with antrostomies through the natural maxillary sinus ostia (*arrows*). More complete ethmoid bullectomy has been performed on the left, and the basal lamella, denoting the location of the sinus lateralis, is visible (*small arrows*). **D:** Coronal CT image in a third patient showing type 4 changes on the left with uncinectomy and middle antrostomy, complete ethmoidectomy, and middle turbinectomy. Postoperative scarring is present within the ethmoid cavity (*small arrows*) along with a defect of the fovea ethmoidalis (*large arrow*). It is very important to document bony dehiscences in the radiologic report to prevent complications if further surgery is necessary.

ning at the OMC. The approach the author uses in looking at the postoperative study is to retrace the surgeon's operative steps, using the Anand–Panje classification as a template, beginning with the uncinate process and ethmoidal bulla (Fig. IID-10). The extent of uncinectomy and ethmoid bullectomy should be noted. The patency of the natural ostium, or the size and patency of a middle antrostomy, should be reported along with any residual disease or adhesions. The middle turbinate needs to be examined to determine whether turbinectomy has been performed (Fig. IID-11). Displacement of this structure during surgery can lead to a fracture at the vertical attachment along the cribriform plate or the lateral attachment to the lamina papyracea (Fig. IID-12).

The frontal recess and agger nasi cells are evaluated next. The nasofrontal recesses should be closely examined to determine their patency. A significant, but probably underrecognized, cause of postoperative recurrence is nasofrontal recess obstruction (Fig. IID-13). This recess is the narrowest channel in the anterior ethmoid region. Obstruction may result from recurrent disease in the agger nasi cells after incomplete exenteration or be related to postoperative synechiae. The small dimensions of this area and the close proximity of the anterior ethmoid artery, lamina papyracea, and ethmoid roof make this a technically difficult area to navigate from a surgical standpoint. Unlike MR, postoperative fibrosis can not be easily differentiated from inflammatory disease with CT (Fig.

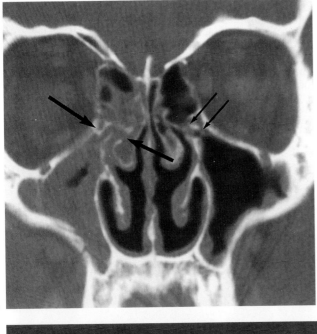

A

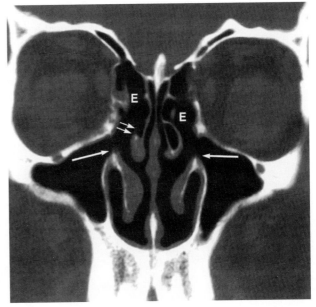

B

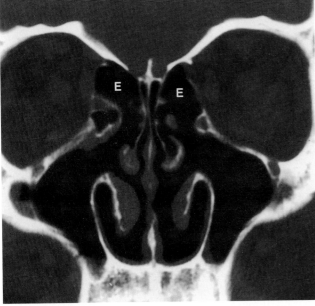

C

FIG. IID-11. Ostiomeatal complex inflammatory disease successfully treated with FESS. **A:** Preoperative coronal CT image through the OMCs reveals inflammatory disease involving the right side (*arrows*). Concha bullosa is also present bilaterally. The right maxillary sinus is completely opacified, and there is associated disease involving the anterior ethmoid sinuses and nasofrontal recess. The left ethmoid infundibulum is also obstructed (*small arrows*). **B:** Postoperative scan at the same level as **A** shows postoperative changes including bilateral uncinectomies (*arrows*). Bilateral ethmoidectomies (E) have also been performed, as well as partial resection of the right concha bullosa (*small arrows*). **C:** Postoperative CT more posteriorly shows the bilateral middle antrostomies. Middle ethmoidectomies have been performed (E), with a single air cell remaining on the right (From Scuderi et al., ref. 23, with permission.)

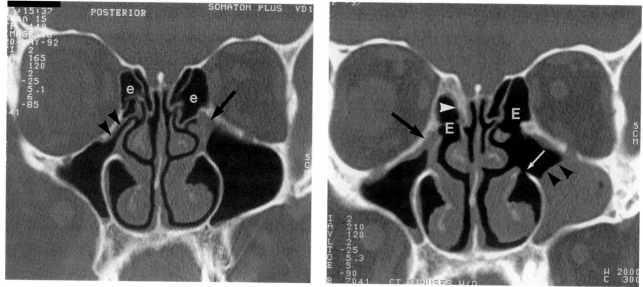

FIG. IID-12. Failed functional endoscopic sinus surgery. **A:** Preoperative coronal CT scan shows mild mucosal thickening within the right ethmoid infundibulum (*arrowheads*) and obstruction of the left infundibulum (*arrow*). The anterior ethmoid air cells (e) are unremarkable. **B:** Postoperative coronal CT image after FESS at the same level shows a left uncinectomy (*small white arrow*) and bilateral ethmoidectomies (E). The right infundibulum is obstructed (*black arrow*), and membrane formation on the left (*arrowheads*) has resulted in maxillary sinus opacification. There is thickening of the right fovea ethmoidalis at the attachment of the middle turbinate (*white arrowhead*). This change usually results from manipulation of the middle turbinate during FESS to improve exposure. If the dura is torn during this maneuver, a CSF leak can result.

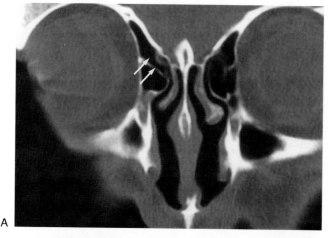

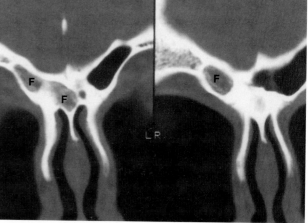

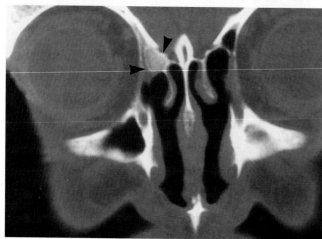

FIG. IID-13. Complication from FESS. **A:** Preoperative coronal CT scan demonstrates a normal nasofrontal recess on the right (*arrows*). **B,C:** Coronal CT images obtained after FESS reveal opacification of the right frontal sinus (F) and obliteration of the nasofrontal recess (*arrows*). Manipulation of the middle turbinate during FESS may lead to a fracture at the junction of the superior strut and the ethmoidal roof (*arrowhead*), in this case resulting in nasofrontal recess occlusion. (From Scuderi et al., ref. 23, with permission.)

IID-14) (8). However, the presence of abnormal soft tissue in this area, in conjunction with persistent symptoms not responsive to medical therapy, probably warrants revision surgery, regardless of whether the tissue is fibrotic or inflammatory in nature. The additional cost of MR in making this determination is probably not justified.

Finally, it is important to inspect carefully the entire course of the lamina papyracea, fovea ethmoidalis (ethmoid roof), cribriform plate, and sphenoid sinus margins. Postoperative dehiscences of the lamina are not infrequently present, usually seen just posterior to the nasolacrimal duct. As noted above, overzealous resection of the anterior uncinate process can lead to nasolacrimal duct injury or penetration into the orbit. Dehiscences of the ethmoid roof and sphenoid sinus walls should also be noted. A soft tissue mass adjacent to a bony defect may require further investigation with MR imaging. In order to avoid complications with revision surgery, it is imperative that the radiologist convey any findings of bony dehiscence in an accurate manner to the otolaryngologist. In instances in which imaging is performed soon after surgery, it is important for the radiologist to realize that opacification of remaining air cells and the nasal cavity

is an expected postoperative finding and should not be construed as abnormal.

Postoperative Complications of FESS

Complications with FESS are uncommon when the procedure is performed by experienced surgeons, but they occur nonetheless. They are similar to the complications encountered with traditional sinus surgery. With FESS, however, the operating surgeon is further removed from the operative field and has a smaller field of view that is limited to the mucosal surface. The presence of anatomic variants and excessive bleeding in the operative field can significantly contribute to complications. In cases of sinonasal polyposis and revision surgery, the loss or distortion of normal anatomic landmarks makes the surgeon's task even more difficult. These facts underscore the important role of the radiologist in helping the otolaryngologist avoid operative complications.

In general, complications from FESS can be divided into major and minor categories (Table IID-3). The incidence of minor complications excluding synechiae varies

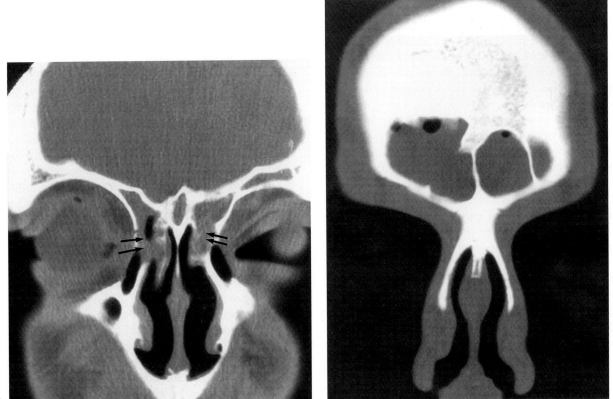

FIG. IID-14. Nasofrontal recess scarring after FESS. **A:** Coronal CT image at the level of the nasofrontal recesses (*arrows*) shows abnormal soft tissue bilaterally after FESS. The left middle turbinate has been removed. **B:** The frontal sinuses are opacified bilaterally. It is frequently not possible to distinguish scar tissue from recurrent inflammatory disease with CT. Scar tissue was found in this particular case. (Case courtesy of H. Ric Harnsberger, M.D.)

TABLE IID-3. *Complications of functional endoscopic sinus surgery*

Minor	Major
Sinonasal	**Orbital**
Synechiae	Persistent diplopia
Ostial stenosis and occlusion	Severe emphysema
Minor hemorrhage	Abscess
Tooth numbness and pain	Hematoma and severe hemorrhage
Nasolacrimal duct injury	Blindness
Olfactory disturbance	**Intracranial**
Orbital	Cerebrospinal fluid leak
Periorbital ecchymosis	Acquired cephalocele
Orbital emphysema	Meningitis and empyema
Transient diplopia	Brain abscess
	Intracranial hemorrhage
	Carotid artery injury
	Frontal lobe injury and stroke

but has been reported in the range of 7% to 12% (31). Postoperative synechiae between the lateral wall and the middle turbinate are a relatively common minor complication that can lead to middle meatal and ostial stenosis. Some authors believe the incidence is increased with partial middle turbinectomy, but others advocate turbinectomy to prevent this complication. Isolated stenosis or occlusion of a middle meatal antrostomy can also occur secondary to scarring. The nasolacrimal duct lies 3 to 6 mm anterior to the maxillary ostium and may be injured during surgical enlargement of the ostium. Evaluation for possible injury to the duct requires imaging in the axial plane. Computed tomographic dacrocystography has been advocated for further investigation (32). The other more minor orbital complications that are listed in Table IID-3 seldom require imaging.

Major complications, fortunately, are much less common. Intracranial hemorrhage after endoscopic surgery is the most serious complication, sometimes resulting in death (15,33,34). Subarachnoid hemorrhage may result from injury to the anterior cerebral artery, internal carotid artery, or cerebral veins. The potential for internal carotid artery injury becomes a major concern in removing bony septa in the sphenoid sinus. Kennedy et al. (21) found an apparent bony dehiscence over the carotid artery in 22% of CT studies. When internal carotid artery injury with hemorrhage is recognized, intraoperative management consists of packing and carotid artery compression. Emergency angiography should be performed in order to identify the type and site of injury. If the injury in not easily amenable to surgical repair, permanent balloon occlusion is the treatment of choice, but only following temporary test occlusion to ensure that adequate collateral circulation is present.

Cerebrospinal fluid (CSF) leak is the most common major complication with FESS, accounting for approximately 66% of all major complications; this has a reported

incidence ranging from less than 0.1% to 0.9% (31). Contributing factors include surgeon inexperience, prior surgery, severe sinonasal polyposis, a low-lying ethmoid roof, and general anesthesia. Prior sinonasal surgery and sinonasal polyposis both result in distortion of the normal landmarks the surgeon uses during FESS. Patients under general anesthesia appear to be at increased risk for development of a CSF leak, as opposed to those patients managed with local anesthesia. The skull base is extremely sensitive to manipulation. Sudden or severe pain reported by the patient during the procedure will lead the surgeon to reevaluate the position of his or her instrumentation, thus avoiding potential inadvertent penetration of the skull base dura. Unfortunately, most patients with sinonasal polyposis require general anesthesia because of the extent of surgery needed in this population. The low-lying ethmoid roof, a normal variation, also predisposes to skull base perforation. Dessi et al. (35) reported that the right side was lower than the left in 8.6% of cases, whereas the reverse was true in only 1.2%. It is important for the radiologist to convey to the surgeon any variation in the height of the ethmoid roof. Most CSF leaks have been reported on the right side (36). Some authors believe this is because of reduced visibility on the right side for a right-handed surgeon (33).

Leaks of CSF can occur anywhere along the anterior skull base but are more common along the anterior cribriform plate, where the vertical plate of middle turbinate attaches to the lateral cribriform plate. This is the site where the anterior ethmoidal artery enters the nasal cavity and is the weakest site of the ethmoid bone. Therefore, it is important for the surgeon to stay lateral to the middle turbinate during endoscopy. Fracture of the turbinate, sometimes done to improve exposure, can potentially tear the dura, resulting in CSF rhinorrhea. Many times CSF leaks are recognized at the time of surgery and can be repaired endoscopically, using a septal mucoperichondrial graft or temporalis fascia. However, they can present any time from the immediate postoperative period to 2 years later (36). Presenting symptoms include CSF rhinorrhea (most common), headache related to pneumocephalus, and meningitis or meningoencephalitis. Many leaks will cease with conservative measures. If one is persistent, however, then evaluation is indicated (Fig. IID-15). The following protocol reflects the one used at the University of Minnesota. If the patient is actively leaking clinically, CT with intrathecal water-soluble contrast medium is the procedure of choice. A precontrast CT scan, done in the coronal plane with 2- to 3-mm slice thickness, is initially performed, and the anterior skull base is evaluated for areas of bony dehiscence. The patient is then taken to the fluoroscopy suite, where 5 to 6 ml of nonionic contrast medium (180 to 240 mg/dl) is placed in the lumbar subarachnoid space. The prone patient is placed in Trendelenberg position for 2 min and then transported to CT with the patient remaining prone, slightly head-down. The

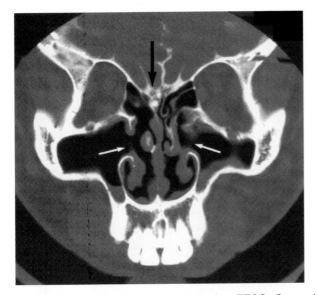

FIG. IID-15. Cerebrospinal fluid leak after FESS. Coronal CT after intrathecal contrast administration, with the patient prone, demonstrates a defect of the right cribriform plate (*arrow*) and contrast medium entering the right ethmoid region. A small amount of contrast medium is also observed between the nasal septum and the right middle turbinate (*small arrow*). Middle antrostomies are present bilaterally (*white arrows*).

coronal CT is repeated, and additional 2- to 3-mm axial images are obtained through the sphenoethmoid sinuses. All images are filmed with both soft tissue and bone window settings.

If the CSF leak is intermittent, and a nonenhanced CT is nonrevealing, radionuclide cisternography is performed with 400 to 500 μCi of indium-111-labeled DTPA. Prior to injection, nasal pledgets are placed by the head and neck surgeon. The radionuclide is then injected into the lumbar subarachnoid space, and the patient is imaged at intervals up to 24 hr. Physical activities that may elicit CSF rhinorrhea are encouraged. The pledgets are removed at 24 hr, and the activity within the pledgets is compared to activity in a sample of serum drawn at the same time. If the ratio of pledget activity to serum activity is greater than 1.5, then the study is considered positive. The location of the leak is estimated by the location of the pledgets showing the greatest activity. Radionuclide activity identified over the abdomen, even without activity in the pledgets, is considered a positive test.

In difficult cases in which the CSF leak cannot be demonstrated, CT cisternography can be performed under conditions of increased CSF pressure. After placement of a lumbar drain, a constant infusion of normal saline is begun to increase the intracranial pressure to 25 to 30 mm

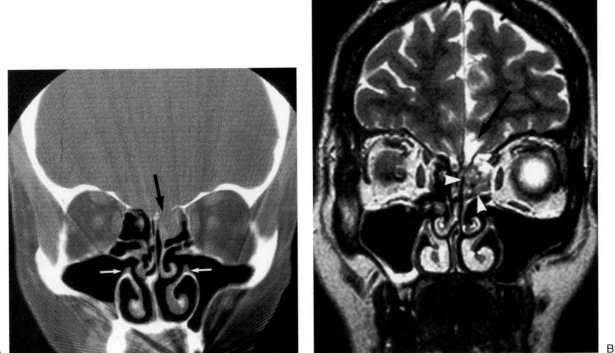

A   B

FIG. IID-16. Frontal lobe injury after FESS. **A:** Coronal CT image reveals focal dehiscence of the left fovea ethmoidalis and cribriform plate (*arrow*) associated with an intraethmoidal soft tissue mass. Bilateral uncinectomies are also present (*white arrows*). **B:** Coronal T$_2$W MR image also shows a hypointense mass (*arrowheads*) within the left ethmoid region. The "mass" represents fascia used to repair an intraoperative CSF leak during FESS. Injury to the frontal lobe is also well visualized on this image (*large arrow*), a recognized but unusual complication after FESS. (Case courtesy of H. Ric Harnsberger, M.D.)

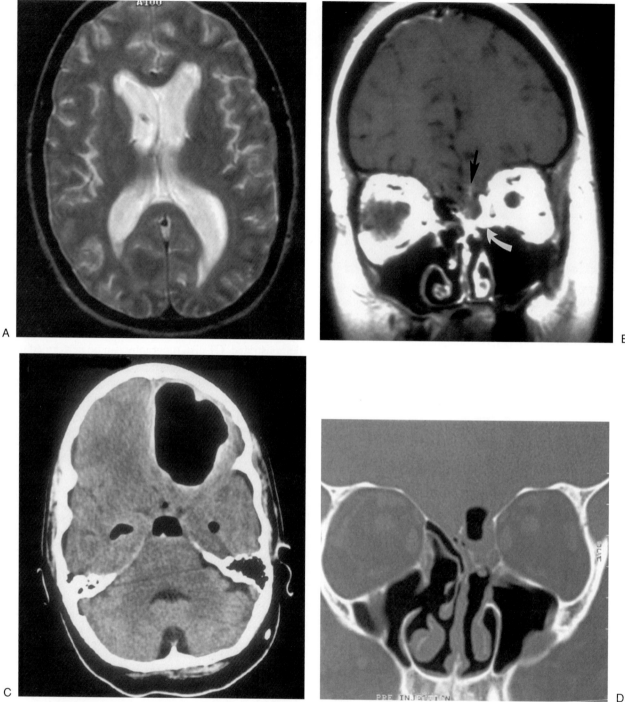

FIG. IID-17. Intracranial complications after FESS. **A:** Axial T$_2$W MR image, obtained 6 weeks follow-ing FESS, shows hydrocephalus resulting from bacterial meningitis. The initial source of the infection was not known. **B:** Coronal T$_1$W contrast-enhanced image shows minor focal enhancement of the left gyrus rectus (*arrow*) with protrusion of frontal lobe into the left ethmoid region. Enhancing mucosa is present inferiorly (*white arrow*). No CSF leak was present at the time of this scan. **C:** Nonenhanced axial CT scan, performed 2 weeks following the MR study, reveals massive pneumocephalus. **D:** Coronal CT image clearly shows air traversing the right fovea ethmoidalis, indicating the origin of the pneumocephalus. The patient had a CSF leak at this time, confirmed by CT cisternography (not shown). (Case courtesy of Daniel J. Loes, M.D.)

H₂O in order to precipitate the leak. Magnetic resonance cisternography has been advocated to detect CSF fistulas noninvasively (37). These techniques include imaging with fast spin echo or fast inversion-recovery sequences to produce very heavily T_2W images with or without video inversion filming. Flow-sensitive techniques are used with very slow flow-sensitive gradient-echo imaging and diffusion-weighted MR imaging. Further study is needed to determine the accuracy and potential applications of these MR techniques.

Other posttherapeutic complications involving intracranial structures that have been reported include frontal lobe injury and infarction (Fig. IID-16), parenchymal hematoma, meningitis, cerebritis, abscess, acquired cephalocele, massive pneumocephalus (Fig. IID-17), and perforation of the ventricular system (31,33,38,39). Postoperative imaging is indicated in any patient with severe post-FESS headaches or mental status changes. Nonenhanced CT imaging in the axial plane is recommended initially to evaluate for intracranial hemorrhage, with 3- to 5-mm-thick sections through the ethmoid sinuses and anterior skull base. Additional coronal images are performed to assess the bony integrity of the ethmoid roof. Thin-section spiral CT of the sinuses and base of skull with reconstructions offers an alternative if direct coronal images are not possible; however, 2- to 3-mm collimation with at least 50% overlap is suggested to optimize the reformations. Even then, small bony defects may be difficult to confirm using spiral technique with multiplanar reformations.

If subarachnoid, intraventricular, or parenchymal hemorrhage is detected, the patient should be evaluated by selective cerebral angiography to investigate possible arterial injury. When no intracranial hemorrhage or pneumocephalus is present, MR imaging may be performed to look for possible stroke or infection. Pre- and postcontrast T_1W images as well as T_2W images are routinely obtained. Imaging in the coronal plane is mandatory in order to detect small subdural or epidural empyemas. The MR is also superior to CT for detecting postoperative acquired cephaloceles. Heavily T_2W images are useful in differentiating encephaloceles from simple meningoceles. Although less definitive, MR angiography may be employed as an alternative to catheter angiography in cases of nonhemorrhagic stroke to exclude a posttraumatic pseudoaneurysm.

Major orbital complications include diplopia, abscess, significant orbital emphysema, orbital hematoma, and optic nerve injury (40). Dehiscences of the lamina papyracea from prior trauma or surgery increase the risk orbital complications and should be brought to the surgeon's attention because herniation of periorbita or orbital fat through the defect may be mistaken for diseased mucosa. Diplopia can result from extraocular muscle injury during ethmoidectomy. The medial rectus and superior oblique muscles are the ones most often injured. Blindness is most often related to the presence of an acute orbital hematoma.

This results in increased intraorbital pressure, optic nerve compression, and optic nerve ischemia. Laceration of the anterior ethmoidal artery with retraction into the orbit is the usual etiology for the hematoma. It is important for the surgeon to check the orbit manually by palpation during surgery if the patient is under general anesthesia, in order to detect this complication early, before irreversible damage occurs. Significant orbital emphysema can also lead to a compromise in orbital blood flow, threatening vision (Fig. IID-18).

Direct injury to the optic nerve is very rare. The nerve lies in close proximity to both the ethmoid and sphenoid sinuses. As mentioned earlier, endoscopic techniques can be used to decompress the optic nerve. The presence of an Onodi cell (an enlarged posterior ethmoid air cell that directly abuts the optic canal) and extensive pneumatization of the anterior clinoid process are anatomic variants that may predispose to optic nerve injury during surgery. They are best demonstrated using both axial and coronal images in combination, and they should be clearly noted in the radiographic report when present. The initial imaging study in a patient with postoperative blindness should consist of thin-section (2 to 3 mm) axial and coronal CT. The lamina papyracea should be closely inspected for disruption. Although opacity in the adjacent ethmoid sinus region is a normal postoperative finding, orbital emphysema, periorbita protrusion through the lamina, retrobulbar fat infiltration, and proptosis are abnormal. The

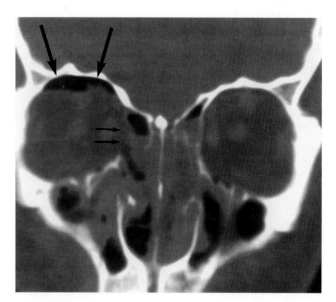

FIG. IID-18. Orbital complication following FESS. There is disruption of the right lamina papyracea (*small arrows*) with emphysema of the right orbit (*large arrows*). One-way entry of air into the orbit (ball-valve mechanism) can lead to significant increases in intraorbital pressure and impair blood flow to the globe. (From Scuderi et al., ref. 23, with permission.)

extraocular muscles and optic nerve should be carefully inspected for signs of injury. Any soft tissue mass or hematoma should be brought to the immediate attention of the surgeon. Contrast-enhanced CT and MR are reserved for cases of possible infection or associated intracranial injury.

NEOPLASTIC DISEASE

The majority of masses involving the paranasal sinuses are inflammatory in nature and are initially investigated using nasal endoscopy; CT is the procedure of choice when imaging is required. On the other hand, if the clinical history and endoscopic findings are suggestive of a neoplastic process, then MR becomes the initial radio-graphic study of choice, and CT is reserved for further evaluation of bony detail and to answer questions raised on the MR study. With the possible exception of small inverted papillomas and other similar benign lesions of the nasal cavity, neoplasms of the sinonasal region require open surgical approaches. The type of surgery depends on the extent of the tumor. Operations for sinonasal neoplasms include maxillectomy, with its various modifications, and craniofacial resection. Whereas the preoperative study is very important in planning the surgical approach, the postoperative study assumes a major role in subsequent patient management.

Maxillectomy

Medial maxillectomy, a procedure popularized over the past 20 years, is indicated for benign and low-grade ma-

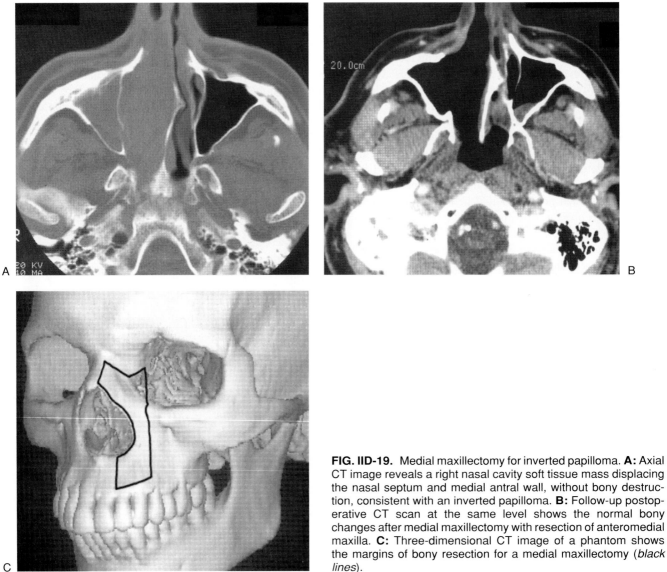

FIG. IID-19. Medial maxillectomy for inverted papilloma. **A:** Axial CT image reveals a right nasal cavity soft tissue mass displacing the nasal septum and medial antral wall, without bony destruction, consistent with an inverted papilloma. **B:** Follow-up postoperative CT scan at the same level shows the normal bony changes after medial maxillectomy with resection of anteromedial maxilla. **C:** Three-dimensional CT image of a phantom shows the margins of bony resection for a medial maxillectomy (*black lines*).

lignant lesions involving the ethmoid sinuses, lateral nasal wall, and maxillary sinus (41). This procedure is utilized if there is no extension of tumor to the lateral maxilla, orbit, or anterior cranial fossa. With the medial maxillectomy procedure, block resection contains the entire lateral nasal wall with the inferior and middle turbinates, the ethmoid labyrinth, and the lamina papyracea (Fig. IID-19). This procedure is widely utilized for management of inverted papilloma. Significant complications after this procedure are rare.

Partial maxillectomy and total maxillectomy are performed for more advanced malignant tumors of the maxillary sinuses (41). Because many maxillary sinus tumors extend into the ethmoid labyrinth, larger tumors with limitation of extension into the lower ethmoid region are also approached with this procedure. Extension to the ethmoid roof or involvement of the orbital apex are contraindications for total maxillectomy. This procedure can be performed with or without orbital exenteration. When total maxillectomy is performed with orbital exenteration, the resection specimen includes the orbital contents, the floor and medial wall of the orbit, the malar bone and anterior aspect of the zygomatic arch, the maxillary antrum, the ethmoid labyrinth, the anterior wall of the sphenoid sinus, the pterygoid plates, and the hard palate on the side of the lesion (Fig. IID-20). If the ethmoid sinuses are involved with the tumor, the nasal septum is also resected. The cavity is lined with a split-thickness skin graft. Orbital wall contour reconstruc-

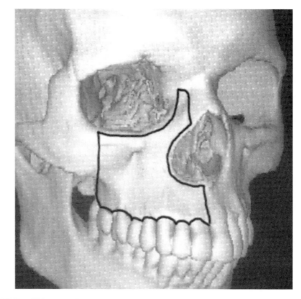

FIG. IID-21. Partial maxillectomy. Three-dimensional CT image demonstrates the margins of bony resection for a partial maxillectomy (*black lines*). The orbit is left intact with this modification.

tion could be performed with the use of pericranial or temporalis muscle flap or a microvascular free flap. Early complications include infection and graft necrosis. More delayed complications involve contraction of the graft and ocular exophthalmos.

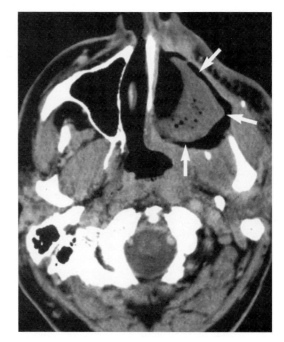

FIG. IID-22. Postmaxillectomy, with prosthesis in place. Axial CT image in a patient after partial maxillectomy shows a prosthetic implant (*arrows*) within the postmaxillectomy cavity. These prosthetic implants should be removed prior to scanning because metal artifact at the palate level can result in significant image degradation on both CT and MR images.

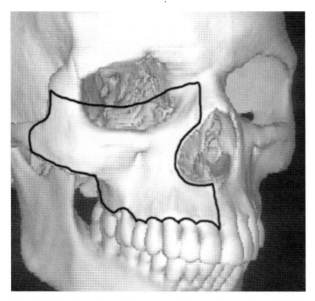

FIG. IID-20. Total maxillectomy. Three-dimensional CT image demonstrates the margins of bony resection for a typical medial maxillectomy procedure (*black lines*). The bone cuts may be modified depending on the extent of the tumor.

When the malignant tumor involves only the lower portion of the maxillary sinus or hard palate, a partial maxillectomy may be performed (41). With this procedure, the orbital floor is preserved. The resected specimen includes the lower two-thirds of the maxilla with the hard palate (Fig. IID-21). The nasal septum and middle turbinate are preserved, and the cavity is lined with a skin graft. With either a partial or total maxillectomy, a preoperatively prepared palatal prosthesis is used to reconstruct the palatal defect and alveolar ridge and maintain proper shape to the face.

Radiologic evaluation of the postmaxillectomy patient for malignant disease begins with a baseline study. This should be obtained no sooner than 6 to 8 weeks after surgery in order to allow any postoperative hemorrhage or edema to subside. The palatal prosthesis, depending on the composition, can cause significant artifacts on both CT and MR if left in place and should be removed prior to imaging (Fig. IID-22). The normal postmaxillectomy cavity should have a smooth, relatively uniform internal lining (Fig. IID-23). Any focal thickening, nodularity, or focus of increased enhancement should be suspicious for recurrent tumor (42). The medical imaging physician can help direct the surgeon in these instances to ensure biopsy of the appropriate site, as recurrent tumor may lie beneath the skin graft or mucosa and be invisible on visual inspection in the early stages. The posterior aspect of the cavity in the region of the pterygoid muscles is a difficult area to evaluate, particularly with CT, because of the distorted anatomy and mildly enhancing nature of the residual musculature (Fig. IID-24). The tendency in this area is often to overcall tumor recurrence. The presence of a baseline or prior comparison study is extremely helpful in evaluating this region in order to critically and correctly analyze posttherapeutic changes.

Craniofacial Resection

Craniofacial resection is an anterior skull base technique initially performed for *en bloc* resection of large frontoethmoid malignancies. The indications for the procedure have been modified to include both benign and malignant tumors originating in the superior nasal cavity, frontal, ethmoid, and sphenoid sinuses, orbits, and olfactory groove with ethmoid extension that extend beyond the limits of resection possible by total maxillectomy (41). Contraindications for craniofacial resection include involvement of the cavernous sinus, intracranial carotid artery, optic chiasm, and temporal

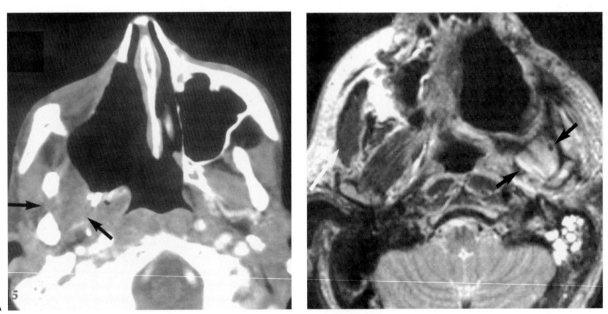

FIG. IID-23. Normal CT and MR after maxillectomy. **A:** Axial CT image after partial maxillectomy demonstrates a smooth surface along the inner margins of the postoperative cavity. The zygomatic prominence is present. In a total maxillectomy, this bone is resected. The masticator space region (*arrows*) can be a difficult area to evaluate for recurrence with CT. **B:** Axial T$_2$W MR scan in a different patient following total maxillectomy shows normal contour to the cavity. Hyperintense signal within the left medial pterygoid muscle from denervation atrophy is present (*arrows*). Enhancement may be observed in the early months after surgery, probably resulting from denervation. The MR is superior to CT in differentiating tumor from denervation changes in this area.

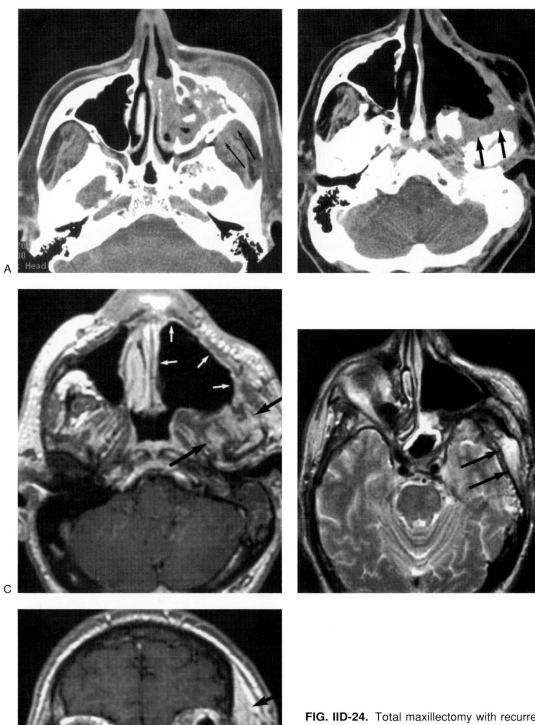

FIG. IID-24. Total maxillectomy with recurrence. **A:** Axial CT reveals a destructive squamous cell carcinoma of the left maxillary sinus with extension into the superficial soft tissues and retromaxillary fat (*arrows*). **B:** Baseline CT after total maxillectomy shows normal postoperative changes anteriorly. Tumor recurrence was suspected posteriorly (*arrows*). **C:** Axial contrast-enhanced T$_1$W MR scan shows normal enhancement of the skin graft (*small arrows*) and some soft tissue enhancement posteriorly (*large arrows*). Biopsy of this tissue yielded fibrosis and muscle denervation atrophy. **D:** Follow-up T$_2$W MR study, 6 months after **C,** again shows a normal appearance of the maxillectomy cavity. However, there is thickening and hyperintensity of the temporalis muscle (*arrows*). **E:** Contrast-enhanced coronal T$_1$W image shows marked enhancement of the temporalis (*arrows*), indicating recurrent tumor. The lining of the maxillectomy cavity remains normal (*small arrows*).

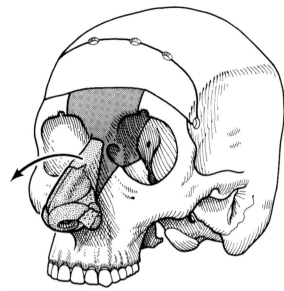

A

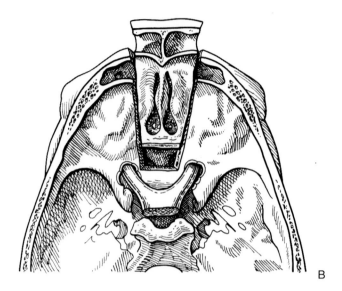

B

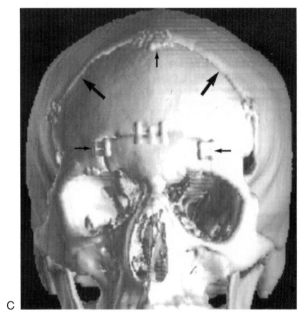

C

FIG. IID-25. Craniofacial resection. **A:** Drawing depicting the location of the orbital and frontonasal osteotomies (*shaded area*). A bifrontal craniotomy is present superiorly. The nasal bones and cartilage are detached during the operation (*curved arrow*), exposing the nasal cavity. **B:** Drawing demonstrating the usual limits of the resection with this approach. The central compartment of the anterior cranial fossa is removed with the lesion *en bloc*. **C:** Three-dimensional CT following craniofacial resection demonstrates the frontonasal osteotomies (*arrowheads*) and the bifrontal craniotomy (*large arrows*). Titanium miniplates (*small arrows*) are visible only as small surface irregularities. (**A** and **B** from Skekar and Janecka, ref. 51, with permission.)

FIG. IID-26. Normal postoperative appearance following craniofacial resection. **A:** Baseline coronal CT image, obtained 3 months after aneurysmal bone cyst resection, shows the bony resection margins (*arrows*). A bone graft has been used to reconstruct part of the anterior cranial fossa floor (*arrowheads*). **B:** Nonenhanced coronal T_1W MR image obtained at the same time as **A** demonstrates the vascularized pericranial graft above the nasal cavity (*white arrows*). The thin bone graft on the left is barely visible (*arrowheads*). **C:** Contrast-enhanced T_1W image at the same level reveals intense enhancement of the graft (*arrows*). **D:** Follow-up T_1W scan 18 months after surgery shows interval thinning of the graft. **E:** T_2W image at the same level shows the hypointense signal of the fascial graft (*arrows*). **F:** Images after contrast administration reveal persistent enhancement (*arrows*). The appearance of the graft should stabilize 12 to 18 months after surgery.

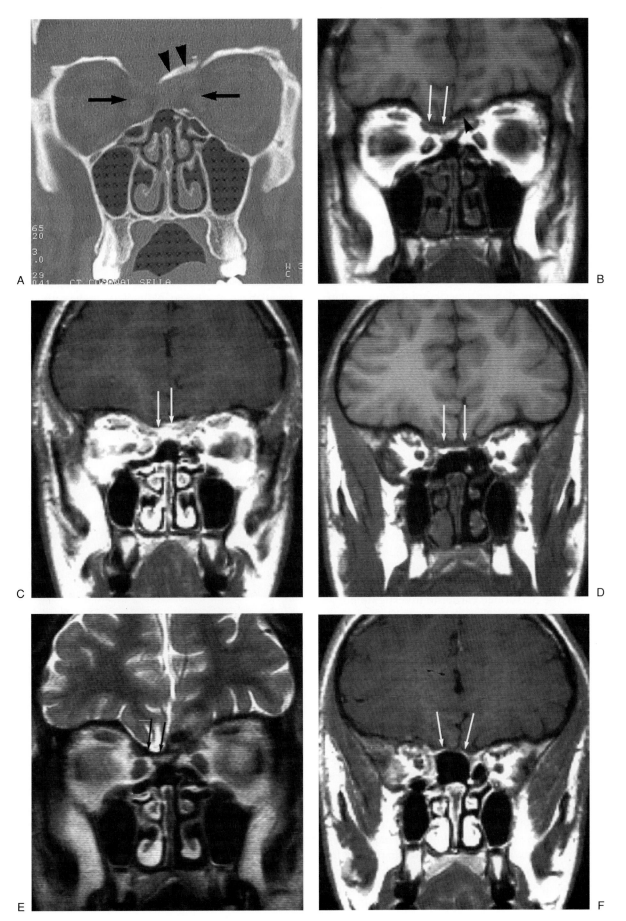

lobe (43). The procedure, performed by a neurosurgical–head and neck surgery team, combines a bifrontal craniotomy with an extended lateral rhinotomy approach (Fig. IID-25). After the craniotomy is performed, the bone and dura are excised to provide adequate margins, and any frontal lobe containing tumor is resected. The facial portion of the tumor is then removed with a medial, partial, or total maxillectomy, including the medial orbital wall.

The *en bloc* bone specimen after resection typically contains the ipsilateral ethmoid labyrinth and ethmoid roof, the cribriform plate, and the superior and lateral walls of the sphenoid. It can be extended to include the posterior wall of the frontal sinuses, the orbital roof, and opposite ethmoid and medial orbital wall. The anterior cranial fossa defect is then closed with an anterior dural flap or pericranial graft and a temporalis musculofascial free flap or a pericranial pedicle flap (44). Occasionally, a bone graft or synthetic materials (e.g., titanium mesh) are needed for anterior cranial floor and orbital reconstruction. The exposed soft tissues of the sinonasal cavity are covered with spit-thickness skin grafts.

The general approach to the postoperative paranasal sinus described previously also applies to patients following craniofacial resection, the only difference being that the anterior cranial fossa and brain will also show postoperative changes that require monitoring. The importance of postoperative baseline comparison studies cannot be overemphasized. Although either CT or MR can be used for follow-up, MR imaging is preferred for the reasons previously mentioned. Additional advantages of MR include increased sensitivity over CT to brain and dural pathology. Therefore, depending on the initial diagnosis, an initial postoperative study is recommended 6 to 12 weeks after surgery. Imaging may be performed earlier to investigate postoperative complications. The most common complications from craniofacial resection are infection and CSF leak: MR is recommended to evaluate possible infection, unless accompanied by CSF rhinorrhea; CT with water-soluble intrathecal contrast is usually the initial study of choice to evaluate for possible CSF leak in these cases.

Most malignant ethmoid tumors tend to recur at the margins of the resection. The lymphatic drainage from this area is not completely known, but the high retropharyngeal lymph nodes, the most likely first-order drainage site, are rarely involved. The diagnostic difficulty most often encountered is the differentiation of tumor at the resection site from postoperative scarring and fibrosis. Normal postoperative dural enhancement and scarring occur at the craniotomy site and can persist almost indefinitely (9). Secondly, the tissue used to reconstruct the anterior cranial floor will also normally enhance to some extent. Finally, reconstruction of the orbital walls and

ethmoid roof with soft tissue usually results in some bulging into the sinonasal cavity. The normal flap appearance remains fairly stable on CT over time. With MR imaging, temporal changes occur, resulting in a reduction in signal intensity on T$_2$W images as the flap matures and becomes more fibrotic (Figs. IID-26 and IID-27). These changes may be less apparent with the vascularized pericranial flaps.

Early detection of tumor recurrence requires careful evaluation of the graft or flap site. The flap appearance usually stabilizes by 8 months after surgery (9). As the flap matures, gradual thinning is usually noted. Because the developing scar tissue is quite vascular, administration of contrast is of little help in detection of recurrent tumor. Furthermore, signal intensity differences on T$_2$W images, although helpful in differentiating tumor from inflammatory tissue, are of less value in separating tumor from vascularized scar tissue, particularly in the early postoperative period. Any new nodularity or focal thickening of the graft or flap should elicit suspicion of tumor recurrence. Similarly, progressive diffuse thickening is also worrisome for tumor. Because chronic infection of hypertrophic scar tissue can produce similar changes at times, biopsy of the area in question is necessary. Tumor recurrence may at times be very indolent, requiring careful comparison with multiple prior studies (Fig. IID-28).

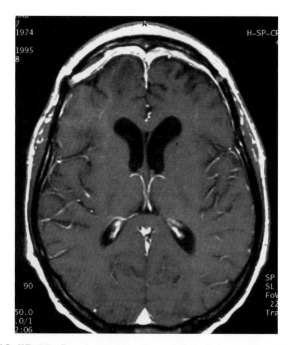

FIG. IID-27. Dural reaction after craniofacial resection. Contrast-enhanced T$_1$W axial image 2 months after craniofacial resection shows marked thickening and enhancement of the dura underlying the frontal craniotomy flap. This type of dural reaction is occasionally normally observed behind the obliterated frontal sinuses following craniofacial resection. It should be viewed with suspicion if it persists or increases on follow-up imaging.

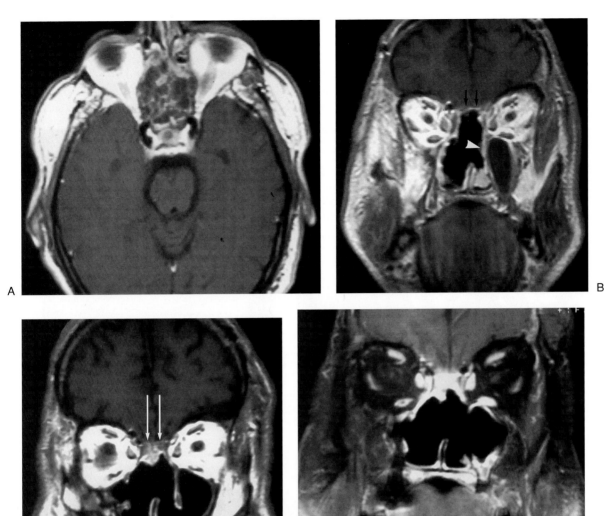

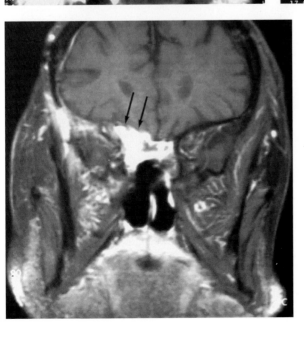

FIG. IID-28. Craniofacial resection for sinonasal adenocarcinoma. **A:** Preoperative contrast-enhanced axial T₁W MR image shows a large heterogeneous tumor occupying the upper nasal cavity and ethmoid sinuses. Multiple low-signal-intensity areas are noted within the mass, representing mucin collections within an unusual mucinous cystadenocarcinoma. **B:** Coronal contrast-enhanced T₁W MR image obtained 1 year after surgery shows a relatively thin, uniformly enhancing, normal-appearing vascularized fascial graft along the roof of the postsurgical cavity (*arrow*). The left maxillary sinus is obstructed secondary to scarring of the maxillary ostium (*arrowhead*). **C:** Coronal T₁W contrast-enhanced scan 2 years after surgery shows interval thickening of the soft tissue along the roof of the common sinonasal cavity (*arrows*). Biopsy revealed recurrent tumor, and the patient was treated with radiation therapy. **D:** MR scan obtained 3 years following initial surgery shows stabilization of the abnormal soft tissue (*arrow*) after radiation therapy. However, a subtle increase in soft tissue thickness was noted more posteriorly (not shown). **E:** Follow-up MR scan 4 months after **D** shows definite tumor recurrence posteriorly (*arrows*). Any areas of increasing soft tissue thickness on follow-up imaging should be presumed to represent recurrent tumor until proven otherwise.

MISCELLANEOUS SINONASAL PROCEDURES, RADIATION, AND CHEMOTHERAPY

Transsphenoidal Pituitary Surgery

Surgical treatment of pituitary tumors is most commonly performed using a transsphenoidal approach to the sella. With the sublabial transseptal approach, a labial incision is made and carried down to the nasal septum. The mucosa is then stripped from the septum, forming a mucoperichondrial or mucoperiosteal tunnel that extends to the sphenoid sinus (45). The cartilaginous septum is separated from its osseous attachment, and the superior

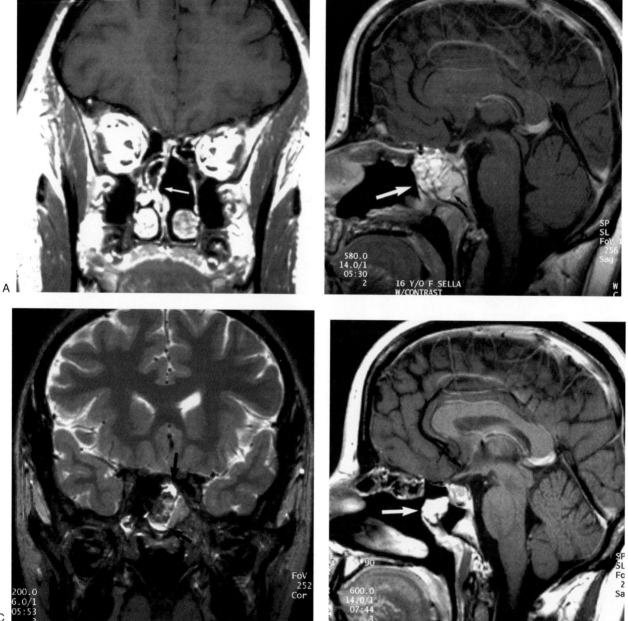

FIG. IID-29. Transsphenoidal pituitary surgery. **A:** Coronal T$_1$W contrast-enhanced MR image demonstrates postsurgical changes within the nasal cavity. The middle and superior turbinates have been resected, and the nasal septum is significantly displaced to the right (*arrow*) from surgical manipulation of the vomer. **B:** T$_1$W contrast-enhanced sagittal image 3 months after surgery shows increased signal within the sphenoid sinus. A fat graft is present anteriorly (*large arrow*), and a hyperintense effusion is present more posteriorly (*small arrows*), almost indistinguishable from the fat graft. **C:** Coronal T$_2$W image from the same study shows mixed signal intensity from the fat graft and a hyperintense postoperative effusion (*arrows*). **D:** Six months after the initial operation, a follow-up scan now shows resolution of the postoperative sphenoid sinus effusion. The position of the fat packing (*arrow*) is clearly visible relative to pituitary floor. A fat graft or other soft tissue is usually placed within the sphenoid sinus if CSF is encountered during surgery, to seal any potential CSF leak.

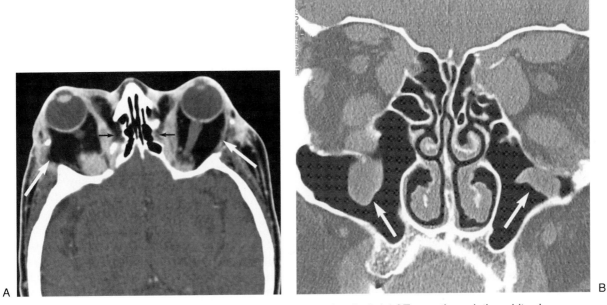

FIG. IID-30. Orbital decompression for thyroid orbitopathy. **A:** Axial CT scan through the orbits shows changes of bilateral lateral orbitotomies (Krönlein's procedure) (*large arrows*). Medial orbital decompressions (*small arrows*) were also performed. **B:** Coronal CT scan of the same patient shows changes from bilateral orbital floor decompression procedures with herniation of fat into the maxillary antra (*large arrows*). When postoperative changes are restricted to the medial and/or inferior orbital walls, the CT findings could be misinterpreted as posttraumatic changes without appropriate history.

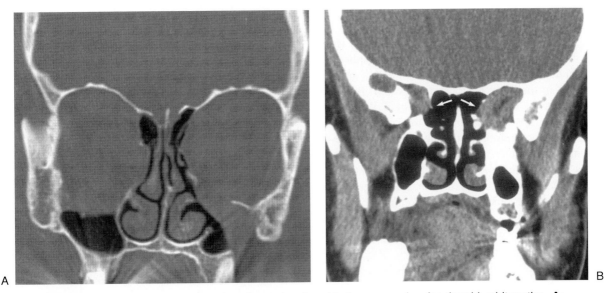

FIG. IID-31. Combined antral and endoscopic ethmoid decompression for thyroid orbitopathy. **A:** Coronal CT image shows orbital floor decompressions bilaterally with protrusion of orbital contents into the maxillary antra. This decompression procedure is performed through a Caldwell–Luc approach. **B:** Coronal CT image more posteriorly shows postsurgical changes involving the posterior ethmoid sinuses (*arrows*). This area was approached endoscopically. Endoscopic techniques have an advantage over the conventional orbital floor approach in decompressing the orbital apex, the location where the optic nerve is often compromised most severely.

bony septum is usually partly resected. The anterior wall of the sinus is resected, and the mucosa removed. The extent of mucosal stripping is variable, but it is usually incomplete. The floor of the sella is then removed, giving access to the pituitary fossa contents. Following tumor removal, the sellar floor defect may be repaired with a small bone graft or fascia lata graft. Fat and/or muscle is often inserted into the sphenoid sinus for graft support and to prevent bleeding.

The appearance of the sphenoid sinuses after transsphenoidal surgery for pituitary disease can be quite varied and complex. Postoperatively, the nasal septum may initially appear thickened by submucosal effusion and/or hematoma. These postoperative collections are eventually replaced by fibrosis. A surgically created defect in the nasal septum can be seen immediately anterior to the sphenoid wall. The sellar floor defect is usually closed by placement of some type of autogenous material into the defect. This tissue may be a single or double layer of fascia lata or a bone graft. Many surgeons use a bone graft to close the defect if a CSF leak is encountered during surgery. Placement of fat in the sphenoid sinus, used to prevent displacement of the graft, is readily detected on the sagittal T_1W images. However, muscle tissue can be used in place of or in addition to fat tissue. The latter tissue will be mildly hypointense on T_1W images relative to brain and will have mildly to moderately hypointense signal on T_2W acquisitions.

An effusion within the sphenoid sinus is virtually always present in the first 1 to 3 months after surgery (Fig. IID-29). Therefore, the signal intensities within sphenoid sinuses can have a complex appearance on both T_1W and T_2W images in the early postoperative period. Both fat and blood products will be hyperintense on T_1W images. The addition of T_2W images and the use of fat-suppression techniques are helpful in distinguishing the type of tissue within the sinuses. Stickney et al. (46) reported persistent mucosal disease in 78% of their patients after 2 to 3 years. They concluded that these changes most likely represented chronic mucosal thickening from postoperative fibrosis rather than active inflammation. They also found no difference in the appearance of the sphenoid sinus in those patients who had undergone postoperative radiation from those who had surgery alone.

Orbital Decompression

In patients with Graves orbitopathy, orbital decompression may be indicated when the vision-threatening disease is present, either the result of exaggerated corneal exposure because of proptosis or, more commonly, secondary to compressive optic neuropathy. There are several procedures that may be utilized in decompression of the orbit (46). These include lateral orbital wall decompression (Krönlein's procedure), superior orbital wall decompres-

sion, medial wall decompression by either external ethmoidectomy or endoscopic ethmoidectomy, transantral decompression of the orbital floor using a Caldwell–Luc approach, and the transconjunctival–transcaruncular (intraorbital) approaches. The transantral orbital floor decompression (Caldwell–Luc approach) is widely utilized and usually achieves favorable results (Fig. IID-30). However, it must be performed bilaterally to avoid postoperative diplopia and cosmetic deformity. In addition, the ability to achieve satisfactory optic nerve decompression is more limited.

Recently, endoscopic ethmoidectomy has been performed in conjunction with orbital floor decompression to gain further orbital floor decompression (47). With these procedures, the bone is removed from the orbital floor with herniation of fat into the antrum (Fig. IID-31). With the endoscopic ethmoidectomy, a routine uncinectomy is carried out along with resection of the anterior and posterior ethmoid air cells. Once the lamina papyracea is satisfactorily exposed, this bone is removed, and an incision is made in the periorbita to allow herniation of fat into the ethmoidal cavity. Contraindications to the endoscopic approach include the presence of acute or chronic

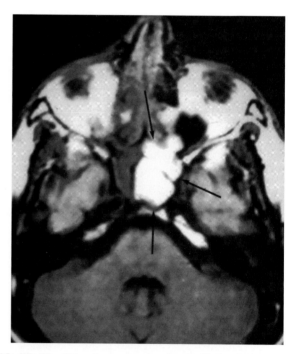

FIG. IID-32. Chronic mucocele after radiation for nasopharyngeal carcinoma. Axial nonenhanced T_1W MR image shows abnormal signal within the sphenoid sinuses. The right sphenoid sinus is mildly hypointense, while the left sphenoid sinus shows marked hyperintensity (*arrows*). On T_2W images (not shown), the right sphenoid sinus was markedly hyperintense, while the left sphenoid sinus demonstrated a decrease in signal intensity. The signal intensity changes within the left sphenoid sinus on T_1W and T_2W images reflect the high protein concentration and viscous secretions within a chronic mucocele, where an obstruction of the right sphenoid sinus occurred more recently.

sinusitis, thickening of the bone of the medial and anterior orbital wall, and maxillary sinus hypoplasia. The advantage of the transconjunctival–transcaruncular (intraorbital) approach is that it allows for safer and more complete decompression of the optic nerve without the need to invade the sinonasal cavity.

Imaging of the sinuses and orbits following orbital decompression will show herniation of orbital fat and extraocular muscle through the bony defect. With inferior orbital decompression, the inferior rectus muscle and adjacent fat herniate into the maxillary sinus. Similarly, herniation of fat and muscle is noted through the lamina papyracea. Without the appropriate history, these changes may be misinterpreted as old orbital blow-out fractures. Additionally, the antral changes may be misinterpreted as the soft tissue process. If the changes are limited to the orbital floor, the soft tissue within the maxillary sinuses may be misinterpreted as inflammatory disease.

Radiation Therapy

Radiation therapy for neoplasms of the sinonasal area is most commonly utilized as adjunctive therapy in high-risk patients following surgical resection, but it may be used as a primary treatment modality for patients with advanced disease, frequently in conjunction with chemotherapy. The long-term effects of radiation therapy may take years to reveal themselves, and objective evidence regarding the incidence of bony and soft tissue effects of radiation therapy is very limited (48). The same soft tissue and bone changes that affect other areas of the body can be seen within the face. Mucosal atrophy, fibrosis, and telangiectasias of the sinonasal mucosa do not have specific imaging manifestations. Fibrosis seldom produces any difficulty with interpretation unless it causes obstruction of the sinus ostium (49). This can lead to recurrent inflammatory disease that may interfere with monitoring for tumor recurrence. Infrequently, chronic obstruction can result in mucocele formation (Fig. IID-32). Craniofacial radiation during childhood, usually performed in children with rhabdomyosarcoma or retinoblastoma, can retard the growth of the facial bones (Fig. IID-33). Progressive fibrosis of the pterygoid muscles occurs in patients receiving radiation for maxillary sinus, nasopharyngeal, and oropharyngeal carcinomas.

Osteoradionecrosis is less commonly seen involving the facial bones today as a result of improvement in radiation therapy equipment and planning (50). The mandible is the most frequently affected facial bone, with the maxilla and zygoma affected less commonly. Radiation osteitis may not become clinically evident until one or two

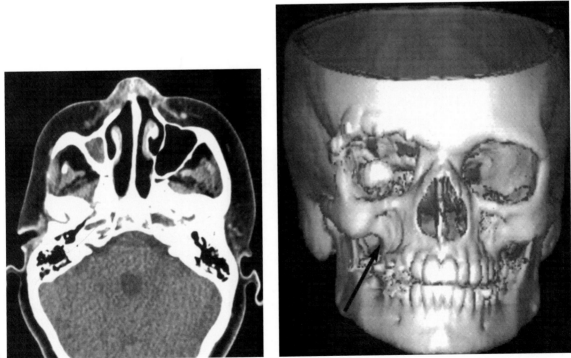

FIG. IID-33. Midface growth retardation following radiation therapy. **A:** Axial CT image of the midface shows opacification of the maxillary sinus with significant reduction in size compared to the left. The depression of the anterior wall indicates growth retardation rather than simple antral contraction from chronic sinusitis. **B:** Three-dimensional CT image readily demonstrates the midface asymmetry with hypoplasia of the right maxilla (*arrow*).

decades after treatment. It is often suspected when a patient complains of increasingly severe pain, usually accompanied by soft tissue swelling and inflammation in a region that has been previously irradiated. The clinical differential diagnosis almost always includes tumor recurrence and/or osteomyelitis. Radionuclide bone scanning is not particularly helpful in differentiating among these entities, but indium-labeled white blood cell scans can be used to exclude infection. Computed tomography is the preferred imaging modality for investigation of osteoradionecrosis. In such cases, the mandible usually appears atrophic and has a mixed lytic–sclerotic appearance. Pathologic fractures are not uncommon, and there may be evidence of a nonunion. The absence of any adjacent soft tissue mass or reaction favors osteoradionecrosis. The maxilla and other facial bones may also demonstrate a mixed lytic–sclerotic appearance with greater fragmentation (Fig. IID-34). Although the fragmentation may mimic tumor destruction, the changes with osteoradionecrosis are typically more diffuse and usually not associated with a discrete soft tissue mass. Furthermore, the densely sclerotic bony fragments seen with advanced postradiation osteitis indicate dead bone rather than bony destruction. If there is limited involvement, chronic osteomyelitis should also be considered. Circumscribed areas of osteonecrosis may heal spontaneously. More advanced or clinically refractory disease requires surgical intervention and resection, with or without reconstruction (48). In the future,

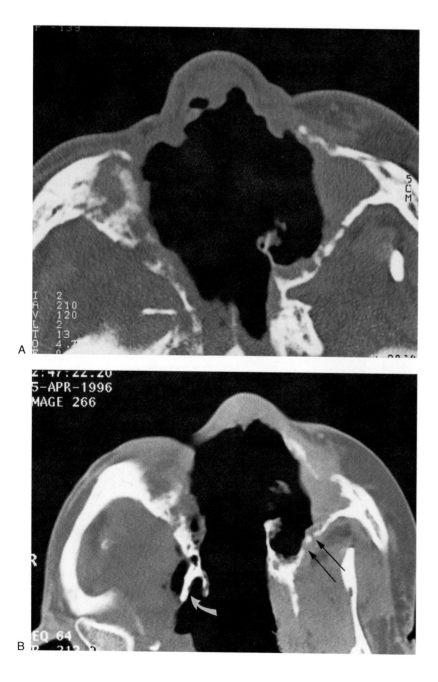

FIG. IID-34. Osteoradionecrosis of the facial bones. **A:** Axial CT image through the maxillary sinuses shows mixed lytic and sclerotic changes involving the facial bones with fragmentation. Mucosal thickening is identified bilaterally in this patient with a history of adenoid cystic carcinoma of the hard palate and multiple previous surgical resections. **B:** Axial CT image obtained 1 year later shows some increased fragmentation and bone loss of the left maxilla (*arrows*) and denuded pterygoid plates on the right (*curved arrow*). Biopsy on both occasions revealed osteoradionecrosis without evidence of tumor.

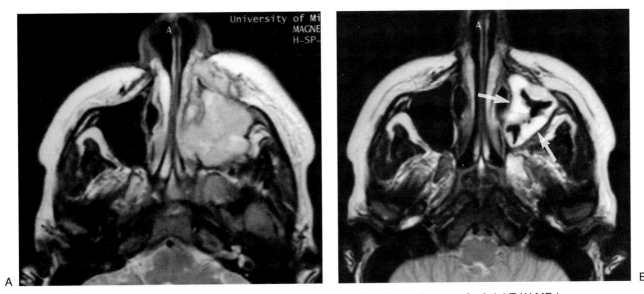

FIG. IID-35. Posttherapeutic inflammatory disease following chemotherapy. **A:** Axial T$_2$W MR image shows a large soft tissue mass involving the left maxillary sinus with extension through the anterior wall into the subcutaneous soft tissues. There is an area of central hyperintensity (*arrows*) indicating trapped secretions secondary to obstruction of the sinus ostium. Biopsy revealed rhabdomyosarcoma in this child. **B:** Following two cycles of chemotherapy, there is dramatic interval reduction in tumor mass. Mucoperiosteal thickening (*arrows*) and mucus retention cyst formation are frequent findings following rapid tumor response to chemotherapy. The hyperintensity of the mucosal changes on the T$_2$W images is helpful in differentiating inflammatory disease from residual tumor.

as more aggressive radiation therapy regimens are used with head and neck cancer, osteoradionecrosis may become more common.

Chemotherapy

There is limited information available regarding the changes that take place within the paranasal sinuses after chemotherapy for malignant tumors of the sinonasal region. Combination chemotherapy alone, or in combination with radiation therapy, is usually reserved for treatment of rhabdomyosarcoma and other soft tissue sarcomas, osteogenic sarcoma, Ewing's sarcoma, unresectable esthesioneuroblastoma, multiple myeloma (plasmacytoma), and lymphoma. The soft tissue sarcomas, particularly rhabdomyosarcoma, are often quite large at the time of diagnosis as a result of very rapid growth. The response after initiation of chemotherapy is frequently dramatic. As the tumor recedes, inflammatory tissue is commonly seen within the involved sinus or sinuses (Fig. IID-35). Characteristics differentiating tumor from inflammatory disease with MR imaging have been described in the preceding sections. The importance of carefully evaluating the T$_2$W images in these instances cannot be overemphasized, so that inflammatory mucosal hypertrophy is not mistaken for residual tumor, and vice versa.

CONCLUSIONS

Pretherapeutic imaging currently occupies a very important role in evaluating inflammatory and neoplastic diseases of the paranasal sinuses. As endoscopic procedures and more aggressive surgical and nonsurgical treatment become widespread for neoplastic disease, it will become increasingly important for radiologists as well as other physicians involved with the care of these patients to gain familiarity with the posttherapeutic imaging appearance of the sinonasal region. Cost-containment issues will put increasing pressure on physicians to eliminate ''unnecessary'' imaging studies. A key part of this is stressing the importance of the posttherapeutic baseline examination with regard to subsequent critical patient follow-up. Awareness on the part of the radiologist of the issues facing the head and neck surgeon in postoperative management will allow the radiologist to be a more valuable consultant, leading to more clinically meaningful exam interpretation and, ultimately, improved patient management.

REFERENCES

1. Bolger WE, Butzin CA, Parsons DS: Paranasal sinus bony anatomic variations and mucosal abnormalities: CT analysis for endoscopic sinus surgery. *Laryngoscope* 1991;101:56–64.
2. Mafee MF: Endoscopic sinus surgery: Role of the radiologist. *Am J Neuroradiol* 1991;12:855–860.
3. Zinreich SJ, Kennedy DW, Rosenbaum AE, Gayler BW, Kumar AJ, Stammberger H: Paranasal sinuses; CT imaging requirements for endoscopic surgery. *Radiology* 1987;163:709–715.
4. Som PM, Lawson W, Biller HF, Lanzieri CF: Ethmoid sinus disease: CT evaluation in 400 cases. II. Postoperative findings. *Radiology* 1986;159:599–604.
5. Lund VJ, Howard DJ, Lloyd GAS, Cheesman AD: Magnetic reso-

nance imaging of paranasal sinus tumors for craniofacial resection. *Head Neck* 1989;11:279–283.

6. Som PM, Urken ML, Biller H, Lidov M: Imaging the postoperative neck. *Radiology* 1993;187:593–603.

7. Som PM, Shapiro MD, Biller HF, Sasaki C, Lawson W: Sinonasal tumors and inflammatory tissues: differentiation with MR imaging. *Radiology* 1988;167:803–808.

8. Som PM, Brandwein M: Sinonasal cavities; Inflammatory diseases, tumors, fractures, and postoperative findings. In: Som PM, Curtin HD, eds. *Head and Neck Imaging*, 3rd ed. St. Louis: Mosby-Year Book, 1996:287–315.

9. Som PM, Lawson W, Biller HF, Lanzieri CF, Sachdev VP, Rigamonti D: Ethmoid sinus disease: CT evaluation in 400 cases. III. Craniofacial resection. *Radiology* 1986;159:605–609.

10. Messerklinger W: *Endoscopy of the Nose.* Baltimore: Urban & Schwarzenberg, 1978.

11. Kennedy DW, Zinreich SJ, Rosenbaum AE, Johns ME: Functional endoscopic sinus surgery: theory and diagnostic evaluation. *Arch Otolaryngol* 1985;111:576–582.

12. Stammberger H: Endoscopic endonasal surgery: concepts in treatment of recurring rhinosinusitis. *Otolaryngol Head Neck Surg* 1986; 94:143–156.

13. Roithmann R, Witterick I, Cole P, Hawke M: Sinusitis in adults. Principles of surgical management and overview of techniques. In: Gershwin ME, Incaudo GA, eds. *Diseases of the Sinuses. A Comprehensive Textbook of Diagnosis and Treatment.* Totowa, NJ: Humana Press, 1996:513–526.

14. Unger JM, Dennison BF, Duncavage JA, Toohill RJ: The radiological appearance of the post-Caldwell–Luc maxillary sinus. *Clin Radiol* 1986;37:77–81.

15. Maniglia AJ, Dodds BL: A safe technique for frontal sinus osteoplastic flap. *Laryngoscope* 1991;101:908–910.

16. Catalano PJ, Lawson W, Som P, Biller HF: Radiographic evaluation and diagnosis of the failed frontal osteoplastic flap with fat obliteration. *Otolaryngol Head Neck Surg* 1991;104:225–234.

17. Loevner LA, Yousem DM, Kennedy DW, Lanza DC, Hayden RE, Goldberg A: MR and osteoplastic frontal sinus flaps [abstract]. In: *American Society of Head & Neck Radiology—29th Annual Scientific Conference and Post Graduate Course in Head & Neck Imaging, May 17–21, 1995.*

18. Friedman WH: Ethmoid sinus. In: Blitzer A, Lawson W, Friedman WH, eds. *Surgery of the Paranasal Sinuses.* Philadelphia: WB Saunders, 1985:146–155.

19. Maniglia AJ: Fatal and major complications secondary to nasal and sinus surgery. *Laryngoscope* 1989;99:276–283.

20. Buus DR, Tse DT, Farris BK: Ophthalmic complications of sinus surgery. *Ophthalmology* 1990;97:612–619.

21. Kennedy DW, Zinreich SJ, Hassab MH: The internal carotid artery as it relates to sphenoethmoidectomy. *Am J Rhinol* 1990;4:7–12.

22. Mafee M: Preoperative imaging anatomy of the nasal–ethmoid complex for functional endoscopic sinus surgery. *Radiol Clin North Am* 1993;31(1):1–20.

23. Scuderi A, Babbel R, Harnsberger H: The sporadic pattern of inflammatory sinonasal disease including postsurgical changes. *Semin Ultrasound CT MR* 1991;12(6):575–591.

24. Kennedy DW, Zinriech SJ: The functional endoscopic approach to inflammatory sinus disease: current perspectives and technique modifications. *Am J Rhinol* 1988;2(3):89–93.

25. Panje WR, Anand VK: Endoscopic sinus surgery indications, diagnosis, and technique. In: Anand VK, Panje WR, eds. *Practical Endoscopic Sinus Surgery.* New York: McGraw-Hill, 1993:68–86.

26. Clerico DM, Kennedy DW, Henick D: Functional endoscopic sinus surgery. In: Gershwin ME, Incaudo GA, eds. *Diseases of the Sinuses: A Comprehensive Textbook of Diagnosis and Treatment.* Totowa, NJ: Humana Press, 1996:547–561.

27. Kennedy DW, Josephson JS, Zinreich SJ, Mattox DE, Goldsmith

28. MM: Endoscopic sinus surgery for mucoceles: a viable alternative. *Laryngoscope* 1989;99:885–895.

28. Levine HL: Functional endoscopic sinus surgery: evaluation, surgery, and follow-up in 250 cases. *Laryngoscope* 1990;100:79–84.

29. Rice DH: Endoscopic sinus surgery: results at 2-year follow-up. *Otolaryngol Head Neck Surg* 1989;101:476–479.

30. Katsantonis GP, Friedman WH, Sivore MC: The role of computed tomography in revision sinus surgery. *Laryngoscope* 1990;100: 811–816.

31. Mackay IS, Cumberworth VL: Complications and long-term sequelae of functional endoscopic sinus surgery in children and adults. In: Gershwin ME, Incaudo GA, eds. *Diseases of the Sinuses. A Comprehensive Textbook of Diagnosis and Treatment.* Totowa, NJ: Humana Press, 1996:563–575.

32. Massoud TF, Whittet HB, Anslow P: CT-dacryocystography for nasolacrimal duct obstruction following paranasal sinus surgery. *Br J Radiol* 1993;66:223–227.

33. Hudgins P, Browning D, Gallups J: Endoscopic paranasal sinus surgery: radiographic evaluation of severe complications. *Am J Neuroradiol* 1992;13:1161–1167.

34. Hudgins P: Complications of endoscopic sinus surgery: the role of the radiologist in prevention. *Radiol Clin North Am* 1993;31(1): 21–31.

35. Dessi P, Moulin G, Triglia JM, Zanaret M, Cannoni M: Radiology in focus—difference in the height of the right and left ethmoidal roofs: a possible risk factor for ethmoidal surgery. Prospective study of 150 CT scans. *J Laryngol Otol* 1994;108:261–262.

36. Stankiewicz JA: Cerebrospinal fluid fistula and endoscopic sinus surgery. *Laryngoscope* 1991;101:250–256.

37. Levy LM, Gulya AJ, Davis SW, LeBihan D, Rajan SS, Schellinger D: Flow-sensitive magnetic resonance imaging in the evaluation of cerebrospinal fluid leaks. *Am J Otol* 1995;16:591–596.

38. Maniglia A: Fatal and other major complications of endoscopic sinus surgery. *Laryngoscope* 1991;101:349–354.

39. Stankiewicz JA: Complications in endoscopic intranasal ethmoidectomy: an update. *Laryngoscope* 1989;99:668–670.

40. Neuhaus RW: Orbital complications secondary to endoscopic sinus surgery. *Ophthalmology* 1990;97:1512–1518.

41. Clement P, Halama AR: Soft tissue masses of the paranasal sinuses. Principles of surgical management and overview of techniques. In: Gershwin ME, Incaudo GA, eds. *Diseases of the Sinuses. A Comprehensive Textbook of Diagnosis and Treatment.* Totowa, NJ: Humana Press, 1996:527–545.

42. Som PM, Shugar JMA, Biller HF: The early detection of antral malignancy in the postmaxillectomy patient. *Radiology* 1982;143: 509–512.

43. Shah JP, Kraus D, Arbit E, Galicich JH, Strong EW: Craniofacial resection for tumours involving the anterior skull base. *Otolaryngol Head Neck Surg* 1992;106:387–393.

44. Janecka IP: Surgical approaches to the skull base. *Neuroimag Clin North Am* 1994;4(3):639–656.

45. Eisele DW, Flint PW, Kelly WA, Cummings CW, Janas JD, Weymuller EA Jr: The sublabial transseptal transsphenoidal approach to sellar and parasellar lesions. *Laryngoscope* 1988;98:1301–1308.

46. Stickney KO, Weymuller EA Jr, Mayberg M: MRI evaluation of the sphenoid sinus after transsphenoidal approach to the pituitary. *Laryngoscope* 1994;104:1–4.

47. Metson R, Shore JW, Gliklich RE, Dallow RL: Endoscopic orbital decompression under local anesthesia. *Otolaryngol Head Neck Surg* 1995;113(6):661–667.

48. Larson DL: Management of complications of radiotherapy of the head and neck. *Surg Clin North Am* 1986;66(1):169–182.

49. Som PM, Lawson W, Biller HF, Lanzieri CF: Ethmoid sinus disease: CT evaluation in 400 cases. I. Nonsurgical patients. *Radiology* 1986;159:591–597.

50. Som PM: Radiation osteitis of the facial bones. *Am J Otolaryngol* 1992;13:310–311.

51. Skekar LN, Janecka IP, eds: *Surgery of Cranial Base Tumors.* New York: Raven Press, 1993.

Posttherapeutic Neurodiagnostic Imaging,
edited by J.R. Jinkins,
Lippincott-Raven Publishers, New York © 1997.

CHAPTER **IIE**

The Posttherapeutic Neck

Pamela Van Tassel and Suresh K. Mukherji

Treatment of malignant neoplasms of the upper aerodigestive tract includes surgery, radiation therapy (RT), and, at times, induction (neoadjuvant) chemotherapy (1–9). The exact treatment depends on the histology, location, and staging of the tumor and may also be influenced by institutional preferences. Both radiation therapy and surgery alter the underlying normal anatomic structures, thereby making interpretation of posttreatment imaging studies challenging. Familiarization with the expected imaging changes following therapy allows accurate radiologic evaluation and may prevent misinterpretation of posttreatment changes as recurrent disease.

Computed tomography (CT) and magnetic resonance (MR) imaging are the most frequently utilized imaging modalities for evaluating the head and neck cancer patient before and after treatment. There is controversy over which is the better overall modality, and each has its strong points. Computed tomography is still more widely available, and there is often faster and more convenient scheduling than for an MR study. The CT examination is also performed more rapidly, is cheaper, and leads to fewer failures than MR with respect to claustrophobia and artifacts in motion-sensitive areas such as the larynx and oro- and hypopharynx. The extreme sensitivity of MR images to patient motion is probably the greatest limitation of this modality for head and neck imaging. By the nature of their disease, these patients typically have respiratory difficulty and trouble managing secretions, resulting in coughing, frequent swallowing, and labored respirations, which severely degrade the images. Because scan times are shorter, and individual slices can be easily repeated on CT, patient motion is less of a problem with this modality. In the future, echo planar imaging, with its extremely rapid imaging times, may

contribute to imaging the head and neck cancer patient. There are no definite data yet to show that MR can equal the accuracy of CT for nodal staging and detection of extracapsular extension of metastatic tumor (10–12).

On the other hand, many of the familiar advantages of MR imaging in other areas of the body apply also to the neck: there is no ionizing radiation, images are easily obtained in three planes without moving the patient or needing computerized reconstructions, and there is excellent contrast discrimination between adjacent tissues. Vascular patency can be easily assessed without the necessity of intravenous contrast. Contrast-enhanced, fat-suppressed images are sensitive in detecting tumor. Of importance, MR imaging has an advantage over CT in distinguishing mature scar tissue from adjacent muscle and tumor (13,14).

Positron-emission tomography is also emerging as a powerful means of differentiating recurrent tumor from posttreatment changes; however, its limited availability and high cost are disadvantages.

IMAGING OF POSTRADIATION CHANGES

The radiographic appearance of the irradiated neck is significantly altered from pretreatment imaging studies (15,16). The effects of RT are seen in multiple structures of the larynx, pharynx, and superficial soft tissues of the neck included within the radiation portal. The histologic changes and the associated radiographic changes that occur as a result of radiation have been previously described and result mainly from edema and fibrosis (17). Histologically, RT results in an acute inflammatory reaction within the deep connective tissues characterized by leukocytic infiltration, histiocyte formation, necrosis, and hemorrhage. Microscopic examination of the small arteries, veins, and lymphatics demonstrates detachment of the lining endothelial cells, causing increased permeability and resulting in interstitial edema. Within 1 to 4 months, there is deposition of rich collagenous fibers with sclerosis and hyalinosis of connective tissues. This inflammatory

P. Van Tassel: Department of Radiology, Medical University of South Carolina, Charleston, South Carolina 29425.

S. K. Mukherji: Department of Radiology, University of North Carolina School of Medicine, Chapel Hill, North Carolina 27599.

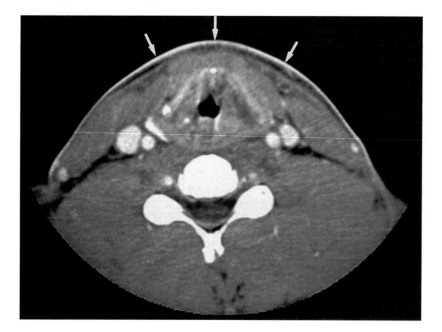

FIG. IIE-1. Postradiation skin thickening. Axial CT image at the level of the false vocal cords in a patient radiated for nasopharyngeal carcinoma shows thickening of the skin of the anterior neck (*arrows*) as well as thickening of the false cords.

process eventually results in obstruction of the small arteries, veins, and lymphatics. By 8 months, there is advanced sclerosis, hyalinosis, and fragmentation of the collagen fibers within connective tissues. Eventually, there may be a reduction in interstitial fluid as a result of the formation of collateral neocapillary and lymphatic channels (17).

The extent of the observed changes in the area included within the radiation port is mainly dependent on the total dose, with the most severe and significant changes occurring after 6800 to 7000 cGy (18). Doses of 4500 to 5000 cGy often do not produce any CT or MR findings (13). Fraction size and time between fractions also con-

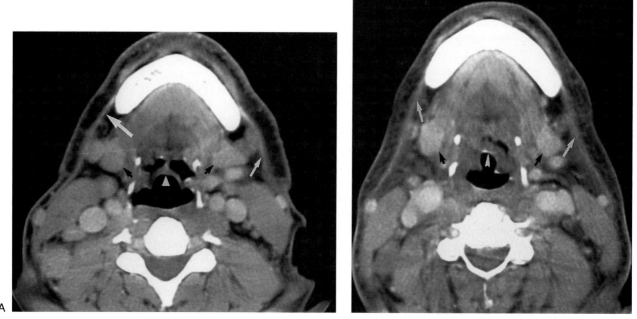

FIG. IIE-2. Postradiation changes in the subcutaneous fat, epiglottis, platysma, and submandibular glands. (**A**) Preradiation scan. (**B**) Postradiation scan shows multiple linear densities in the subcutaneous fat, thickening of the suprahyoid epiglottis (*arrowhead*) and platysma muscle (*long arrows*), and increased enhancement of the submandibular glands (*short arrows*) relative to the pretreatment scan.

tribute to the degree of radiation-induced injury. More advanced and persistent changes may be seen in patients who continue to smoke after RT.

Skin, Subcutaneous Fat, Lymph Nodes, and Muscle

Within 4 months after the completion of RT, reactive changes can be visualized within the skin and subcutaneous tissues in the majority (60% to 90%) of patients (15). These changes include thickening of the skin (Fig.IIE-1) and reticulation of the subcutaneous and deep investing fat. The subcutaneous linear stranding represents lymphedema and perilymphatic fibrosis (Fig. IIE-2) (13,19). Resolution of these changes occurs in about 50% of treated patients (15), but with doses of 6500 cGy and above, these superficial changes are usually permanent in all patients (13).

Lymph node atrophy occurs in the vast majority of pretreatment CT-negative nodes (13,15). Treated nodes involute to about 25% of their original pretreatment size (Fig. IIE-3) (15). Consequently, enlarging lymph nodes after RT are an ominous sign in patients treated with definitive radiotherapy for squamous cell carcinoma (SCCA) of the upper aerodigestive tract.

The platysma muscle lying superficially in the anterior neck and submandibular region commonly demonstrates a thickened, shaggy appearance after RT (Fig. IIE-2). Skeletal muscle in the head and neck exposed to higher than usual doses of RT has been reported to exhibit necrosis. On CT, this has been illustrated as enlargement of the muscle with low density and no significant enhancement (20). Uniform enhancement of prevertebral muscles in an irradiated patient has also been reported as a radia-

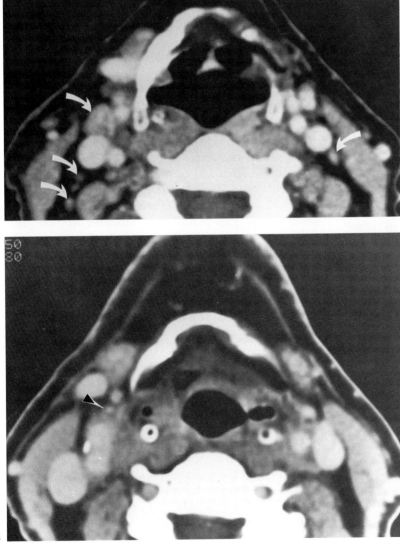

FIG. IIE-3. Postradiation lymph node atrophy. **(A)** Pretreatment CT scan shows several normal-appearing level II and V nodes (*arrows*). **(B)** Scan 15 months after RT demonstrates complete shrinkage of the left level II node and the level V nodes bilaterally and approximately 75% reduction in size of the right level II node (*arrowhead*). (From Mukherji et al., ref. 15, with permission.)

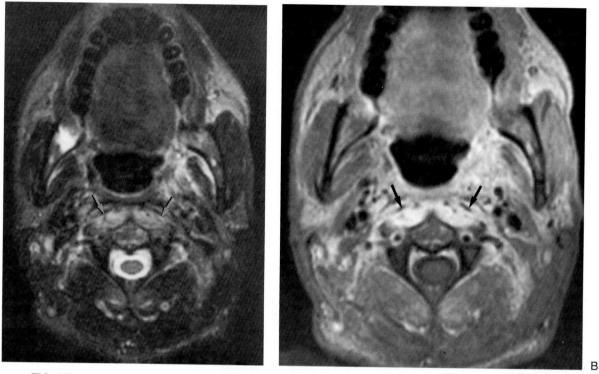

FIG. IIE-4. Radiation-therapy-induced muscle injury. (**A**) Axial T_2-weighted and (**B**) postcontrast T_1-weighted MR images demonstrate abnormal signal intensity and enhancement in the longus capitus and colli muscles bilaterally (*arrows*) in a patient who received a cumulative dose of 140 Gy for treatment of nasopharyngeal carcinoma.

tion effect (Fig. IIE-4) (16).

Salivary Glands

Irradiation may result in acute sialadenitis of the salivary glands after the first treatment. These acute effects are transient and usually resolve within 1 to 2 days (21). Increased size and enhancement of the gland may be seen if imaging is performed within 1 week following the completion of RT. Because imaging is usually performed at least 2 months after completion of therapy, the radiographic changes most commonly observed are those of chronic sialadenitis. These changes include increased enhancement and atrophy (Fig. IIE-5). Fatty replacement of salivary tissue may also be seen (Figs. IIE-6 and IIE-7). Doses above 3500 cGy result in loss of salivary function in most patients, which is usually not recovered (21). The clinical effects of radiation in the major salivary glands (parotid and submandibular) are xerostomia (dry mouth), thick, tenacious saliva, and dental caries from a lowered salivary pH (21).

Pharynx and Larynx

Within the pharynx, postradiation mucositis is observed clinically and is reflected on imaging studies as thickening of the pharyngeal mucosal space, increased CT density

and T_2-weighted MR signal intensity, and increased enhancement of the pharyngeal mucosa (Fig. IIE-8). These changes usually commence after delivery of 2000 to 3000 cGy, with edema and soft tissue thickening reaching a maximum at 2 to 5 weeks after termination of RT (16,18,22). Mucosal enhancement and thickening of the posterior pharyngeal wall were observed in more than half of the 61 patients in the series of Mukherji et al. (15) and resolved in 69% and 56%, respectively (15). Patients treated to a high dose or retreated may be prone to develop pharyngeal mucosal ulceration, which otherwise is unusual (Fig. IIE-9). Lymphedema in the retropharyngeal space has been reported in 50% of patients with neck RT for squamous cell cancer, with resolution in one-third (Fig. IIE-10) (15). This finding is thought to be secondary to obstruction of lymphatic channels in the neck by the effects of radiation and has also been reported in jugular vein thrombosis, ligation, or compression (23).

Mucosal and submucosal reaction to RT is also seen in the structures of the larynx. When feasible, treatment of laryngeal cancers with RT allows the patient to retain a functioning larynx, whereas surgical cure would require partial or total laryngectomy. Radiation of the larynx results in thickening of the supra- and infrahyoid epiglottis (Fig. IIE-2) (15,16,18,24,25). In the series by Mukherji et al. (15), this was detected on CT in 63% by 3 months after completion of RT. All patients will also have sym-

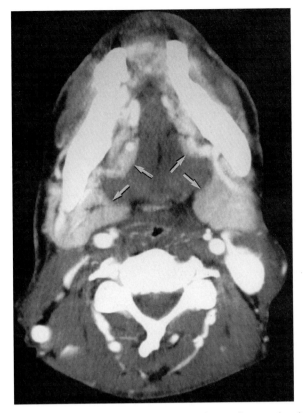

FIG. IIE-5. Postradiation change in the salivary glands. There is dense enhancement of submandibular and sublingual salivary tissue (*arrows*) on this postcontrast CT.

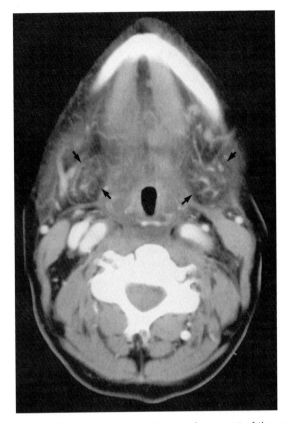

FIG. IIE-6. Radiation-induced fatty replacement of the submandibular glands. Note the similar density of the submandibular glands (*arrows*) to subcutaneous fat in this patient who had RT for laryngeal cancer 7 years earlier.

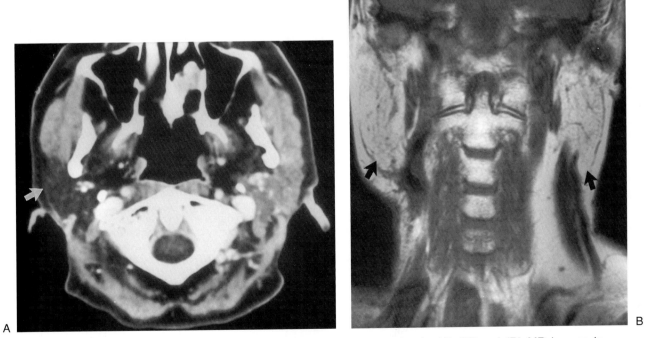

A

B

FIG. IIE-7. Radiation-induced fatty change in the parotid glands: (**A**) CT and (**B**) MR images in different patients showing chronic postradiation fatty replacement in parotid tissue (*arrows*).

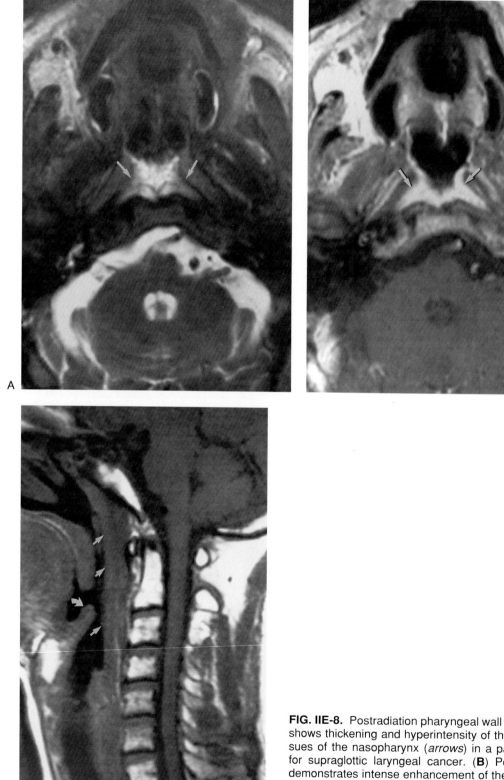

A

B

C

FIG. IIE-8. Postradiation pharyngeal wall thickening. (**A**) T$_2$-weighted MR shows thickening and hyperintensity of the mucosal and submucosal tissues of the nasopharynx (*arrows*) in a patient irradiated 3 years earlier for supraglottic laryngeal cancer. (**B**) Postcontrast T$_1$-weighted image demonstrates intense enhancement of the same regions. (**C**) Sagittal T$_1$-weighted image in a different patient shows postradiation thickening of the posterior pharyngeal wall (*straight arrows*) and of the epiglottis (*curved arrow*).

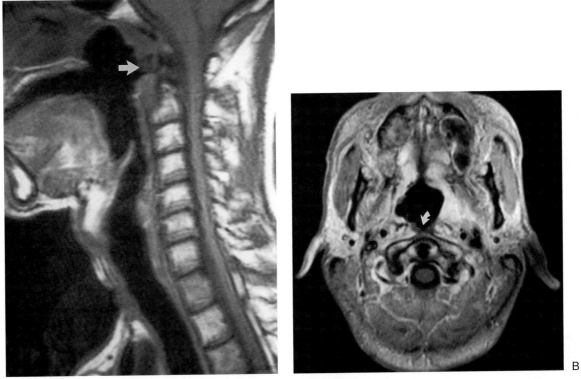

A   B

FIG. IIE-9. Nasopharyngeal ulceration. (**A**) Sagittal precontrast and (**B**) axial postcontrast T_1-weighted MR images show an ulceration in the posterior nasopharyngeal wall (*arrows*). This patient was treated over several years for nasopharyngeal carcinoma with external beam and interstitial RT and surgical resection. The ulcer was probably produced by a palatal obturator contacting the friable nasopharyngeal mucosa. Biopsies showed no tumor.

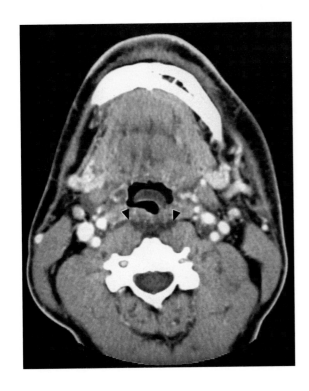

FIG. IIE-10. Retropharyngeal space edema. Postcontrast CT shows abnormal hypodensity anterior to the prevertebral space (*arrowheads*) after RT for nasopharyngeal cancer. Enlargement of the epiglottis and platysma muscle is also seen, along with salivary gland enhancement.

metric thickening of the aryepiglottic folds and false vocal cords (Fig. IIE-11). Increased attenuation of fat in the paralaryngeal and preepiglottic spaces is also frequently seen. In the majority of patients, these postradiation changes in the supraglottic larynx do not resolve (15), and there may be diffuse subclinical lymphedema in the supraglottic larynx for years (13,22). Persistant severe laryngeal mucosal edema may occur several months after RT (Fig. IIE-12) and may indicate recurrent tumor or laryngeal necrosis.

An early postradiation change that may be seen in the glottis is increased attenuation of the limited paraglottic fat. In Mukherji's series (15), this was seen in 50% of patients within 2 months of RT and resolved in 71%. As a rule, mild swelling is seen at the level of the true vocal cords, in contrast to the changes described above for the supraglottic laryngeal structures. Late changes at the glottic level in a minority of patients may include thickening of the anterior and posterior commissures, which tends not to resolve (Fig. IIE-13) (15). Atrophy of the thyroarytenoid muscle may also be seen as a late finding (22). Symmetric subglottic mucosal thickening will be seen in about 80% of patients and resolve in approximately half of these (Fig. IIE-14) (15,22).

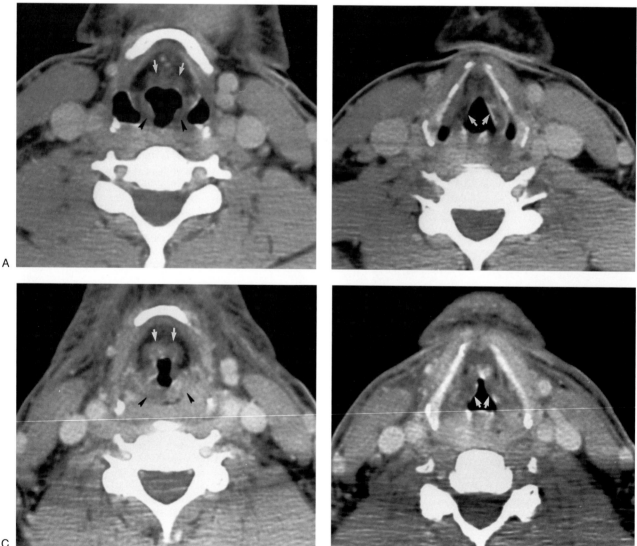

FIG. IIE-11. Postradiation supraglottic edema. Preradiation scans at the level of the infrahyoid epiglottis (**A**) and false vocal cords (**B**). Postradiation scan (**C**) at same level as **A** shows thickening of epiglottis (*arrows*) and aryepiglottic folds (*arrowheads*) and stranding and increased density of the subcutaneous and preepiglottic fat. (**D**) Image at same level as **B** shows thickening of false vocal cords (*arrows*) and increased density of paraglottic fat.

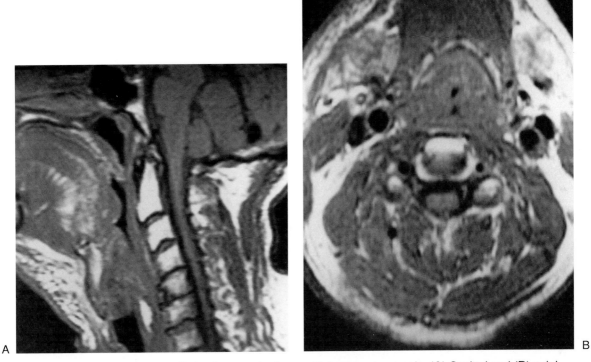

FIG. IIE-12. Severe postradiation laryngeal edema with laryngeal necrosis. **(A)** Sagittal and **(B)** axial T₁-weighted MR images several months after RT for supraglottic cancer show severe edematous changes within the larynx. Biopsies were negative for tumor.

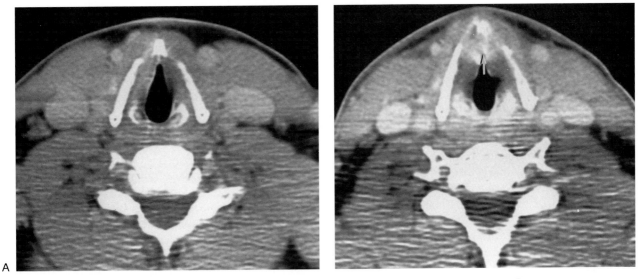

FIG. IIE-13. Postradiation effects at the glottic level. **(A)** Axial pretreatment CT. **(B)** Posttreatment image shows thickening of the true vocal cords and anterior commissure (*arrow*).

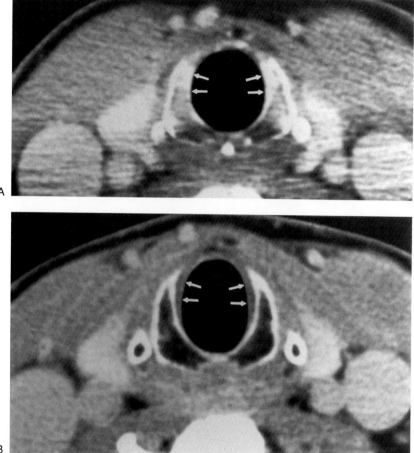

FIG. IIE-14. Postradiation effects at the subglottic level. (**A**) Pretreatment CT shows the normal negligible mucosa (*arrows*) in the subglottic larynx. (**B**) Scan 2.5 months after RT reveals symmetric, bilateral mucosal thickening (*arrows*). (From Mukherji et al., ref. 15, with permission.)

The laryngeal cartilages are relatively unresponsive to the acute effects of RT because of their hypocellularity (26). Thickening and fibrosis of the perichondrium occurs by 8 months following treatment (17). Vascular damage within the perichondrium by radiation results in perichondritis or chondritis, which may lead to chondronecrosis (26). The irradiated larynx is more susceptible to infection because of breakdown of the laryngeal mucosa, and even a mild viral laryngitis may cause a severe perichondritis (26,27). Infection, combined with poor vascularization from RT, can lead to chondronecrosis (18,26). Previous surgery or tumor invasion into cartilage also predisposes to persistent edema and chondronecrosis in the irradiated larynx (22,26). The soft tissue changes associated with chondronecrosis mimic laryngeal tumor both clinically and on imaging studies. Biopsy of the irradiated larynx for documentation of recurrent tumor should not be lightly entertained, as it further compromises the laryngeal cartilages by possibly introducing bacterial infection and causing or aggravating chondronecrosis. Often, many biopsies are required to detect recurrent tumor, which tends to occur in multiple tiny nests (26,28).

The epiglottic cartilage is the laryngeal cartilage most frequently affected by chondronecrosis. It often heals well without significant functional impairment (29,30). The arytenoid cartilages are the second most frequently involved by this form of radiation injury (18,29). Typically, there is a great deal of associated soft tissue swelling, which may extend into the true vocal cords and paralaryngeal spaces. There may be sclerosis of cartilages, and, in advanced cases, cartilage fragmentation and destruction will be seen (Fig. IIE-15) (18). The necrotic cartilage may slough, leaving defects and possibly causing aspiration pneumonia (22,29). When the thyroid cartilage is affected, CT may demonstrate inward bowing or infracturing of one or both thyroid laminae near the midline, with associated soft tissue swelling (Fig. IIE-16). This may progress to laryngeal collapse and narrowing of the airway, with a laryngectomy required in advanced cases despite the absence of persistent or recurrent tumor (18,22). Changes in laryngeal cartilage mineralization on follow-up CT may offer important information. Progressive sclerosis of a cartilage may indicate tumor recurrence with cartilage invasion or chondronecrosis, whereas resolution of pretreatment cartilage sclerosis is indicative of successful control (Fig. IIE-17) (15,31).

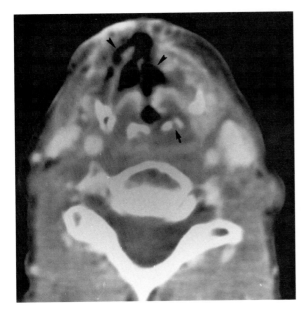

FIG. IIE-15. Postradiation laryngeal chondronecrosis. Axial CT demonstrates bilateral edema in the true vocal cords and postcricoid area with airway narrowing. There is destruction of the anterior thyroid cartilage with extraluminal and extralaryngeal gas (*arrowheads*) and early destruction of the left arytenoid cartilage (*arrow*).

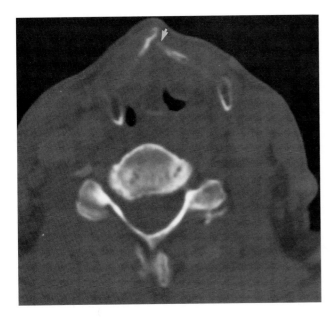

FIG. IIE-16. Postradiation laryngeal chondronecrosis. Axial CT shows sclerotic reaction in the anterior thyroid cartilage bilaterally and a fracture with inward displacement of the left lamina (*arrow*). Note the severe supraglottic edema and narrowed airway. (Case courtesy of Ya-Yen Lee, M.D., Houston, TX.)

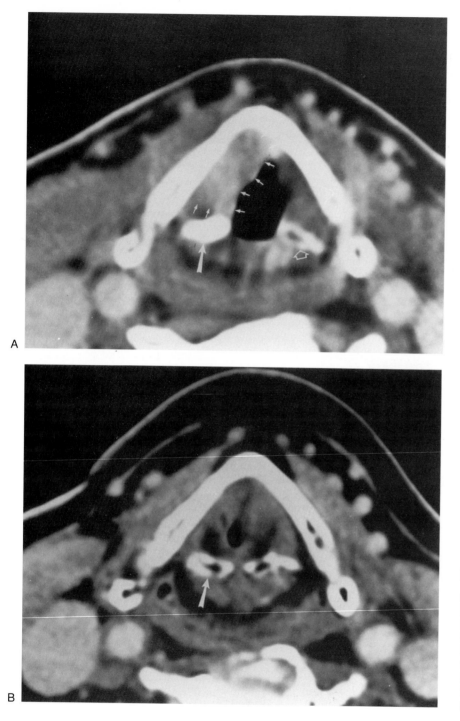

FIG. IIE-17. Favorable change in laryngeal cartilage. (**A**) Pretreatment CT of a T2 right glottic tumor (*small arrows*) also shows sclerosis of the arytenoid cartilage on that side (*large solid arrow*). Note normal appearance of the left arytenoid (*open arrow*). (**B**) Scan 20 months after RT demonstrates reduction of sclerosis of the right arytenoid (*arrow*) and successful treatment of the vocal cord tumor. (From Mukherji et al., ref. 15, with permission.)

Arteries

Injury to the carotid artery within the field of radiation for head and neck cancer is uncommon. Its precise incidence is not known, as stenosis or occlusion of the carotid may be clinically silent if there are good collaterals, and naturally occurring atherosclerotic arterial narrowing is a common occurence in this age group of patients (21). Radiation-induced arterial stenoses are often atypical in location and are characterized by intimal thickening, atheroma, fragmented internal elastic membrane, fibrosis of the media and adventitia, and thrombosis (16,21,32). The radiation dose can be quite variable, and the appearance of symptoms is usually after one or many years from treatment (33). Contributing factors may include diabetes, hypertension, hyperlipidemia, and smoking. Treatment includes carotid endarterectomy and arterial bypass, and surgery is more technically difficult in these patients because of the prior RT (21). A rare, acute form of injury is also known, occurring weeks to months after RT, that results in arterial rupture (33). Carotid thrombosis has been reported in three young adults within months of treatment and in the absence of atherosclerosis (34). Signs and symptoms of cerebral ischemic disease in patients with head and neck radiation should be promptly investigated.

Brachial Plexus

Radiation therapy injury to the brachial plexus is seen much more often after treatment of breast cancer than malignancies of the head and neck and has been correlated with fractions of 300 cGy or larger (21,35). Symptoms may include paresthesia, hypesthesia, and hand weakness and are seen several months to 2 years after treatment (21). In one series, the mean time for presentation was 43 months (35). This injury is characterized by supraclavicular and axillary fibrosis affecting the brachial plexus, especially in patients who have received a high dose or multiple courses of RT (Fig. IIE-18) (16,21,35). On microscopic examination, endarteritis and thickening of the epi- and endoneurium have been observed (35).

Spinal Cord and Brain

Permanent injury to the spinal cord following RT to the neck is, fortunately, rare. With conventional fractions of 180 to 200 cGy/day and five treatments per week to a total dose of 5000 cGy, the risk of cord injury is probably zero if only a short segment of the cord is radiated (21). A conservative estimate of radiation myelopathy occurring after 6000 cGy over 7 weeks is less than 5% (21). Fractions larger than 200 cGy and greater lengths of the spinal cord within the portal correlate with a greater chance for injury. Most centers exclude the cervical cord from the radiation portal after a dose of 4500 cGy is reached and treat the posterior neck with electrons if there are palpable nodes or rely on surgical neck dissection.

Signs and symptoms of radiation myelopathy usually occur within 6 months to 2 years after RT, commonly beginning with paresthesias and numbness. Eventually, paraplegia or quadriplegia and bowel and bladder dysfunction may occur. The deficits are usually permanent, as there is no effective therapy, although steroids may give some improvement in symptoms. Radiation myelopathy is a diagnosis of exclusion, and other entites, particularly recurrent or metastatic tumor, should be ruled out.

Before the era of MR imaging, myelography was performed. Results would usually be normal, but sometimes an atrophic or enlarged cord was demonstrated (36). Magnetic resonance imaging has since shown T_1 and T_2 signal prolongation and areas of focal intramedullary enhancement in patients with radiation myelopathy (36–38). Edematous enlargement of the cervical cord, frequently with focal enhancement at C2, has been seen in several cases imaged within 8 months from onset of symptoms after RT for nasopharyngeal carcinoma (37,38). When scans were obtained beyond 8 months from onset of symptoms, cord atrophy was seen (37,38). The injury is predominantly to the white matter, and the pathologic correlate is demyelination, vacuolization, gliosis, and edema for short-latency lesions and predominant vascular, as well as white matter, damage for long-latency lesions (37).

The temporal lobes may be injured by RT for nasopharyngeal carcinoma (21,39,40). This result is usually seen when more than one course of radiation is given or large fractions are used, which is often necessary for control of carcinoma in this region (21,40). Small volumes of radiated brain appear to tolerate 6000 to 6500 cGy, and 5500 cGy in 30 fractions over 6 weeks is generally felt to be the maximum safe dose for radiating the entire brain (21). Sites of injury and necrosis in the brain are principally in the white matter, as with spinal cord injury. Histologically, there are interstitial fibrinous exudate, fibrinoid vascular necrosis, demyelination, and multiple coalescing foci of white matter necrosis (41).

The imaging findings of late delayed RT injury (occurring several months to many years after RT) have been described as diffuse and focal white matter lesions, and the two may occur together (42). The more common diffuse form produces areas of increased T_2-weighted MR signal intensity in the periventricular white matter, which may become extensive and reach the subcortical white matter, but generally there is no focal mass effect. When these imaging findings are mild in degree, the patients are usually asymptomatic; severe changes are often associated with cognitive impairment. When the temporal lobes are the sites of injury after treatment of nasopharyngeal cancer, temporal lobe seizures,

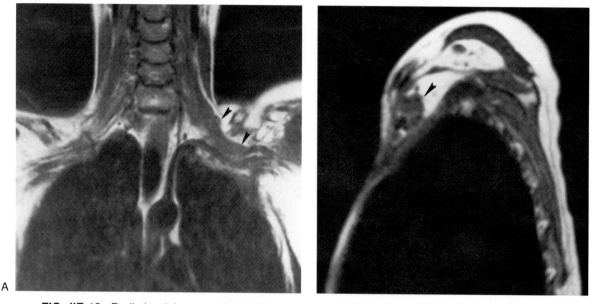

FIG. IIE-18. Radiation injury to the brachial plexus. (**A**) Coronal and (**B**) sagittal T$_1$-weighted MR show thickening of the left brachial plexus (*arrowheads*). The patient was treated for breast cancer with external beam RT and later with brachytherapy for a chest wall recurrence. Biopsies in the supraclavicular region showed no tumor.

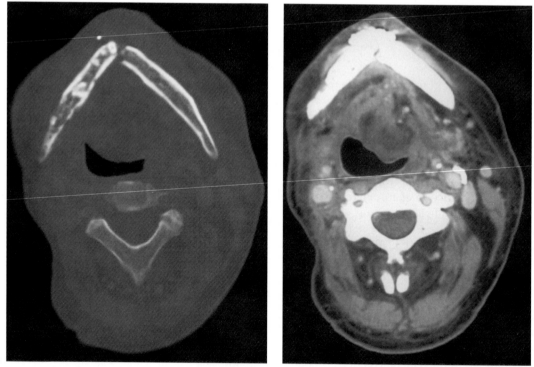

FIG. IIE-19. Radiation osteitis of the mandible. The patient failed RT with 66 Gy for carcinoma of the right tonsil and tongue base. Afterward, resection was done via anterior mandibulotomy (with non-union). (**A**) A CT with bone window setting 2 years after RT shows cortical thinning and abnormal lucency and trabecular pattern in the right posterior mandibular body. (**B**) Soft tissue window shows myocutaneous graft in the right oral cavity and submandibular region and radical neck dissection.

impaired memory, personality change, and nonspecific signs of increased intracranial pressure have been reported (40). Focal radiation necrosis on imaging studies is seen as an area of parenchymal enhancement, often ring enhancing, with surrounding edema and sometimes with associated hemorrhage or calcification (42). Mass effect and focal neurologic deficits are associated with these lesions. The diagnosis is more obvious when the primary radiated tumor was extracranial rather than intracranial in the area of new abnormality.

Bone

Radiation osteitis, or osteoradionecrosis, is an inflammatory reaction in the bone marrow, with death of blood-forming cells as well as osteoblasts and osteoclasts (43). Endarteritis also occurs in the periostium and bone. Radiographs are initially normal. At about 1 year after RT, osteoporosis is seen as the areas of dead bone and necrotic tissue are replaced by ingrowth of cells from adjacent nonischemic bone. Focal areas of lucency appear in the cortex and medullary bone. New bone is gradually laid down on unresorbed trabeculae, creating areas of coarse

trabeculae with sclerosis, seen many years after RT. Irradiated bone is more susceptible to fracture and infection. Fractures and severe cases of radiation osteitis were seen more frequently in survivors of orthovoltage therapy, which delivered nearly twice the soft tissue dose to bone (43). Current megavoltage therapy delivers approximately equal doses to soft tissue and bone. The fractures are most often seen in weight-bearing bones or ones with strong muscle pull (43). They are often spontaneous and slow healing, and nonunion is common.

In the head and neck, the mandible is the most common bone to be injured by RT (Fig. IIE-19). Generally, this is seen with doses over 5000 cGy, and interstitial radiation carries a greater risk of bone necrosis (21). Removal of carious teeth prior to RT decreases the likelihood of this complication. About 95% of mandibular radiation osteitis begins with mucosal necrosis and ulceration (21). The radiated mucosa of the oral cavity becomes thin with telangiectatic vessels and is more susceptible to the effects of alcohol and tobacco and trauma from eating and wearing dentures and prostheses. Many mucosal ulcerations heal completely without bone involvement, and up to 90% of bone necroses will heal with conservative therapy (21). Because bone exposed to oral cavity contents is likely

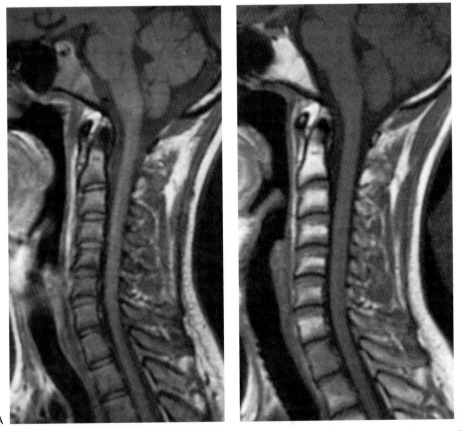

A   B

FIG. IIE-20. Effect of RT on bone marrow. **(A)** Sagittal MR prior to RT for a small invasive nasopharyngeal carcinoma in a 16-year-old patient. **(B)** An MR 1.5 years posttreatment shows the change from red to fatty marrow in the clivus and cervical spine.

to become infected, antibiotics are administered. Bony sequestra may be spontaneously extruded. Hyperbaric oxygen therapy is often helpful for larger areas of disease, and surgical resection is required for advanced cases.

Radiation therapy produces fatty replacement of bone marrow, which is now a well-known finding on MR imaging. High signal intensity is seen in the bone marrow within the radiation portal on T_1-weighted scans in all patients receiving therapeutic doses (Fig. IIE-20). This signal change may be seen as early as after 1600 cGy and is believed to be irreversible (16,43).

Radiation-Induced Neoplasia

Postirradiation sarcoma (PIS) is an unfortunate complication in long-term survivors of cancer treatment. As with radiation osteitis, PIS is more frequently seen in patients with prior orthovoltage treatment. Other risk factors for developing PIS include a young age at treatment, high doses, and multiple treatments over months to years (Fig. IIE-21) (21). Radiation of abnormal bone (fibrous dysplasia and Paget disease) is also associated with an increased risk of sarcoma induction. The incidence of PIS is approximately 0.1% to 0.2% in 5-year cancer survivors and represents 1% to 5% of all sarcomas in various institutions (21,43,44). The mean latency period is 10 years or longer. Osteosarcoma (skeletal and extraosseous), malignant fibrous histiocytoma, and fibrosarcoma predominate in most series, with different percentages reported for osseous and extraosseous sarcomas (43–46). Postirradiation sarcoma most frequently affects bones of the shoulder and pelvic regions, reflecting the large numbers of patients with breast cancer, gynecologic malignancies, and Hodgkin disease treated with RT with long survival (44–46). Female patients are thereby predominantly affected. These sarcomas are usually high grade, large when diagnosed, and difficult to treat. For osteosarcoma of bone, adjacent changes of radiation osteitis may be seen (44). The PIS usually arises at the edge of the treated field, where the radiation dose was high enough to induce mutations but not to cause cell death (46). Computed tomography greatly facilitates the diagnosis, compared to conventional radiographs. A soft tissue mass adjacent to an area of bone destruction is commonly seen, and bone expansion and tumor matrix mineralization may be noted (46).

The occurrence of thyroid carcinoma years after radiation of the neck in childhood is well known (47,48). It is associated with small doses of radiation (under 2000 cGy) that are not lethal to follicular tissue of the thyroid gland (Fig. IIE-21) (21). In the past, such radiation was given for enlarged tonsillar tissue in Waldeyer's ring and for an enlarged thymus and cervical lymph nodes. Well-differentiated papillary and mixed papillary and follicular carcinoma are the most common malignancies associated with RT (48). Benign adenomatous thyroid nodules are also associated with low-dose RT to the thyroid and occur more frequently than carcinoma (48).

IMAGING OF POSTSURGICAL CHANGES

A variety of anatomic alterations may be encountered on imaging studies of patients who have had surgical therapy for head and neck cancer. These findings may relate to the pharynx, larynx, neck, or a combination thereof. Surgical changes are rarely encountered in the nasopharynx, as radiation therapy is the treatment of choice for nasopharyngeal carcinoma. Elsewhere, surgical defects, absence of normal structures, and loss of expected tissue planes may be seen, possibly along with reconstruction of tissue defects with regional myocutaneous or free tissue flaps.

Laryngectomies

There are several surgical approaches for laryngeal carcinoma, the choice of which depends on the location and extent of the primary lesion, presence of nodal metastases, and the preference of the otolaryngologist. A description of the basic types of laryngectomies is given below, but there are several variations on these operations that are beyond the scope of this text.

Vertical hemilaryngectomy is a form of voice conservation surgery for T1 and T2 true vocal cord carcinomas. It is not suitable for patients who have false vocal cord involvement, a fixed cord, or cartilage invasion. Tumors with sufficient extension into the subglottic larynx to imply involvement of the anterior or posterior cricoid cartilage are usually not candidates for this operation, although some surgeons perform limited cricoid resection as part of an extended vertical hemilaryngectomy (49). The true and false cords and intervening laryngeal ventricle are removed, along with the ipsilateral thyroid cartilage ala (49,50). Up to one-third of the opposite true cord and all of the arytenoid and a small portion of the cricoid cartilage can be removed if necessary (51). The perichondrium of the thyroid cartilage or the aryepiglottic fold or omohyoid or sternohyoid muscles may be used to construct a pseudocord on the operated side (51). DiSantis et al. (51) reviewed CT scans in 22 patients who had vertical hemilaryngectomy and found that the larynx is characteristically tilted toward the operated side (Fig. IIE-22). The thyroid ala may regenerate in a patchy fashion, mimicking tumor with cartilage destruction. They also found that the pseudocord had a straight or concave border at the level of the glottis in the absence of recurrent tumor but was normally convex at the supraglottic level. The residual true cord on the opposite side was often partially convex, particularly in its anterior portion. Recurrent laryngeal cancer increased the width of the residual true vocal cord and produced a convex contour of the pseudocord at the glottic level (51).

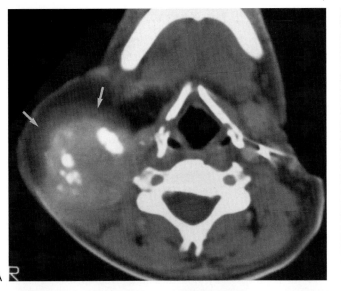

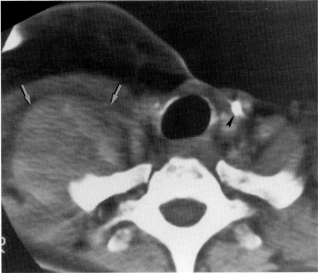

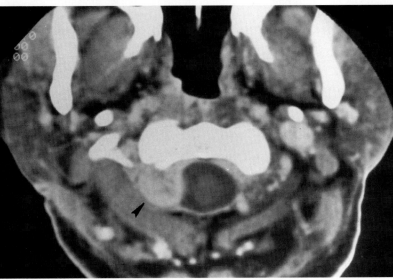

FIG. IIE-21. Recurrent radiation-induced osteosarcoma. This 39-year-old patient was radiated at the age of 1 year for enlarged tonsils. At age 12 years, he developed papillary carcinoma of the thyroid and received 44 Gy after thyroidectomy. Extraskeletal osteosarcoma developed in the lower right neck at age 35. This was resected, and a trapezius flap was placed. Four years later the sarcoma recurred under the flap. (**A** and **B**) Large mass with calcifications (*arrows*) in the right lateral neck under the trapezius flap. Note thyroidectomy and clip in the left neck (*arrowhead*). (**C**) Same patient, probable radiation-induced schwannoma or meningioma on the right at C2 (*arrowhead*). (Case courtesy of Ya-Yen Lee, M.D., Houston, TX.)

Supraglottic laryngectomy is performed for low-volume tumors arising in the supraglottic larynx. Primary sites that may be suitable for treatment with this form of partial laryngectomy include the epiglottis, aryepiglottic fold, and false vocal cord. This procedure involves bilateral resection of endolaryngeal structures above the laryngeal ventricle, including the aryepiglottic folds, false vocal cords, epiglottis, and preepiglottic fat. There is also excision of the thyroid cartilage ipsilateral to the tumor. The hyoid bone may need to be resected for those tumors that invade the preepiglottic space (52). Imaging studies at the level of the glottis usually appear normal unless one of the arytenoid cartilages has been partially resected (25). Above the glottis, absence of the thyroid cartilage is evident, and the soft tissues around the airway may have a slightly irregular appearance (25). For small tumors of the suprahyoid epiglottis, a modified supraglottic laryngectomy may be done, in which not all of the supraglottic

structures mentioned above are resected (Fig. IIE-23). Aspiration is expected for a time after supraglottic laryngectomy, and if a contrast swallow examination is required, barium is used instead of gastrografin.

Total laryngectomy is the surgical procedure of choice for treating advanced laryngeal cancers and is performed for glottic tumors that cause vocal cord fixation, invade the laryngeal cartilages, involve the interarytenoid region, extend subglottically more than the limits for conservation surgery, or have extension outside of the larynx. Total laryngectomy is preferred over hemilaryngectomy for transglottic lesions, even small ones, that have crossed the ventricle to involve the false cord and thereby have greater access to the paraglottic space and lymphatics (49). Total laryngectomy is also used as a salvage operation for patients who fail partial laryngectomy or radiation therapy, with residual or recurrent tumor, and for patients who have severe posttreatment complications in the lar-

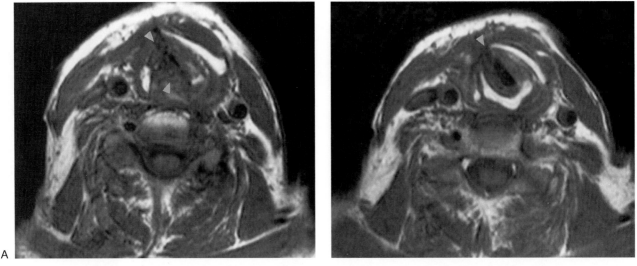

FIG. IIE-22. Vertical hemilaryngectomy. Resection of right-sided endolaryngeal structures was done elsewhere 15 years earlier, with an unknown type of repair. A new tumor at the anterior commissure was treated with RT 9 months earlier. (**A** and **B**) T$_1$-weighted axial images show partial resection of the right side of the thyroid cartilage and absence of the arytenoid cartilage (*arrowheads*). There is tilting of the larynx to the right.

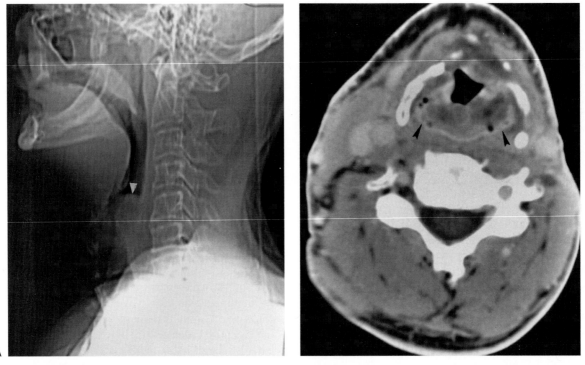

FIG. IIE-23. Modified supraglottic laryngectomy. (**A**) Lateral scout view from CT shows absence of the epiglottis and postradiation swelling of residual aryepiglottic folds and arytenoid mucosa (*arrowhead*). (**B**) Axial CT image also shows mucosol swelling (*arrowheads*) and demonstrates resection of the anterior thyroid cartilage. There was no recurrent tumor. (Case courtesy of Ya-Yen Lee, M.D., Houston, TX.)

ynx, such as cartilage necrosis associated with infection, airway obstruction, or aspiration. This procedure entails complete resection of all endolaryngeal structures including the epiglottis, aryepiglottic folds, true and false vocal cords, and subglottis. There is also removal of the hyoid bone and thyroid, cricoid, and arytenoid cartilages. The pyriform sinuses are also resected. The postoperative defect in the anterior hypopharynx is closed and sutured to the tongue base, forming a new passageway for food and liquids called the neopharynx (53). Typically, there is appreciable enhancement of the neopharynx on postcontrast CT and MR imaging, which should not be confused with recurrent tumor. On postoperative imaging studies, the neopharynx and cervical esophagus have an anterior location just deep to the subcutaneous fat of the neck (Fig. IIE-24) (54). When the pharyngoesophagus contains air, it may be mistaken for the trachea; however, the actual trachea and trachesotomy will be seen in the lower anterior neck. One lobe of the thyroid gland is often removed at the time of total laryngectomy and neck dissection. The remaining lobe is often somewhat anteriorly displaced from its normal location (Fig. IIE-25). This asymmetry may be confusing, and the thyroid may be mistaken for a vascular structure, as it is intensely enhancing.

Tumor recurrence after total laryngectomy is seen at the tracheostoma in about 5% of cases (Fig. IIE-26). A stomal recurrence is associated with tumors larger than 2 cm, a transglottic tumor with subglottic extension, large tumors requiring emergency tracheostomy, and tumors with vascular or perineural invasion and positive surgical margins (55). The cause may be metastatic tumor to paratracheal and pretracheal nodes, tumor implantation of the tracheostomy wound, or incomplete resection of the primary tumor. Less commonly, recurrence may be found at the site of the proximal anastomosis. Disease may also recur in the cervical lymph nodes.

Speech rehabilitation is an important part of the overall management of the patient with laryngeal cancer undergoing total laryngectomy. This can be achieved with an external artificial larynx, esophageal speech, or with tracheoesophageal phonation. The latter gives a more normal laryngeal quality voice than the other options and is produced by creating a fistula between the trachea and esophagus at the level of the tracheostoma. A small prosthesis is inserted into the fistula, typically a Blom–Singer (duckbill) or Panje device (56,57). These devices contain a valve that opens to the positive airway pressures but closes when air flow stops, preventing digestive tract contents from entering the airway. The inflowing air from the lungs causes vibration of pharyngoesophageal mucosal membranes, which permits speech. The prosthesis itself, or air contained within it, can be imaged on CT or MR (Fig. IIE-27). Complications of the surgically created fistula include aspiration pneumonia, enlargement of the fistula, leakage of saliva and food around the prosthesis, aspiration of the prosthesis itself, and infection (56,57).

Teflon Injection of the Vocal Cord

A surgical mode for treatment of a paralyzed true vocal cord that may have striking radiographic findings is injection of Teflon paste (polytetrafluoroethylene). The Teflon is injected into the paraglottic space at the level of the midportion of the true cord for the purpose of bringing a paramedian nonmobile cord more to a midline position to permit contact with the other cord and vocalization. This procedure is done for nontumoral causes of cord paralysis and sometimes for restoring bulk after vertical hemilaryngectomy. The Teflon is hyperdense on CT (Fig. IIE-28) and causes a granulomatous reaction (25,58).

Pharyngolaryngectomy

This procedure, also known as an extended total laryngectomy, is done for tumors of the hypopharynx not managable by conservation operations (59). A typical tumor requiring this type of resection is a pyriform sinus carcinoma with extension to the paraglottic space and transglottic growth. Tumors in the apex of the pyriform sinus, postcricoid area, and hypopharyngeal lesions associated with cord fixation usually require this type of radical surgery. In cases in which there is adequate pharyngeal mucosa remaining, the pharyngeal defect can be closed primarily. For larger defects, closure is achieved most

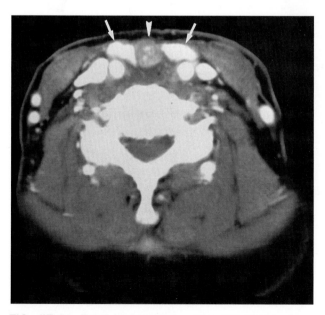

FIG. IIE-24. Total laryngectomy. The CT image shows changes of a total laryngectomy without neck dissection. Note the anterior location of the neopharynx (*arrowhead*). Thyroid gland indicated by *arrows*.

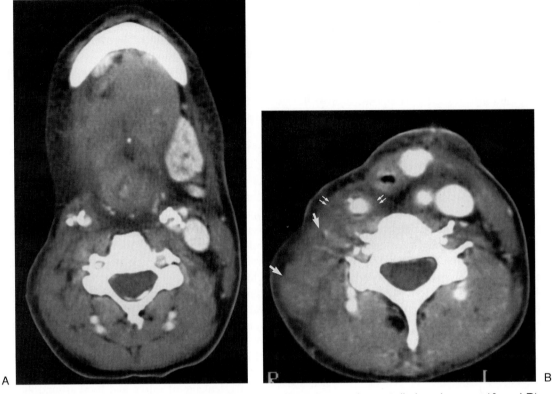

FIG. IIE-25. Total laryngectomy, right radical neck dissection, and postradiation changes. (**A** and **B**) Postcontrast CT. Note the soft tissue defect in the neck and absence of the submandibular gland, sternocleidomastoid muscle, internal jugular vein, and thyroid on the right. The levator scapulae muscle is hypertrophied (*arrows*), and there is scar tissue around the right carotid sheath (*double arrows*).

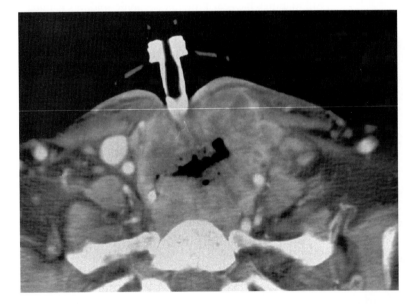

FIG. IIE-26. Recurrent tumor after total laryngectomy. The CT image shows a large heterogeneously enhancing mass lesion around the tracheostoma and esophagus that has ulcerated into the trachea.

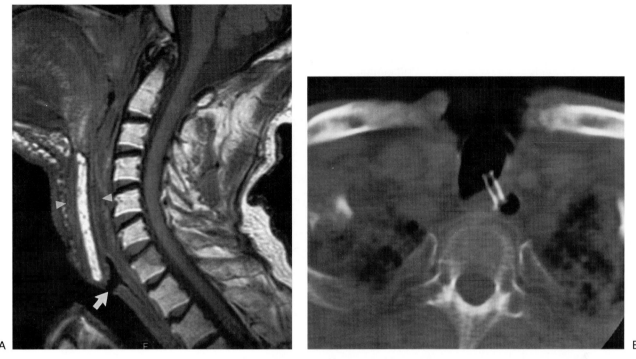

FIG. IIE-27. Tracheoesophageal (TE) prosthesis. **(A)** Sagittal MR image showing surgically created TE fistula for speech rehabilitation (*arrow*). Flap reconstruction of the pharynx is also present (same patient as Fig. IIE-29). **(B)** Axial CT in a different patient shows the Blom−Singer prosthesis itself connecting the trachea and esophagus.

frequently with a pectoralis major myocutaneous flap with a pedicled blood supply (59). Trapezius and latissimus dorsi flaps can also be used. The flap can also provide coverage for the carotid artery if a radical neck dissection is done. The flap is mobilized and tunneled subcutaneously over the clavicle and brought up to the area of the pharyngeal defect. It is then tubed on itself with the skin surface forming the pharyngeal lumen. Both CT and MR images demonstrate this surgical anatomy well, revealing a rounded central soft tissue structure that forms the wall of the pharyngeal lumen, with a variable amount of surrounding adipose tissue (Figs. IIE-29 and IIE-30). The muscular component of the flap usually becomes atrophic because of denervation. Complications of this surgery include development of a stricture at the pharyngeal anastomosis (Fig. IIE-31) and pharyngocutaneous fistulas. An example of tumor recurrence after laryngopharyngectomy is shown in Fig. IIE-32.

Tumors that significantly involve the postcricoid area or cervical esophagus require esophagectomy as well as laryngopharyngectomy if surgical treatment is elected. Reconstruction can be done with a reversed gastric tube, gastric transposition, colonic interposition, or an intestinal microvascular free graft (59). Imaging studies in these patients show larger air-filled lumens in the neck and chest than seen with the normal esophagus, representing the gastric or intestinal structures (Fig. IIE-33).

Oral Cavity and Oropharyngeal Surgical Changes

The anterior two-thirds of the tongue is second only to the lip in frequency of oral cavity squamous cell carcinomas, with most arising on the lateral and ventral borders (60). T1 and T2 stage tumors can usually be managed by partial or hemiglossectomy perorally with primary closure, even with *en bloc* technique resection of normal tissue margins. A portion of the residual tongue may be used to close the defect, or a tissue graft may be placed (Fig. IIE-34) (61). T3 and T4 lesions usually must be approched via a mandibulotomy for adequacy of resection, and a near total or total glossectomy is done. Wound closure is with a split-thickness skin graft or tissue flap (60). Tumors near or superficially extending onto the gingiva require a marginal mandibulectomy, and larger lesions or those with gross or radiographically evident mandibular invasion require segmental mandibulectomy along with removal of the oral cavity tumor and a neck dissection (composite resection) (Fig. IIE-35) (61). A hemimandibulectomy is done when the inferior alveolar canal is involved with perineural extension of tumor (Fig. IIE-36).

Resection of the posterior body or ramus of the mandible produces little deformity but does result in a functional deficit (Fig. IIE-35) (61). Removal of the body or anterior arch produces great deformity and functional compro-

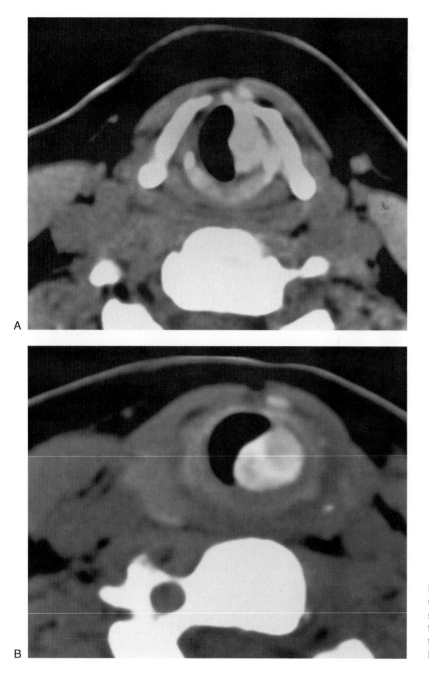

FIG. IIE-28. Teflon injection of vocal cord. The CT images at the levels of the glottis (**A**) and subglottis (**B**) show high-attenuation Teflon material in the left true vocal cord and in the subglottic larynx after treatment of abducted, paralyzed left true vocal cord.

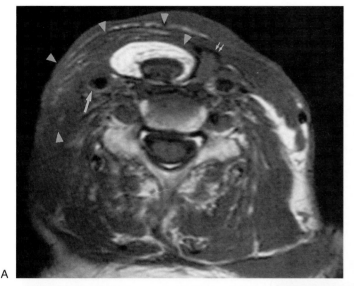

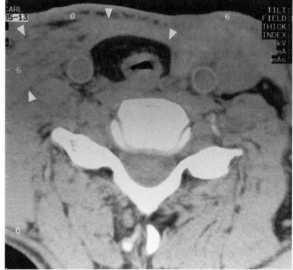

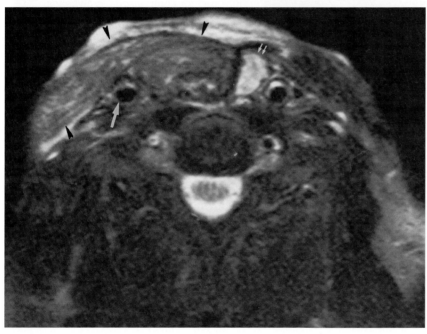

FIG. IIE-29. Pharyngolaryngectomy with myocutaneous flap. (**A**) T$_1$-weighted and (**B**) T$_2$-weighted images showing pectoralis major flap (*arrowheads*) for reconstruction of the hypopharynx after laryngopharyngectomy. The flap contains fat and its bulk in the right neck also protects the carotid artery (*arrow*) following radical neck dissection. Left lobe of thyroid, *double arrows*. (**C**) A CT image for correlation.

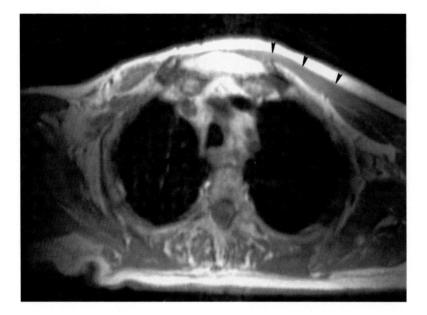

FIG. IIE-30. Pectoralis major muscle donor site. Patient has undergone pharyngolaryngectomy, radical neck dissection, and pectoralis flap reconstruction. Axial T_1-weighted MR at level of upper thorax shows absence of the pectoralis major muscle on the right. Left side included for comparison (*arrowheads*).

mise, and the defect should be reconstructed (61,62). However, immediate reconstruction at the time of mandibulectomy carries a significant risk of failure, especially if alloplastic materials are used (62,63). This is because of entry into the oral cavity and salivary contamination of the graft. Temporary fixation of mandibular fragments with a pin is usually done to prevent muscles from pulling the segments into grossly malaligned positions until a delayed repair can be done. This second surgery, months to years after the oncologic operation, is done via an extraoral approach and results in better success when nonvascularized bone autografts, metallic compression plates, or perforated prosthetic trays filled with autogenous cancellous bone are used. If a vascularized graft is utilized, immediate reconstruction may be done at the time of oncologic surgery, as these grafts are less likely to fail (62). These grafts may be pedicled flaps such as the trapezius/scapular spine osteomyocutaneous flap or microvascular free flaps utilizing iliac crest, rib, scapular spine, or metatarsal bone. These flaps have their own arterial and venous supply, which is anastomosed to vessels in the recipient bed.

Small resection defects in the tongue may not be apparent on imaging studies. Larger resections will demonstrate reduced tongue volume, contour, and position (Fig. IIE-34). If a myocutaneous tissue flap has been used for reconstruction after extensive surgery, fatty composition of the flap may be noted (Fig. IIE-37). Operative defects in the mandible are easily recognizable at imaging, and repair with an osteomyocutaneous graft or alloplastic material will be readily noted. Metallic rods, trays, plates, and screws, whether titanium or stainless steel, will produce artifacts on CT and MR imaging, obscuring visualization of the adjacent soft tissues (Figs. IIE-36 and IIE-38).

Neck Dissections

In patients with squamous cell carcinoma of the upper aerodigestive tract and clinically palpable cervical lymph nodes, the treatment is usually surgical, with the ipsilateral neck dissected in conjunction with removal of the primary tumor. The traditional operation by which all other neck dissections are compared is the radical neck dissection (RND). This procedure entails *en bloc* removal of all the lymph nodes in one side of the neck from the inferior mandible to the clavicle and from the lateral border of the sternohyoid muscle, hyoid bone, and contralateral anterior belly of the digastric muscle to the anterior border of the trapezius muscle (14,64). The nodes that are resected include the submental and submandibular groups (level I), the internal jugular chain (levels II to IV), and the spinal accessory chain (level V). The sternocleidomastoid muscle, spinal accessory nerve, internal jugular vein, and submandibular gland are also removed. This form of lymphadenectomy is performed for cases of obvious multiple nodal metastases, especially when the location is near the spinal accessory nerve (65). Recognition of changes of a RND on postoperative CT or MR imaging studies is straightforward, in that there is an obvious contour deformity of the neck and absence of the sternocleidomastoid muscle and internal jugular vein (Figs. IIE-25 and IIE-39). Atrophy of the trapezius muscle from loss of cranial nerve 11 is usually noted, and there may be compensatory hypertrophy of the levator scapulae muscle (Fig. IIE-39) (14). Comparison with a normal contralateral neck is usually possible, although some patients have undergone bilateral neck dissections, even RNDs, but not usually simultaneously.

The surgical extirpation of disease from RND also re-

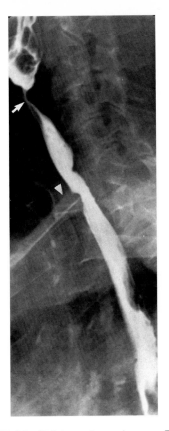

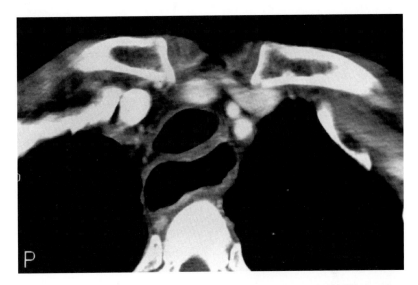

FIG. IIE-31. Stricture of neopharynx. Barium esophagram in a patient with laryngopharyngectomy shows stenosis of lumen near the proximal anastomosis (*arrow*). Blom–Singer speech prosthesis also seen (*arrowhead*), and there is slight leakage or aspiration of barium into the trachea.

FIG. IIE-33. Gastric transposition for esophageal cancer. Axial CT showing a large air density between the tracheal airway and the spine, representing the stomach, which has been relocated into the chest and anastomosed to the cervical esophagus.

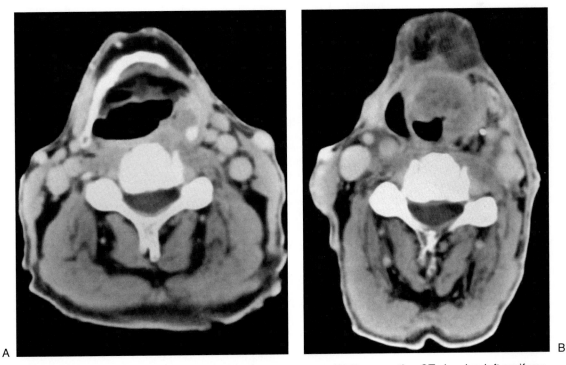

FIG. IIE-32. Recurrent tumor after laryngopharyngectomy. (**A**) Preoperative CT showing left pyriform sinus tumor. (**B**) Postoperative scan reveals large recurrent tumor near the proximal pharyngeal anastomosis.

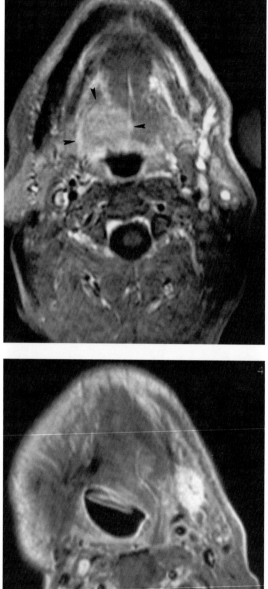

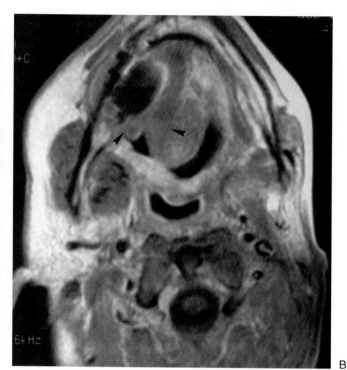

FIG. IIE-34. Partial glossectomy. (**A**) Preoperative T$_1$-weighted MR image demonstrates enhancing tumor in the right tongue base and posterior oral tongue (*arrowheads*). (**B** and **C**) Postoperative MR 16 months later shows changes of partial glossectomy and radical neck dissection. A rectus free flap was placed in the defect in the right tongue (*arrowheads*). No recurrent tumor is seen. There is metal artifact from a surgical clip.

sults in cosmetic deformity and shoulder dysfunction (pain, shoulder drop, and limited abduction because of trapezius muscle atrophy) (66). With this consideration in mind, and with accumulation of knowledge in recent years as to predictable patterns of nodal spread of cancer, many modifications of the standard RND have arisen. These operations are classified as modified radical neck dissection, selective neck dissection, and extended radical neck dissection (64). In a modified radical neck dissec-

tion, there is resection of the cervical nodes removed in the RND (levels I to V), but with preservation of one or more of the following structures: sternocleidomastoid muscle, spinal accessory nerve, or jugular vein. The decision as to which structures to preserve is based on the extent and location of the involved lymph nodes. In the past, the terms functional and conservation neck dissection have also been used to describe this procedure. However, the term modified radical neck dissection has been

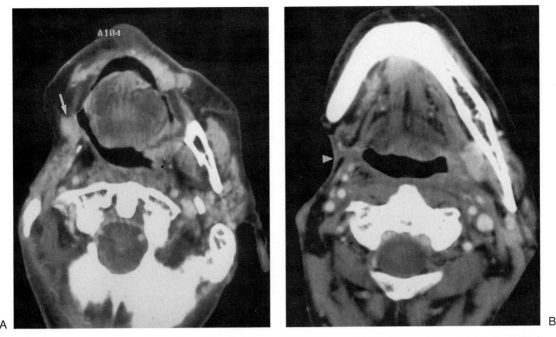

FIG. IIE-35. Composite resection with partial mandibulectomy. Surgical resection of the ramus and posterior body of the mandible for retromandibular trigone cancer. (**A**) Note absence of these segments of the right mandible, soft tissue defect externally, and surgical changes in the right tonsillar pillar. *Arrow* indicates residual masseter muscle. (**B**) Nonenhancing soft tissue compatible with scar (*arrowhead*).

proposed as the most appropriate and specific terminology and is recommended for uniform nomenclature (64). Radiographically, one can determine this type of neck dissection by the structures that are resected and preserved (Fig. IIE-40) (65), but at times the surgical changes are subtle. A CT evaluation for tumor in the postoperative neck may be difficult after a modified radical and some selective (see below) neck dissections. This is because the sternocleidomastoid muscle lies against the paraspinous muscles with the carotid artery and internal jugular vein in between, without intervening fat to provide helpful tissue contrast (10). In this context, MR imaging may be better than CT because of improved contrast between adjacent tissues of different origin.

A selective neck dissection entails resection of only the positive lymph nodes and those at highest risk of containing metastases based on the location of the primary tumor, preserving other nodal groups normally removed with RND. The sterocleidomastoid muscle, spinal accessory nerve, and internal jugular vein are also perserved. A variety of different procedures are included under the category of selective neck dissections. They include anterolateral, lateral, and posterolateral neck dissections. For the anterolateral, or supraomohyoid, neck dissection, nodes in levels I to III are removed, with preservation of level IV and V nodes (Fig. IIE-41). The lateral neck dissection entails resection of level II to IV nodes, sparing levels I and V. The posterolateral dissection removes nodes in levels II to V. When there are deviations from

these standardized selective neck dissections, with resection of additional nodal levels, the specific procedure should be described by the surgeon.

The extended radical neck dissection entails removal of one or more additional nodal groups and/or nonnodal structures not resected in the classical RND (14,64). Such structures include retropharyngeal, superior mediastinal, and paratracheal lymph nodes, the carotid artery, hypoglossal nerve, vagus nerve, and paraspinal muscles (Fig. IIE-42) (64). Removal of the retropharyngeal lymph nodes may be performed when the primary tumor arises from the pharyngeal wall or there is secondary involvement of the pharyngeal wall from an adjacent tumor. Resection of the pretracheal and paratracheal nodes may be performed for transglottic, subglottic, esophageal, and thyroid carcinomas. The carotid artery may be resected in patients in whom the tumor is fixed to the artery, although the long-term benefits of this procedure are not clear (65). Preoperative arteriography and balloon test occlusion are typically done when this operative strategy is anticipated.

Thyroid Gland Resection

Thyroidectomy is performed for malignant disease of the gland after a preoperative work-up, which may include fine-needle aspiration (FNA), ultrasonography, and radionuclide scans. Lobectomy is generally

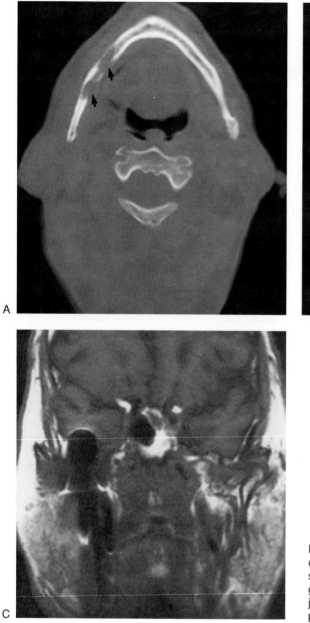

A

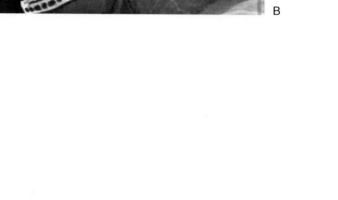

B

C

FIG. IIE-36. Hemimandibulectomy. (**A**) Widening of the inferior alveolar canal and bone destruction (*arrows*) in a patient with recurrent squamous cell carcinoma of the lip. (**B**) Postoperative lateral radiograph showing titanium prosthesis in place with temporomandibular joint articulation. (**C**) Coronal T$_1$-weighted MR showing artifact from prosthesis.

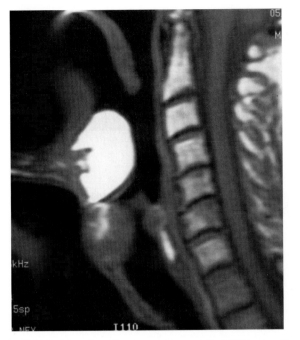

FIG. IIE-37. Free flap. Postoperative sagittal MR in a patient with resection of tongue base tumor and rectus abdominis graft, which contains a large fatty component.

done for a solitary well-differentiated papillary carcinoma. Unilateral surgery may also be done for lymphoma with limited extent of disease, for thyroid nodules that are benign on FNA and cold on the technetium-99m scan but remain stable or enlarge during thyroid suppression, and for cystic lesions that re-form after two aspirations (67). Complete removal of the gland is indicated for well-differentiated cancer under the following circumstances: a high-grade follicular cancer; papillary cancer with a history of neck RT (because of multicentric disease); multicentric disease in one lobe, bilateral disease, and lesions larger than 1.5 cm; tumors with regional or distant metastases; and for Hürthle cell carcinoma (67). Total thyroidectomy is also done for medullary carcinoma. A subtotal thyroidectomy may be performed for Graves disease. Complications of thyroid surgery include recurrent laryngeal nerve paralysis and hypoparathyroidism.

Examples of a lobectomy and total thyroidectomy are shown in Fig. IIE-43. The normal thyroid gland is readily identified on CT because of intrinsic beam attenuation as a result of its high iodine content, and the gland also enhances. Absence of this normal paratracheal structure in the lower anterior neck should be noted.

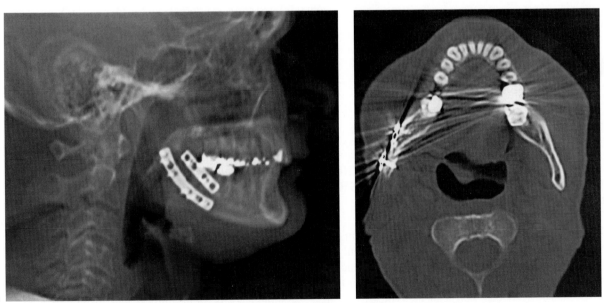

A

B

FIG. IIE-38. Mandibular plating. (**A**) Lateral radiograph and (**B**) axial bone window setting. Two metallic compression plates span a defect at the angle of the mandible after surgery for adenocarcinoma of the tonsil. Streak artifacts are present on the CT image.

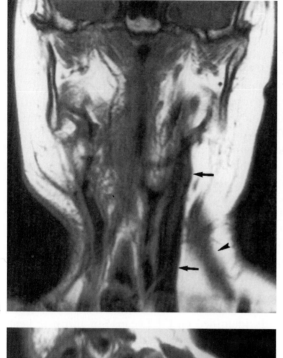

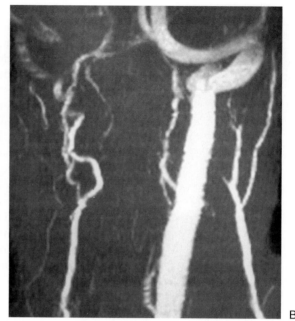

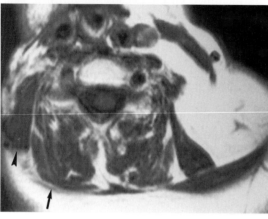

FIG. IIE-39. Radical neck dissection. (**A**) T$_1$-weighted MR shows soft tissue defect in the right neck and absence of the right internal jugular vein (IJV) and sternocleidomastoid (SCM) muscle. Normal structures indicated in left neck (SCM, *arrowhead;* IJV, *arrows*). (**B**) The MR venogram illustrates no flow in the right IJV. (**C**) Axial image demonstrates atrophy of the right trapezius muscle (*arrow*) and slight hypertrophy of the levator scapulae muscle (*arrowhead*) and anterior surgical mobilization of this structure.

DIFFERENTIATION OF RECURRENT TUMOR FROM POSTRADIATION AND POSTSURGICAL CHANGES

Detection of recurrent tumor is the most common indication for imaging the head and neck cancer patient who has been irradiated or operated on. These patients undergo close clinical follow-up during the first 5 years after treatment because squamous cell cancer typically recurs within this time frame, and often by 2 years posttreatment. Tumor may recur at the primary site, in lymph nodes, or at both locations. A new second primary lesion may also arise. Signs suggesting tumor recurrence include local pain, otalgia, trismus, cranial neuropathy, otitis, a new mass, increasing edema, new or worsened hoarseness or dysphagia, and fixation of a previously mobile vocal cord.

With definitive radiation therapy, there is transient swelling of the tumor and appearance of peritumoral edema along with thickening and lymphedema in normal mucosal tissues, as described previously. These changes usually peak at the end of the course of radiation. Most tumors responding well to radiation therapy shrink completely, with a small area of fibrosis remaining by 6 to 12 weeks after therapy (13). Posttreatment baseline imaging should not be done until at least 3 months after therapy to allow for confusing posttreatment inflammatory changes to have diminished. Unfortunately, some degree of mucosal thickening and disturbance of soft tissue planes persists indefinitely in many patients. Often, patients are treated with both surgery and RT and, in these cases, it can be difficult to distinguish changes induced by one from the other at imaging (24).

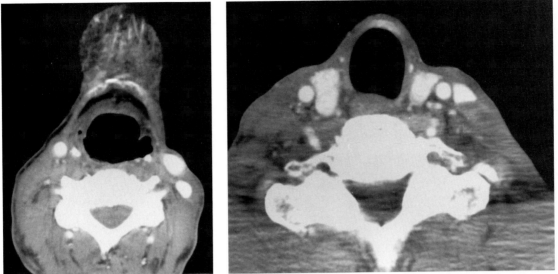

FIG. IIE-40. Bilateral modified radical neck dissection: CT images through the upper (**A**) and lower (**B**) neck demonstrate loss of the fatty tissue plane of the posterior cervical triangle. There has been resection of the right internal jugular vein. Both sternocleidomastoid muscles are present, although the one on the left is atrophic.

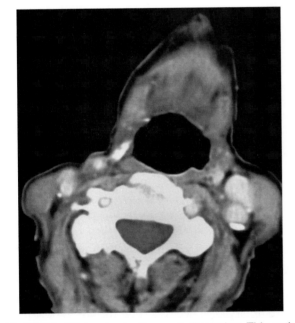

FIG. IIE-41. Bilateral selective neck dissection. This patient has been treated for multiple primaries of the oral cavity and shows changes of bilateral supraomohyoid neck dissections with resection of nodes in levels I to III. Note the loss of soft tissues bilaterally in the submandibular regions.

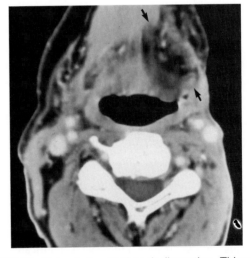

FIG. IIE-42. Extended radical neck dissection. This patient had a supraglottic laryngectomy and extended radical neck dissection for epiglottic tumor and positive level II nodes on the left with extracapsular extension. The hypoglossal nerve was sacrificed with resultant fatty atrophy of the left side of the tongue (*arrows*).

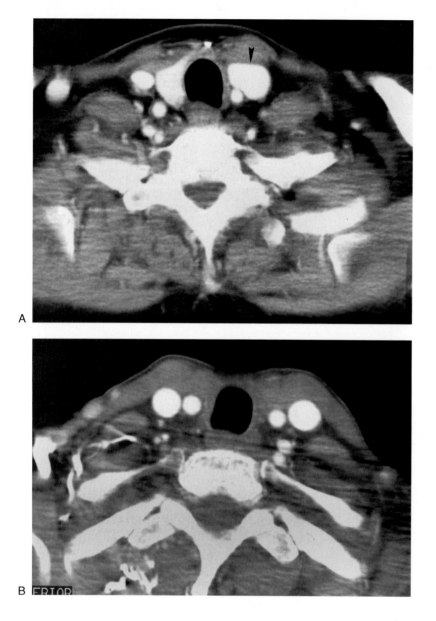

FIG. IIE-43. Surgical changes in the thyroid gland. (**A**) A CT scan in a patient with a left hemithyroidectomy. The left internal jugular vein now lies in the operative bed, mimicking the left lobe of the thyroid gland (*arrowhead*). (**B**) Scan of a different patient showing a total thyroidectomy with absent thyroid tissue on either side of the trachea.

Postradiation edematous changes in the mucosa of the pharynx and larynx and woody induration in the neck frequently limit the physical examination, making identification of recurrent tumor difficult clinically. Computed tomography has been shown to make a significant contribution to the clinical examination of the posttreatment patient. In the series of Harnsberger et al. (68), CT provided important information in 59% of cases of recurrent squamous cell carcinoma by detecting tumor when no mass was felt or seen and revealing deeper extension of disease than was appreciated clinically. At present, CT plays an important role in the follow-up of patients with laryngeal carcinoma treated with definitive RT. Complete resolution of tumor on a postradiation CT scan strongly suggests a successfully controlled primary site (Fig. IIE-44), whereas a persistent mass at the primary site that is unchanged in radiographic appearance correlates with

treatment failure (Fig. IIE-45) (69). Partial resolution of a mass on the posttreatment CT study is an indeterminate finding. These patients require further imaging and close clinical observation. Interval enlargement of a focal mass or persistent severe radiation edema suggests recurrent disease or laryngeal necrosis (Fig. IIE-46) (69). A recent study reports that laryngeal tumors larger than 5 cm^3 with MR findings of thyroid cartilage invasion prior to radiation therapy are more likely to recur than smaller tumors with cartilage invasion (70).

Two papers have compared CT and MR imaging in patients treated surgically and with RT for head and neck tumors (71,72). In the series of Gussack and Hudgins (72), MR imaging was found to be better than CT for recurrent tumors of the nasopharynx (Fig. IIE-47), skull base, paranasal sinuses, and parotid glands, whereas CT was more helpful in detecting pharyngeal and laryngeal

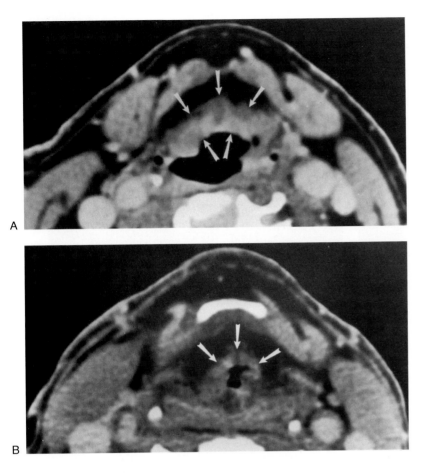

FIG. IIE-44. Tumor response to RT. (**A**) Pretreatment CT shows a carcinoma of the infrahyoid epiglottis (*arrows*). There is minimal invasion of the preepiglottic space on the left. (**B**) This CT 8 months after RT demonstrates complete resolution of the tumor at the primary site (*arrows*). (From Mukherji et al., ref. 69, with permission.)

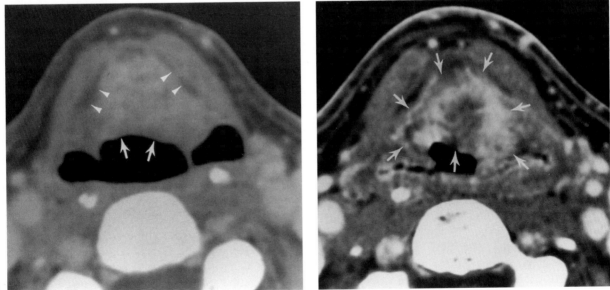

FIG. IIE-45. Radiotherapy failure of tumor control. (**A**) Pretreatment CT shows a large epiglottic tumor (*arrows*) invading the preepiglottic space (*arrowheads*). (**B**) Scan at 4 months after RT demonstrates a persistent heterogeneously enhancing mass (*arrows*), proved to be carcinoma. (From Mukherji et al., ref. 69, with permission.)

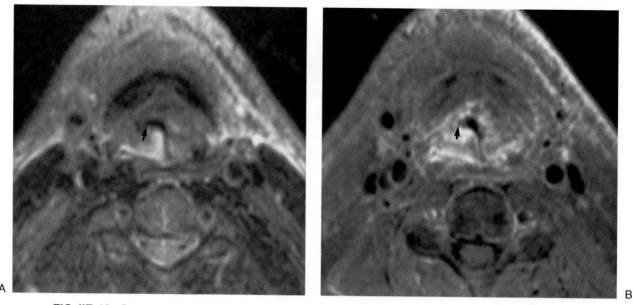

FIG. IIE-46. Severe laryngeal edema masking recurrent tumor. (**A**) Axial T$_2$-weighted and (**B**) postcontrast T$_1$-weighted MR images 6 months after RT for a T2N0M0 lesion of the right infrahyoid epiglottis demonstrate marked diffuse supraglottic swelling. An ulcer containing a small residual or recurrent tumor was found at endoscopy on the right above the false cord (*arrow*), not readily appreciated on MR.

recurrences (72). The experience of Glazer et al. (71) with a larger number of posttreatment patients having MR scans was different. They found MR to be better than CT in the neck for identifying muscular landmarks when normal anatomy had been distorted by treatment. MR was also better for separating tumor from muscle. Recurrent tumor was typically hyperintense to muscle on T$_2$-weighted images, whereas tumor and muscle were approximately isodense on CT. Magnetic resonance imaging has also been shown to have an advantage over CT in distinguishing recurrent tumor and fibrosis (11,14,71). Mature fibrous scar is of intermediate to low signal intensity on T$_1$- and T$_2$-weighted images, being iso- or hypointense to muscle (Fig. IIE-48), whereas recurrent tumor is usually hyperintense on T$_2$-weighted scans (Fig. IIE-49). Mature scar tissue also typically has a linear configuration (71) and does not enhance (13). In cases in which a tumor was treated by RT, a persistent mass that has higher T$_2$-weighted signal intensity than muscle and enhances with gadolinium-based contrast should be presumed to be tumor (13). However, in the postsurgical patient, immature, vascularized scar can also have this appearance, and neither CT nor MR can distinguish tumor from vascularized scar. This tissue is edematous and fibroareolar in nature and usually evolves into more compact dehydrated mature scar (11,13,14). A gradual decrease in size of such tissue on consecutive scans or stability on follow-up is a helpful observation, indicating that one is dealing with resolving scar tissue and not tumor (Fig. IIE-50) (14). However, biopsy is sometimes necessary.

In the patient who has had surgical treatment only, there are expected changes of hemorrhage and lymphedema in the tissues of the neck localized to the area of surgery (14). Most of these changes have resolved significantly by 6 weeks, and a baseline postoperative CT or MR scan can be obtained 6 to 8 weeks after surgery (14). Additional healing occurs slowly over the ensuing months and is delayed if postoperative radiation is given. If CT is done in the immediate postsurgical period, areas of hemorrhage may suggest residual infiltrating tumor, but typical signal intensities from blood products are usually recognized on MR imaging (14). These areas generally resolve or are transformed into sites of fibrosis. Several complications to the surgical procedure may occur in the immediate postoperative period that can mimic a mass on imaging studies; however, the clinical context usually suggests the appropriate diagnosis (14). These entities include hematoma, lymphocele, and abscess (Figs. IIE-51 and IIE-52). If imaging is done, it is mainly to define the extent of the abnormality or to assist with drainage.

For detection of recurrent tumor within or beneath myocutaneous flaps, it is likewise helpful to have a baseline postoperative scan for comparison. As noted earlier, pedicled or free tissue transfer flaps will often be seen in the context of resection of tumors of the tongue, floor of mouth, tonsil, and hypopharynx. Because the innervation of the muscle is not able to be preserved along with the vascular supply, the muscular component of the flap usually atrophies, leaving linear strands of soft tissue within otherwise fatty stroma (73). Recurrent tumor be-

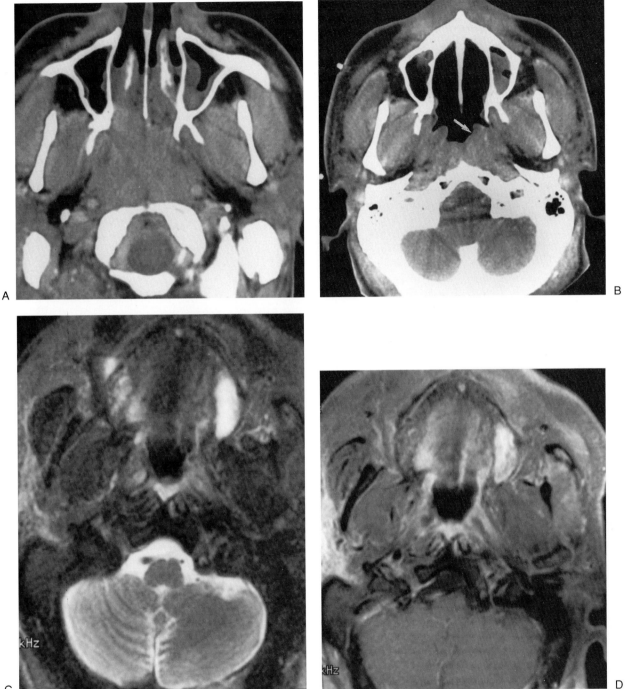

FIG. IIE-47. Recurrent tumor versus postradiation changes. (**A**) Pretreatment CT shows a large bilateral nasopharyngeal carcinoma. (**B**) Eight months after RT, CT demonstrates asymmetric thickening of the left posterolateral nasopharynx (*arrow*). (**C**) T$_2$-weighted and (**D**) postcontrast T$_1$-weighted MR images show mild thickening of the left lateral nasopharyngeal wall with asymmetric signal and enhancement but no discrete mass. Biopsies showed no tumor.

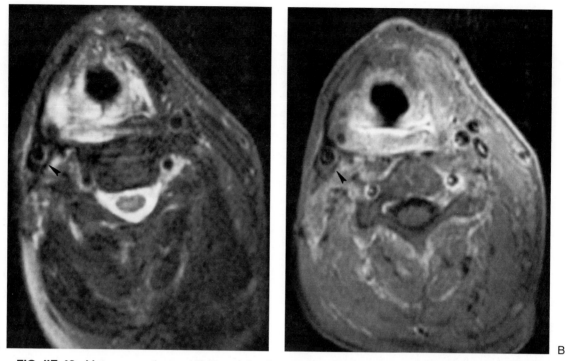

FIG. IIE-48. Mature scar tissue. **(A)** T_2-weighted and **(B)** postcontrast T_1-weighted MR images illustrate hypointense, nonenhancing tissue relative to muscle in the right neck (*arrowhead*) at the site of removal of malignant lymph nodes.

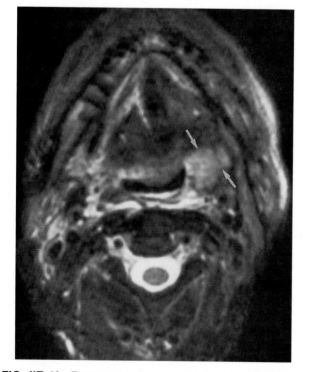

FIG. IIE-49. Recurrent tumor. T_2-weighted image demonstrates a rounded area of signal hyperintense to muscle in the left glossotonsillar sulcus (*arrows*), representing recurrent retromolar trigone tumor after surgical resection.

neath the flap can have a nodular or infiltrative appearance (Fig. IIE-21) and may also mimic infection (72,73).

Metabolic imaging techniques have recently been applied to the evaluation of head and neck cancer, including the posttreatment neck. Studies with 2-^{18}F-fluoro-2-deoxy-D-glucose positron-emission tomography (FDG-PET) have shown that this modality consistently detects squamous cell carcinoma for staging purposes (74–78). Tumor at the primary tumor site and in lymph nodes is reported to demonstrate greater metabolic activity than pharyngeal lymphoid tissue, salivary glands, and skeletal muscle (76,78). In one study, nontumoral tissues were found not to change significantly in metabolic activity after RT as compared to the pre-RT scan, but responding primary tumors and nodal metastases demonstrated significantly decreased isotope uptake (76). Rege et al. (77) have reported their experience in FDG-PET imaging of 60 patients with head and neck cancer. They found FDG-PET to be more accurate than MR imaging in detecting recurrent tumor after RT or surgery and RT and also better able to identify the primary tumor, surgically positive lymph nodes, and unknown primary tumors than MR. Others have also shown the usefulness of FDG-PET in distinguishing between benign and malignant tissues in the head and neck after RT or surgery and RT (79,80). The FDG-PET has been used during the course of RT for head and neck cancer, along with the clinical examina-

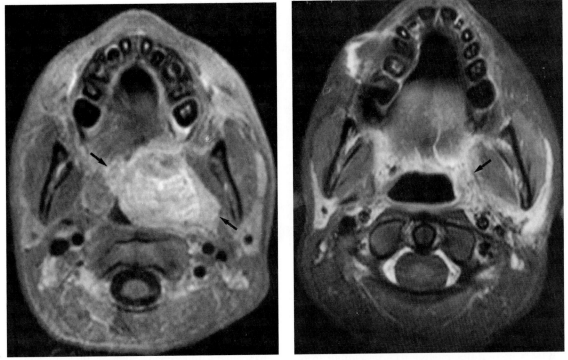

FIG. IIE-50. Probable vascularized scar. (**A**) Pretreatment MR image of a large rhabdomyosarcoma (*arrows*). (**B**) Scan following gross total resection and RT reveals mild thickening and enhancement in the left lateral pharyngeal wall (*arrow*), which has shown interval decrease in size since a previous posttreatment scan.

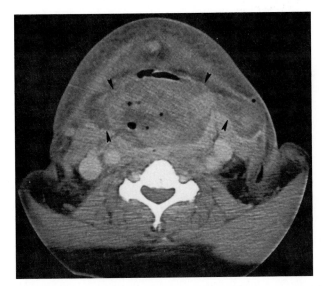

FIG. IIE-51. Infected hematoma. Total laryngectomy had been performed 10 days earlier. A huge anterior neck mass is seen (*arrowheads*). Air was likely introduced at aspiration of the mass prior to scanning. Thickening of the platysma muscle and subcutaneous fat reticulation probably represent combined postoperative changes and cellulitis.

tion, to identify tumors responding to therapy versus non-responders (75).

Fluorodeoxyglucose single-photon-emission computed tomography (SPECT) imaging has also been studied in posttreatment head and neck patients (80). Results showed that a negative scan correlated with absence of tumor. Positive FDG-SPECT scans were ambiguous, however, and could represent tumor recurrence or postradiation changes (Fig. IIE-53).

CONCLUSIONS

Without a doubt, interpretation of CT and MR images of patients with prior radiation therapy and/or surgery in the neck is very challenging because posttreatment changes often mimic or obscure residual or recurrent tumor. In most instances, radiation changes are bilateral and symmetric, and familiarity with the structures usually exhibiting an alteration from normal after RT, as described in this chapter, will aid in image interpretation. With increasing refinements in surgical techniques, more patients with regional or free tissue flap reconstructions

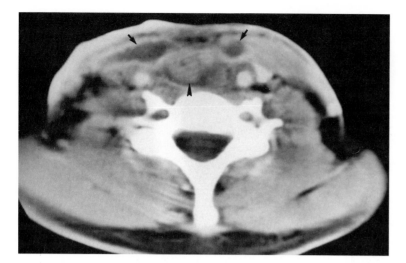

FIG. IIE-52. Neck abscesses (*arrows*) following total laryngectomy and right neck dissection. Neopharynx indicated by *arrowhead*.

after cosmetically deforming surgery will be seen on postoperative imaging studies. These surgical changes may run the gamut from being rather subtle to bizarre in appearance on imaging.

The crucial issue of differentiating recurrent tumor from posttherapeutic change remains problematic. Magnetic resonance imaging offers more specificity than CT in distinguishing among mature fibrous scar, neoplasm, and normal soft tissues because of significant signal intensity differences and enhancement characteristics. The greater sensitivity of enhanced MR images with gadolinium-based contrast as compared to postcontrast CT may permit more accurate detection of minimally enhancing recurrent tumor. These advantages will not apply, however, if the patient is unable to refrain from coughing or excessive swallowing during

MR scanning, a not infrequent situation. Unfortunately, neither enhanced MR nor CT is able to provide differentiation between immature vascularized scar and tumor, as both exhibit hyperintense signal on T$_2$-weighted images and enhancement. Fluorodeoxyglucose PET imaging is showing great promise for distinguishing between recurrent tumor and posttreatment changes in the neck; however, this modality is very expensive and limited in availability. Experience with more accessible FDG-SPECT imaging is less extensive, but this technique does not appear to be as specific as FDG-PET. Communication between the head and neck radiologist and radiation and surgical oncologist is important to facilitate accurate interpretation of posttherapeutic scans and for decision-making on continuing to follow a patient with imaging or intervening with biopsy.

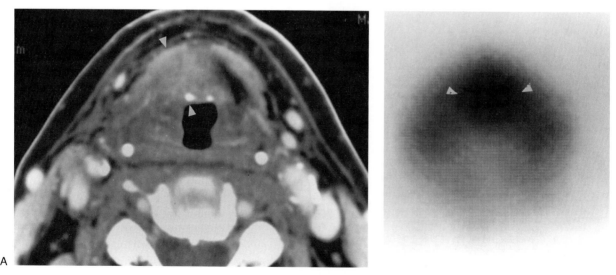

FIG. IIE-53. Recurrent tumor on FDG-SPECT. (**A**) Computed tomographic image of biopsy positive residual infrahyoid carcinoma 1.5 months after RT (*arrowheads*). (**B**) FDG-SPECT image at the same level shows increased activity in the area of the mass on CT.

REFERENCES

1. Wenig BL: The role of surgery in head and neck cancer: standard care and new horizons. *Semin Oncol* 1994;21:289.
2. Sweeney PJ, Haraf DJ, Vokes EE, Dougherty M, Weichselbaum RR: Radiation therapy in head and neck cancer: indications and limitations. *Semin Oncol* 1994;21:296.
3. Amdur RJ, Parsons JT, Mendenhall WM, Million RR, Stringer SP, Cassisi NJ: Postoperative irradiation for squamous cell carcinoma of the head and neck: an analysis of treatment results and complications. *Int J Radiat Oncol Biol Phys* 1989;16:25.
4. Mirimanoff RP, Wang CC, Doppke KP: Combined surgery and postoperative radiation therapy for advanced laryngeal and hypopharyngeal carcinomas. *Int J Radiat Oncol Biol Phys* 1985;11:499.
5. Kramer S, Gelber RD, Snow JB, et al: Combined radiation therapy and surgery in the management of advanced head and neck cancer: Final report of Study 73-03 of the Radiation Therapy Oncology Group. *Head Neck Surg* 1987;10:19.
6. Peters LJ, Goepfert H, Ang KK, et al: Evaluation of the dose for postoperative radiation therapy of head and neck cancer: first report of a prospective randomized trial. *Int J Radiat Oncol Biol Phys* 1993;26:3.
7. Laramore GE, Scott CB, Al-Sarraf M, et al: Adjuvant chemotherapy for resectable squamous cell carcinomas of the head and neck: report on intergroup study 0034. *Int J Radiat Oncol Biol Phys* 1992;23:705.
8. Jaulery C, Rodriquez J, Brunin F, et al: Induction chemotherapy in advanced head and neck tumors. Results of two randomized trials. *Int J Radiat Oncol Biol Phys* 1992;23:483.
9. Rosenthal DI, Pistenmaa DA, Glatstein E: A review of neoadjuvant chemotherapy for head and neck cancer: partially shrunken tumors may be both leaner and meaner. *Int J Radiat Oncol Biol Phys* 1993;28:315.
10. Million RR, Cassisi NJ, Mancuso AA, Stringer SP, Mendenhall WM, Parsons JT: Management of the neck for squamous cell carcinoma. In: Million RR, Cassisi NJ, eds. *Management of Head and Neck Cancer: A Multidisciplinary Approach,* 2nd ed. Philadelphia: JB Lippincott, 1994:75.
11. Mancuso AA, Dillon WP: The neck. *Radiol Clin North Am* 1989;27:407.
12. Yousem DM, Som PM, Hackney DB, Schwaibold F, Hendrix RA: Central nodal necrosis and extracapsular neoplastic spread in cervical lymph nodes: MR imaging versus CT. *Radiology* 1992;182:753.
13. Mancuso AA: Imaging in patients with head and neck cancer. In: Million RR, Cassisi NJ, eds. *Management of Head and Neck Cancer: A Multidisciplinary Approach,* 2nd ed. Philadelphia: JB Lippincott, 1994:43.
14. Som PM, Urken ML, Biller H, Lidov M: Imaging the postoperative neck. *Radiology* 1993;187:593.
15. Mukherji SK, Mancuso AA, Kotzur IM, et al: Radiologic appearance of the irradiated larynx. Part I. Expected changes. *Radiology* 1994;193:141.
16. Tartaglino LM, Rao VM, Markiewicz DA: Imaging of radiological changes in the head and neck. *Semin Roentgenol* 1994;29:81.
17. Manara M: Histological changes of the human larynx irradiated with various technical therapeutic methods. *Arch Ital Otol* 1966;79:596.
18. Mancuso AA, Hanafee WN: Larynx and hypopharynx. In: Mancuso AA, Hanafee WN, eds. *Computed Tomography and Magnetic Resonance Imaging of the Head and Neck,* 2nd ed. Baltimore: Williams & Wilkins, 1985:241.
19. Stringer SP: Flaps and grafts for reconstruction. In: Million RR, Cassisi, NJ, eds. *Management of Head and Neck Cancer: A Multidisciplinary Approach,* 2nd ed. Philadelphia: JB Lippincott, 1994:157.
20. Redvanly RD, Hudgins PA, Gussack GS, Lewis M, Crocker IR: CT of muscle necrosis following radiation therapy in a patient with head and neck malignancy. *Am J Neuroradiol* 1992;13:220.
21. Parsons JT: The effect of radiation on normal tissues of the head and neck. In: Million RR, Cassisi NJ, eds. *Management of Head and Neck Cancer: A Multidisciplinary Approach,* 2nd ed. Philadelphia: JB Lippincott, 1994:245.
22. Million RR, Cassisi NJ, Mancuso AA: Larynx. In: Million RR, Cassisi NJ, eds. *Management of Head and Neck Cancer: A Multidisciplinary Approach,* 2nd ed. Philadelphia: JB Lippincott, 1994:431.
23. Harnsberger HR, Smoker WRK, Watanabe AS: Retropharyngeal space: evaluation of normal anatomy and diseases with CT and MR imaging. *Radiology* 1990;174:59.
24. Bronstein AD, Nybery DA, Schwartz AN, Shuman WP, Griffin BR: Soft-tissue changes after head and neck radiation: CT findings. *Am J Neuroradiol* 1989;10:171.
25. Curtin HD: The larynx. In: Som PM, Bergeron RT, eds. *Head and Neck Imaging,* 2nd ed. St. Louis: Mosby Year Book, 1991:593.
26. Calcaterra TC, Stern R, Ward PH: Dilemma of delayed radiation injury of the larynx. *Ann Otol Rhinol Laryngol* 1972;81:501.
27. Ward PH, Calcaterra TC, Kagan AR: The enigma of post-radiation edema and recurrent or residual carcinoma of the larynx. *Laryngoscope* 1975;85:522.
28. Goldman JL, Cheren RV, Zak FG, et al: Histopathology of larynges and radical neck specimens in a combined radiation and surgery for advanced carcinoma of the larynx and hypopharynx. *Ann Otol* 1966;75:313.
29. Goodrich WA, Lenz M: Laryngeal chondronecrosis following roentgen therapy. *Am J Roentgenol* 1948;60:22.
30. Chandler JR: Radiation fibrosis and necrosis of the larynx. *Ann Otol* 1979;88:509.
31. Tart RP, Mukherji SK, Lee WR, Mancuso AA: Value of laryngeal cartilage sclerosis as a predictor of outcome in patients with stage T3 glottic cancer treated with radiation therapy. *Radiology* 1994;192:567.
32. Feehs RS, McGuirt WF, Bard MG, Strickland HL, Craven TE, Hiltbrand JB: Irradiation. A significant risk factor for carotid atherosclerosis. *Arch Otolaryngol Head Neck Surg* 1991;117:1135.
33. Chuang VP: Radiation-induced arteritis. *Semin Roentgenol* 1994;29:64.
34. Call GK, Bray PF, Smoker WRK, Buys SS, Hayes JK: Carotid thrombosis following neck irradiation. *Int J Radiat Oncol Biol Phys* 1990;18:635.
35. Cooke J, Powell S, Parsons C: The diagnosis by computed tomography of brachial plexus lesions following radiotherapy for cancer of the breast. *Clin Radiol* 1988;39:602.
36. Zweig G, Russell EJ: Radiation myelopathy of the cervical spinal cord: MR findings. *Am J Neuroradiol* 1990;11:1188.
37. Wang P-Y, Shen W-C, Jan J-S: MR imaging in radiation myelopathy. *Am J Neuroradiol* 1992;13:1049.
38. Melki PS, Halimi P, Wibault P, Masnou P, Doyon D: MRI in chronic progressive radiation myelopathy. *J Comput Assist Tomogr* 1994;18:1.
39. Glass JP, Hwang T-L, Leavens ME, Libshitz HI: Cerebral radiation necrosis following treatment of extracranial malignancies. *Cancer* 1984;54:1966.
40. Lee AWM, Ng SH, Ho JHC, et al: Clinical diagnosis of late temporal lobe necrosis following radiation therapy for nasopharyngeal carcinoma. *Cancer* 1988;61:1535.
41. Berger PC, Boyko OB: The pathology of central nervous system radiation injury. In: Gutin PH, Leibel SA, Sheline GE, eds. *Radiation Injury to the Nervous System.* New York: Raven Press, 1991:191.
42. Valk PE, Dillon WP: Radiation injury of the brain. *Am J Neuroradiol* 1991;12:45.
43. Libshitz HI: Radiation changes in bone. *Semin Roentgenol* 1994;29:15.
44. Huvos AG, Woodard HQ, Cahan WG, et al: Postradiation osteogenic sarcoma of bone and soft tissue. A clinicopathologic study of 66 patients. *Cancer* 1885;55:1244.
45. Wiklund TA, Blomqvist CP, Räty J, Elomaa I, Rissanen P, Miettinen M: Postirradiation sarcoma. Analysis of a nationwide cancer registry material. *Cancer* 1991;68:524.
46. Lorigan JG, Libshitz HI, Peuchot M: Radiation-induced sarcoma of bone: CT findings in 19 cases. *Am J Roentgenol* 1989;153:791.
47. Ried HL, Jaffe N: Radiation-induced changes in long-term survivors of childhood cancer after treatment with radiation therapy. *Semin Roentgenol* 1994;29:6.
48. Favus MJ, Schneider AB, Stachura ME, et al: Thyroid cancer occurring as a late consequence of head-and-neck irradiation: Evaluation of 1056 patients. *N Engl J Med* 1976;294:1019.
49. Lawson W, Biller HF: Surgical therapy of the larynx. In: Thawley

SE, Panje WR, eds. *Comprehensive Management of Head and Neck Tumors*. Philadelphia: WB Saunders, 1987:991.

50. Bailey BJ: Early glottic cancers. In: Bailey BJ, ed. *Head and Neck Surgery*. Philadelphia: JB Lippincott, 1993:1313.

51. DiSantis DJ, Balfe DM, Hayden RE, Sessions D, Sagel SS: Neck after vertical hemilaryngectomy: computed tomographic study. *Radiology* 1984;151:683.

52. Desanto LW: Supraglottic laryngectomy. In: Bailey BJ, ed. *Head and Neck Surgery*. Philadelphia: JB Lippincott, 1993:1334.

53. Disantis DJ, Balfe DM, Hayden RE, Sagel SS, Sessions D, Lee JKT: Neck after total laryngectomy: CT study. *Radiology* 1984; 153:713.

54. Fried MP, Girdhar-Gopal HV: Advanced cancer of the larynx. In: Bailey BJ, ed. *Head and Neck Surgery*. Philadelphia: JB Lippincott, 1993:1347.

55. Marks JE: Tumors of the pharynx. In: Thawley SE, Panje WR, eds. *Comprehensive Management of Head and Neck Tumors*. Philadelphia: WB Saunders, 1987:756.

56. Synderman NL: Surgical vocal rehabilitation. In: Paparella MM, Shumrick DA, Gluckman JL, Meyerhoff WL, eds. *Otolaryngology*. Philadelphia: WB Saunders, 1991:2371.

57. Fuller D: Speech and swallowing rehabilitation for head and neck tumor patients. In: Thawley SE, Panje WR, eds. *Comprehensive Management of Head and Neck Tumors*. Philadelphia: WB Saunders, 1987:100.

58. Willatt DJ, Stell PM: Vocal cord paralysis. In: Paparella MM, Shumrick DA, Gluckman JL, Meyerhoff WL, eds. *Otolaryngology*. Philadelphia: WB Saunders, 1991:2289.

59. Thawley SE, Sessions DG: Treatment of tumors of the hypopharynx. In: Thawley SE, Panje WR, eds. *Comprehensive Management of Head and Neck Tumors*. Philadelphia: WB Saunders, 1987:774.

60. Myers EN, Snyderman CH: Near-total glossectomy and reconstruction for large carcinomas of the tongue. In: Bailey BJ, ed. *Surgery of the Oral Cavity*. Chicago: Year-Book Medical Publishers, 1989:71.

61. Shah JP, Shemen LJ, Strong EW: Surgical therapy of oral cavity tumors. In: Thawley SE, Panje WR, eds. *Comprehensive Management of Head and Neck Tumors*. Philadelphia: WB Saunders, 1987:551.

62. Panje WR: Immediate reconstruction of the oral cavity. In: Thawley SE, Panje WR, eds. *Comprehensive Management of Head and Neck Tumors*. Philadelphia: WB Saunders, 1987:563.

63. Lawson WH, Biller HF: Reconstruction of the mandible. In: Paparella MM, Shumrick DA, Gluckman JL, Meyerhoff WL, eds. *Otolaryngology*. Philadelphia: WB Saunders, 1991:2069.

64. Robbins KT, Medina JE, Wolfe GT, Levine PA, Sessions RB, Pruet CW: Standardizing neck dissection terminology. *Arch Otol Head Neck Surg* 1991;117:601.

65. Medina JE, Rigual NR: Neck dissection. In: Bailey BJ, ed. *Head and Neck Surgery*. Philadelphia: JB Lippincott, 1993:1192.

66. Shah JP, Andersen PE: The impact of patterns of nodal metastasis on modifications of neck dissection. *Ann Surg Oncol* 1994;1:521.

67. Friedman M, Toriumi DM: Malignant diseases of the thyroid gland. In: Paparella MM, Shumrick DA, Gluckman JL, Meyerhoff WL, eds. *Otolaryngology*. Philadelphia: WB Saunders, 1991:2499.

68. Harnsberger HR, Mancuso AA, Muraki AS, Parkin JL: The upper aerodigestive tract and neck: CT evaluation of recurrent tumors. *Radiology* 1983;149:503.

69. Mukherji SK, Mancuso AA, Kotzur IM, et al: Radiologic appearance of the irradiated larynx. Part II. Primary site response. *Radiology* 1994;193:149.

70. Castelijns JA, van den Brekel MWM, Tobi H, et al: Laryngeal carcinoma after radiation therapy: correlation of abnormal MR imaging signal patterns in laryngeal cartilage with the risk of recurrence. *Radiology* 1996;198:151.

71. Glazer HS, Niemeyer JH, Balfe DM, et al: Neck neoplasms: MR imaging. Part II. Posttreatment evaluation. *Radiology* 1986;160:349.

72. Gussack GS, Hudgins PA: Imaging modalities in recurrent head and neck tumors. *Laryngoscope* 1991;101:119.

73. Som PM, Biller HF: Computed tomography of the neck in the postoperative patient: radical neck dissection and the myocutaneous flap. *Radiology* 1983;148:157.

74. Minn H, Joensuu H, Ahonen A, Klemi P: Fluorodeoxyglucose imaging: a method to assess the proliferative activity of human cancer *in vivo. Cancer* 1988;61:1776.

75. Minn H, Paul R, Ahonen A: Evaluation of treatment response to radiotherapy in head and neck cancer with fluorine-18 fluorodeoxyglucose. *J Nucl Med* 1988;29:1521.

76. Rege SD, Chaiken L, Hoh CK, et al: Change induced by radiation therapy in FDG uptake in normal and malignant structures of the head and neck: quantitation with PET. *Radiology* 1993;189:807.

77. Rege S, Maass A, Chaiken L, et al: Use of positron emission tomography with fluorodeoxyglucose in patients with extracranial head and neck cancers. *Cancer* 1994;73:3047.

78. Jabour BA, Choi Y, Hoh CK, et al: Extracranial head and neck: PET imaging with 2-[F-18] fluoro-2-deoxy-D-glucose and MR imaging correlation. *Radiology* 1993;186:27.

79. Lapela M, Grénman R, Kurki T, et al: Head and neck cancer: detection of recurrence with PET and 2-[F-18] fluoro-2-D-glucose. *Radiology* 1995;197:205.

80. Greven KM, Williams DW, Keyes JW, et al: Distinguishing tumor recurrence from irradiation sequelae with positron emission tomography in patients treated for larynx cancer. *Int J Radiat Oncol Biol Phys* 1994;29:841.

81. Mukherji SK, Drone WE, Mancuso AA, McLaughlin MP: Differentiation of recurrent tumor from radiation-induced changes with FDG SPECT in the upper aerodigestive tract. *Radiology* 1994;193(P):263.

Posttherapeutic Neurodiagnostic Imaging,
edited by J.R. Jinkins,
Lippincott-Raven Publishers, New York © 1997.

CHAPTER **IIF**

The Posttherapeutic Craniocervical Junction

Stig Holtås

Surgery directed toward the craniocervical junction can be divided into several main areas, including the treatment of trauma, torticollis, rheumatoid arthritis, congenital and developmental anomalies, and neoplasia. In the majority of patients, there is a need for postoperative evaluation of the result and for monitoring during the course of convalescence. The choice of imaging modality depends in part on the type of tissue pathology of interest (e.g., soft tissue, bone, or joint). In many patients, there is a need to use several different imaging modalities in order to be able to obtain a complete postoperative evaluation. Moreover, surgery often involves fixation of the bone elements with different materials, both autologous and exogenous, and in this situation, the choice of imaging method is restricted because of the potential for MR and CT to produce unique artifacts.

TRAUMA

Following reposition and stabilization with a cervical collar, halo vest, or internal fixation material, there is nearly always a need for posttreatment evaluation. In odontoid and hangman-type fractures, conventional radiographs are usually sufficient and relatively simple to perform for the evaluation of proper bony alignment and healing (Fig. IIF-1). In Jefferson fractures, CT is the modality of choice for both initial diagnosis and postoperative analysis. Conventional radiographic tomography can also be used but is time-consuming and must be performed in two projections (Fig. IIF-2). However, as soon as a stable positioning has been confirmed, further evaluation of position can be performed with conventional radiographs obtained in two projections. This is an economical and practical examination that is possible to perform in any x-ray department.

S. Holtås: Department of Radiology, University Hospital, S-221 85 Lund, Sweden.

TORTICOLLIS

Conventional radiographs are often difficult to interpret in atlantoaxial rotary fixation, especially following surgical manipulation during anesthesia. The neuroradiologic evaluation of this condition is therefore preferably performed with CT, which can be combined with three-dimensional imaging and multiplanar reconstruction.

Thin slices parallel to the C1 and C2 arches should be obtained in order to estimate the degree of motion. A full range of motion between C1 and C2 should be seen on both sides following successful treatment. The image interpretation can be facilitated by a double exposure of the two vertebrae on the same film, using a negative image for one and a positive for the other (Fig. IIF-3).

RHEUMATOID ARTHRITIS

Conventional radiography should always be the first choice for the postoperative evaluation of this disease. This examination will reveal whether or not stability has been achieved and in what position. Furthermore, the integrity of the fixation material can be checked, as well as the underlying bony structure for evidence of new fractures or dislocations (Fig. IIF-4). Vertical dislocation can sometimes be difficult to evaluate using Chamberlain's or McGregor's methods of measurement because the tip of the odontoid is not always well visualized, and sometimes it is eroded. Measurement of vertical dislocation can be facilitated by the method suggested by Redlund-Johnell and Pettersson (Fig. IIF-5) (1).

In rheumatoid arthritis there is often also a need for visualization of the soft tissues so that possible cord or root compression can be evaluated. It is especially difficult to determine the neurologic level by clinical examination in rheumatoid arthritis because of generalized joint deformities and pain. The neuroradiologic examination is therefore especially helpful in this situation (Fig. IIF-6). The neuroradiologic evaluation in this circumstance can

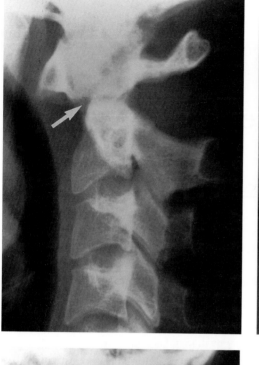

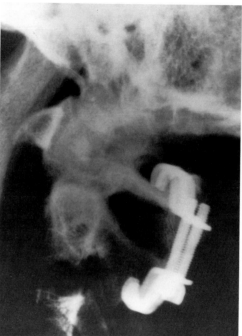

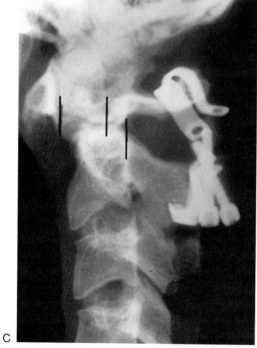

FIG. IIF-1. Odontoid fracture. **A:** Odontoid fracture (*arrow*) with anterior C1-2 subluxation. **B:** Posterior surgical internal fixation performed with vertebral realignment. **C:** One month later, fixation device has spontaneously disconnected, and subluxation has recurred. (Note misalignment of *straight black lines.*)

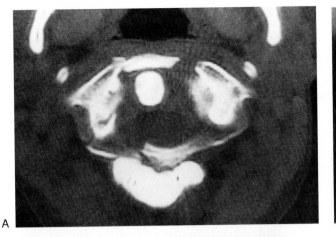

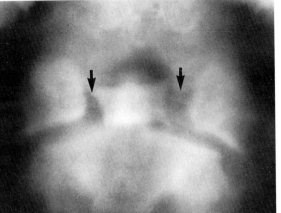

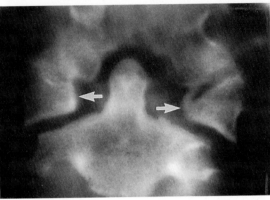

FIG. IIF-2. Jefferson's fracture. **A:** Axial CT of Jefferson's fracture shows dislocations and fixation material posteriorly. **B:** Frontal conventional radiographic tomogram shows the ventral fracture dislocations (*arrows*). **C:** Frontal conventional radiographic tomogram shows the dislocated lateral masses of C1 (*arrow*).

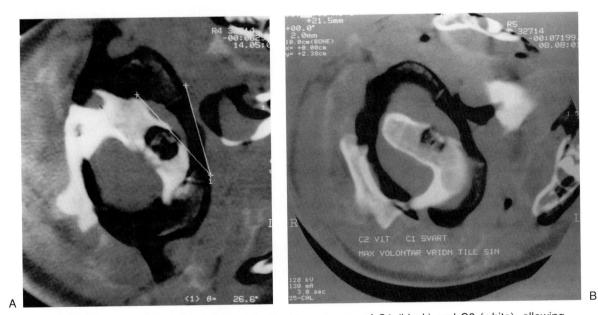

FIG. IIF-3. C1-2 rotational dislocation. **A:** Double exposure of C1 (black) and C2 (white), allowing measurement of the rotation. **B:** Maximum voluntary rotation to the left following successful surgical manipulation during anesthesia. **C:** Maximum voluntary rotation to the right following successful manipulation during anesthesia. The motion range has been normalized by the manipulation. (Courtesy of Dr. Per Grane, Karolinska Hospital, Stockholm, Sweden.)

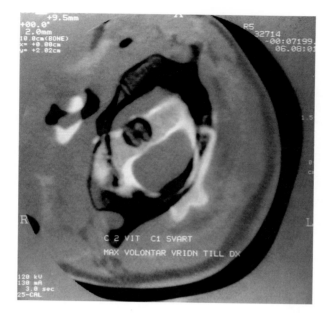

FIG. IIF-3. *Continued*

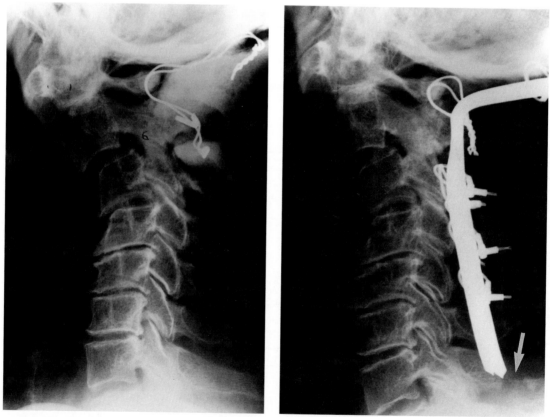

A

B

FIG. IIF-4. Rheumatoid arthritis. **A:** Postoperative evaluation shows subluxation at C1-2 (*black lines*) and also at C2-3 as a result of insufficient surgical fixation. **B:** Following refixation, a reduction of C1-2 and C2-3 subluxation has been achieved, but patient's new pain may be related to a new fracture of the spinous process of C7 (*arrow*).

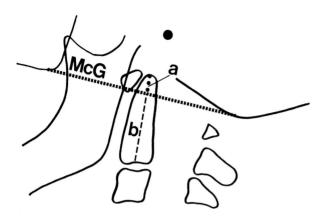

FIG. IIF-5. Measurement of vertical dislocation. Instead of using distance indicated by *a,* which might be difficult to determine, the distance between the lower endplate of C2 and McGregor's line (McG) can be used. (Range of normal: adult men 33.5 to 51 mm; adult women 28 to 50 mm.) (From Redlund-Johnell and Pettersson, ref. 1, with permission.)

be done using computed tomographic (CT) myelography or magnetic resonance (MR) imaging. For CT myelography, approximately 5 ml of nonionic water-soluble iodinated contrast medium (180 mg/ml) is injected into the subarachnoid space, and the contrast is directed to the cervical spinal region. The CT examination can be performed immediately after the introduction of the contrast medium or with a delay of 1 to 2 hr. Thin cuts in the range of 1 to 2 mm should be obtained that will allow sagittal reconstructions. Metallic fixation material may cause artifacts; however, they are often rather limited, so that visualiztion of at least the anterior part of the spinal canal can be obtained. With this method, evaluation for the disappearance of pannus formation surrounding the odontoid process can be evaluated, and the cause of remaining or new symptoms can usually be determined (Fig. IIF-7).

Magnetic resonance can also be used for evaluation of the soft tissues (2,3). However, metallic fixation material may generate artifacts that obscure the posterior spinal

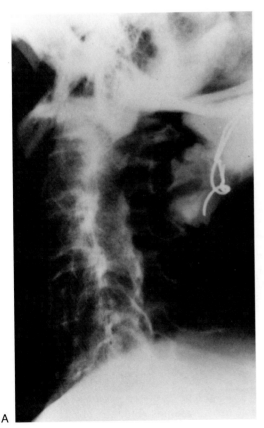

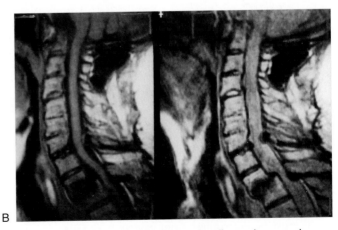

FIG. IIF-6. Rheumatoid arthritis with signs of cord compression. **A:** Conventional radiographs reveal that the fixation material has lost its attachment to C1 and C2 posteriorly. **B,C:** However, MRI (**B,** TR 500, TE 30; **C,** TR 2000, TE 85) reveals that the patient's main subluxation is at the T2-3 level and not at the craniocervical junction.

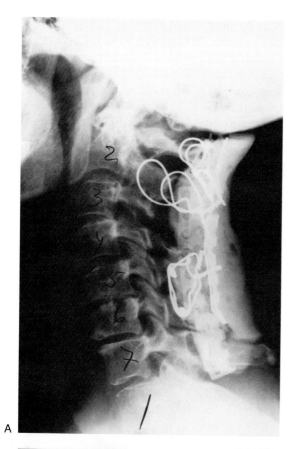

A

FIG. IIF-7. Rheumatoid arthritis with recurrent neurologic symptoms. **A:** Conventional radiography shows good spinal alignment following posterior fixation. **B:** Sagittal reformatted CT myelography excludes cord compression at the craniocervical junction. Only limited metallic artifacts are present. **C:** Coronal reformatted image reveals a schwannoma in the thoracic spine.

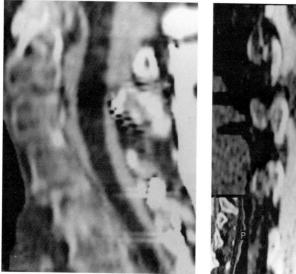

B

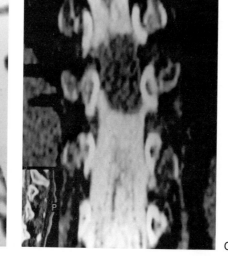

C

canal. To alter the distribution of metallic artifacts favorably in the area of interest, the direction of the frequency encoding gradient can be changed (Fig. IIF-8). The optimal change must be determined from case to case (Fig. IIF-9). It is also important to consider utilizing a high band width because low-band-width techniques increase the size of the artifact (Fig. IIF-10) (4). Gradient-echo

sequences should also be avoided because they are more sensitive to disturbances of the magnetic field produced by ferromagnetic materials (Fig. IIF-11). However, it is usually possible to get a good view of the odontoid region, and the method has been used to study the sequential reduction of pannus formation. In one MR study in nine patients with atlantoaxial instability, pannus reduction or

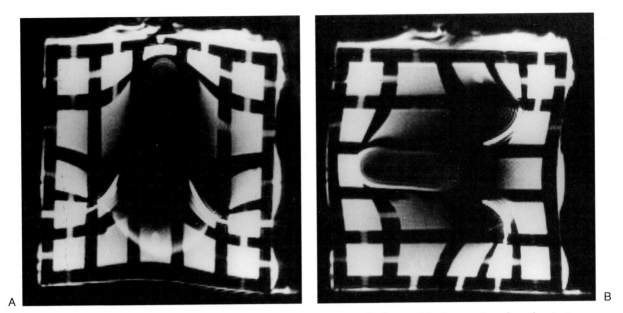

FIG. IIF-8. A frequency-encoding direction. **A:** Aneurysm clip imaged in the center of a phantom encoding direction, bottom to top. **B:** The frequency-encoding direction has been changed left to right. Note altered distortion and visibility of the surrounding boxes.

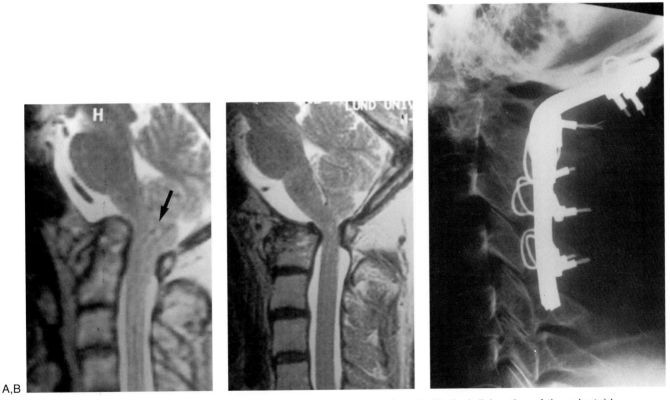

FIG. IIF-9. Rheumatoid arthritis and medullary compression. **A:** Vertical dislocation of the odontoid has occurred, causing compression of the spinal cord at the cervicomedullary junction (*arrow*). **B:** Following transoral removal of the odontoid, the cervicomedullary compression has not improved. **C:** Posterior fixation improves the vertebral alignment. **D:** Magnetic resonance image acquired with frequency-encoding direction in the posterior–anterior direction does not allow evaluation of the spinal cord because of a metallic artifact. **E:** When the frequency-encoding direction changed to the cranio-caudal direction, the cervicomedullary junction anteriorly is visualized, showing resolution of the cord compression.

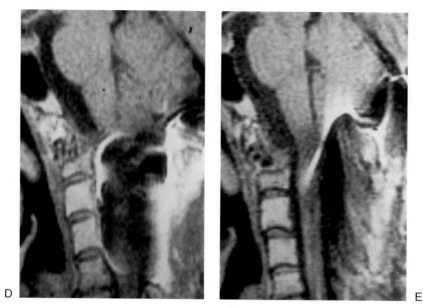

FIG. IIF-9. *Continued.*

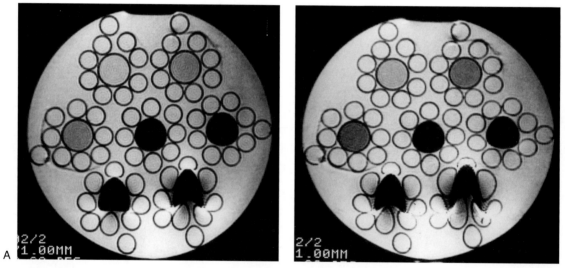

FIG. IIF-10. Cylinders containing increasing concentrations of magnetite. Higher concentrations give lower signals and more image distortion (5 and 7 o'clock). **A:** High band width: 50.86 Hz/mm. **B:** Low band width: 23.43 Hz/mm. Note that the artifacts and distortion are larger than those in **A.**

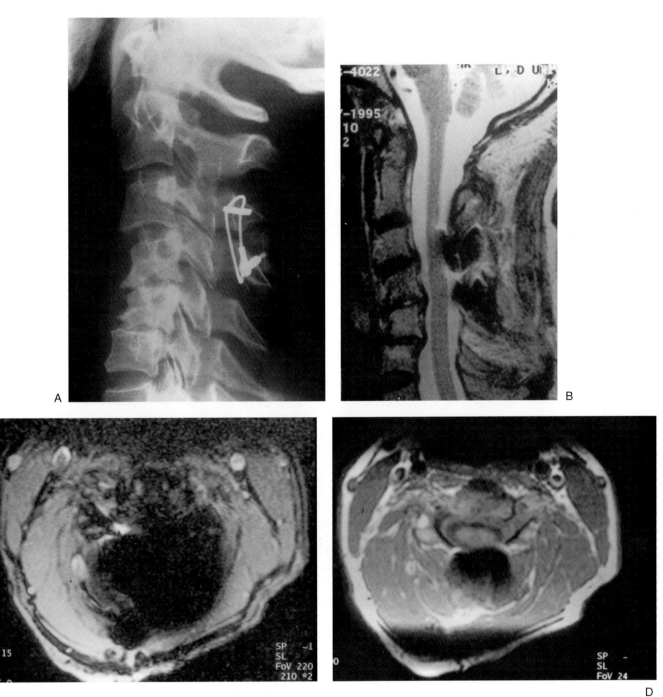

FIG. IIF-11. Patient with trauma and posterior surgical fixation material at the C3-4 level. **A:** Conventional radiograph shows metallic wire fixing the posterior elements at C3-4. **B:** Sagittal T_2-weighted fast spin-echo sequence shows very limited disturbance of the image by the metallic material. **C:** Axial gradient echo axial sequence shows severe distortion and signal drop-out caused by metallic material. **D:** T_1-weighted conventional spin-echo sequence at the same position as in **C** visualizes the cord except in its most posterior aspect.

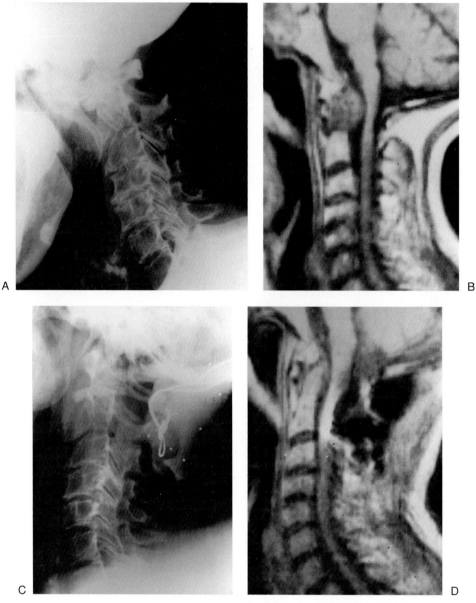

FIG. IIF-12. Rheumatoid arthritis. **A:** Preoperative conventional radiography shows severe craniospinal instability. **B:** Preoperative MRI reveals pannus formation at C1-2 with high cervical cord compression. **C:** Postoperative conventional radiograph shows successful posterior fixation. **D:** Postoperative MRI reveals disappearance of the pannus at C1-2. There are only moderate metallic artifacts posteriorly.

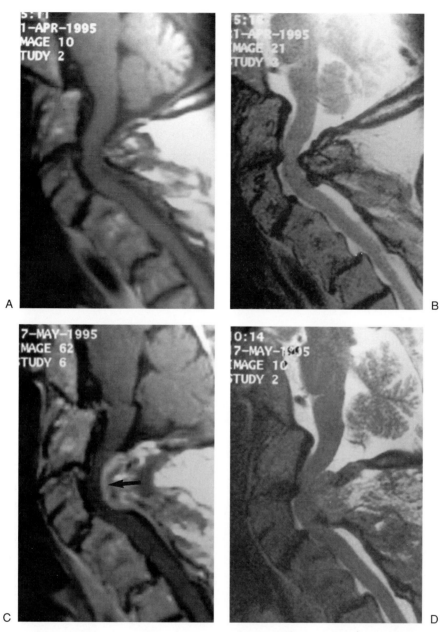

FIG. IIF-13. Patient with rheumatoid arthritis with cord compression at the C2-3 level. **A:** T$_1$-weighted image showing moderate cord compression at C1-2. **B:** T$_2$-weighted image showing moderate cord compression at C1-2. **C:** Unenhanced T$_1$-weighted examination performed postoperatively because of increased clinical symptoms shows postoperative hematoma (*arrow*) with increased cord compression. **D:** Corresponding postoperative T$_2$-weighted image showing no reduction of cord compression caused by the posterior hemorrhage.

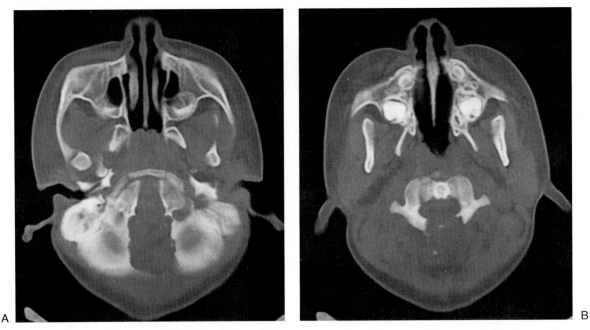

FIG. IIF-14. Postoperative evaluation in a child with achondroplasia. **A:** Postoperative midline defect in occipital bone. **B:** Resection of posterior arch of C1.

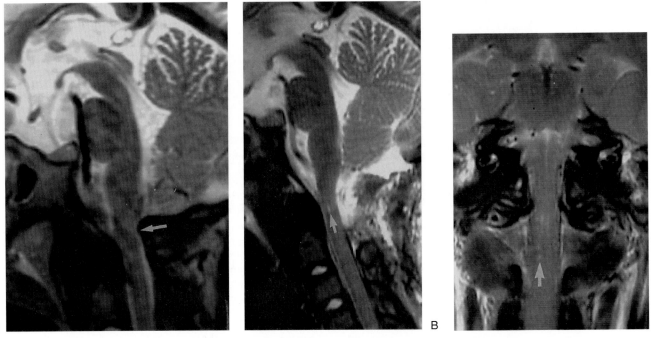

FIG. IIF-15. Child with achondroplasia. **A:** Preoperative MR shows severe narrowing at foramen magnum (*arrow*). **B:** Postoperative MRI performed because of residual or recurrent symptoms shows good width at the foramen magnum area but possible edema (*arrow*) in the cord. **C:** Corresponding postoperative coronal view showing evidence of cord edema (*arrow*). (Courtesy of Dr. Olof Flodmark, Karolinska Hospital, Stockholm, Sweden).

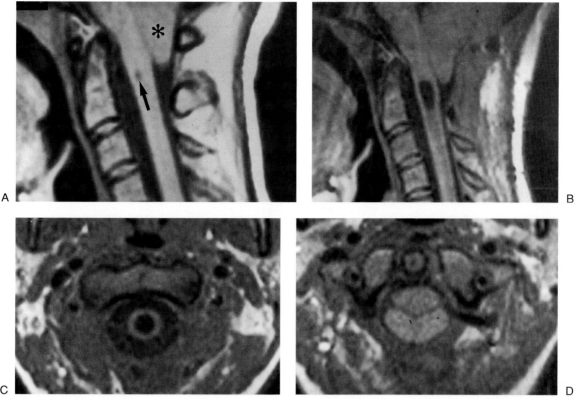

FIG. IIF-16. Chiari I malformation and minimal hydromyelia. **A:** Tonsillar ectopia (*asterisk*) and minimal hydromyelia (*arrow*) are noted. **B:** Postoperative evaluation shows somewhat improved width at the C1-2 level but remaining narrowing at the foramen magnum level. The hydromyelic cavity has increased in size as sign of remaining CSF circulation block. **C:** Axial view at the level of the cord cavity shows good width of the CSF spaces around the spinal cord at the C2 level. **D:** At the foramen magnum level, the tonsillar herniation and the complete obliteration of the CSF spaces are noted. Note: In this case, the only surgery initially performed was resection of bone in the occipital region and the posterior C1 arch. Duraplasty has not been performed; this is probably the reason for the poor result.

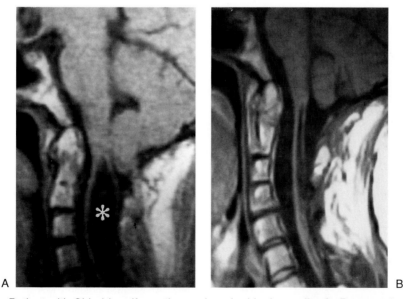

FIG. IIF-17. Patient with Chiari I malformation and marked hydromyelia. **A:** Preoperative MR shows the tonsillar ectopia and the large hydromyelic cavity (*asterisk*). **B:** Postoperative MR shows diminished hydromyelia and good width of the CSF spaces at the foramen magnum level. Note: In this case, duraplasty had been performed, as well as resection of the occipital bone and C1 arch.

disappearance was seen in all patients following successful stabilization (Fig. IIF-12) (5). New fixation materials, such as titanium alloys, cause less disturbance of the magnetic field and therefore result in smaller artifacts than those caused by stainless steel. Composite wires and acrylic bone cement are free from artifacts in both MR and CT. Of course, in patients with rheumatoid arthritis without metallic fixation material, postoperative MR can always be performed for excellent visualization of the soft tissues (Fig. IIF-13).

CONGENITAL AND DEVELOPMENTAL ANOMALIES

Patients with congenital or developmental anomalies, such as the Chiari malformations with disturbed CSF circulation, achondroplasia with a narrow foramen magnum causing cord compression, and odontoideum with instability, may need surgical intervention and postoperative neuroradiologic evaluation. For evaluation of the bony changes of surgery, CT is the best imaging modality (Fig.

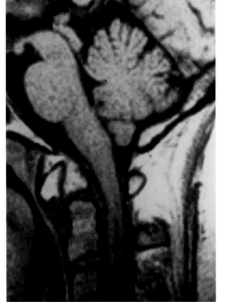

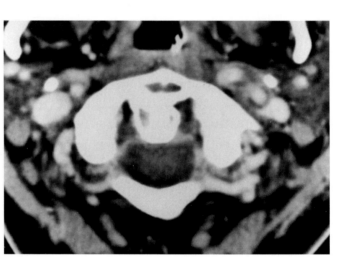

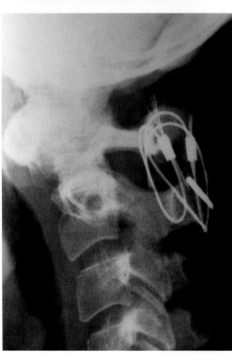

FIG. IIF-18. Patient with os odontoideum threatening cord compression because of instability. **A:** Neutral position MR shows C1-2 subluxation and narrowing of the spinal canal at upper C2 level. **B:** Enhanced axial CT shows the bone elements in better detail and also reveals the flattening of the anterior dural sac. **C:** Postoperative conventional radiography shows fixation and alignment in good position.

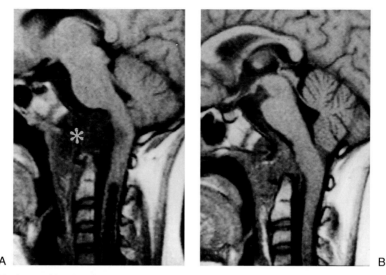

FIG. IIF-19. Patient with chordoma causing disturbed CSF circulation and hydromyelia. **A:** Unenhanced T₁-weighted sagittal MR shows that the relatively low-intensity clival-C1 mass (*asterisk*) results in upper cervical cord compression and syringohydromyelia formation. **B:** Following surgery, there has been a reduction of tumor size and a disappearance of the hydromyelia. (Courtesy of Professor Danielle Baleriaux, Brussels, Belgium.)

IIF-14). Evaluation of the soft tissues may also be required, for instance, to analyze for disappearance of a syringohydromyelic cavity caused by a Chiari malformation or for reduction of cord compression in achondroplasia. This latter is most efficiently accomplished with MR (Figs. IIF-15, IIF-16, and IIF-17). In other patients, gross positional evaluation is sufficient, a judgment that is easily performed with plain films (Fig. IIF-18). In patients with disturbed CSF circulation in this area, the postoperative result following bone resection and duraplasty can

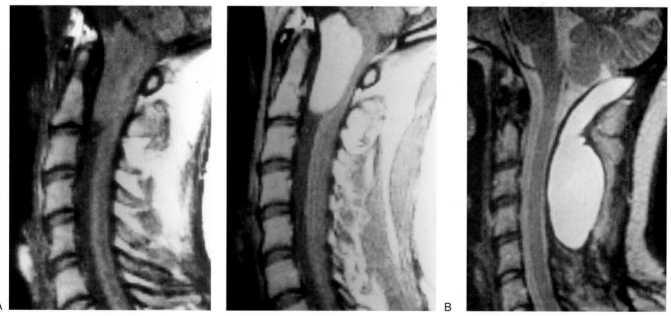

FIG. IIF-20. Paraganglioma of the craniocervical junction. **A:** Unenhanced sagittal T₁-weighted acquisition shows an anteriorly placed tumor at C1-2 compressing the spinal cord posteriorly. **B:** Enhanced T₁-weighted MR shows homogeneous enhancement of the mass. **C:** Sagittal T₂-weighted MR image following surgery shows no remaining tumor or cord compression. However, a postoperative pseudomeningocele has formed posteriorly as a result of a dural leak of CSF.

be evaluated by motion-sensitive MR sequences, and flow velocity can even be measured quantitatively.

TUMORS

A number of tumors can affect this region, including intramedullary tumors such as astrocytomas, ependymomas, and cavernous hemangiomas; intradural extramedullary tumors such as neurinomas or meningeomas; and epidural tumors such as metastases, chordomas, and others. Magnetic resonance is the modality of choice for posttherapeutic evaluation of spinal tumors: MR can reveal residual or recurrent tumors, secondary effects on the cord by the tumor mass, dural herniation, and other complications of surgery (Figs. IIF-19 and IIF-20).

CONCLUSIONS

The type of imaging examination used to evaluate the posttherapeutic craniocervical junction will depend on both the disease mass itself and the type of therapy performed. Posttherapeutic evaluation of the craniocervical junction is often necessary. Conventional radiographs should almost always be obtained for the evaluation of spinal dislocations, and CT should be used to obtain detailed information on bony structure and displacement, especially in cases of torticollis and Jefferson fractures. Magnetic resonance is often necessary for the evaluation of tumors and the soft tissues in rheumatoid arthritis and is invaluable for postoperative analysis of secondary effects such as hydromyelia. Computed tomographic myelography can be used as an alternative to MR in the postoperative evaluation of rheumatoid arthritis.

REFERENCES

1. Redlund-Johnell I, Pettersson H: Radiographic measurements of the craniovertebral region, designed for evaluation of abnormalities in rheumatoid arthritis. *Acta Radiol Diagn* 1984;25:23–28.
2. Pettersson H, Larsson E-M, Holtås S, et al: MRI of the cervical spine in rheumatoid arthritis. *Am J Neuroradiol* 1988;9:573–577.
3. Larsson E-M, Holtås S, Zygmuut S: Pre- and postoperative MR imaging of the craniocervical junction in rheumatoid arthritis. *Am J Neuroradiol* 1989;10:89–94.
4. Holtås S, Wallengren N-O, Ericsson A, Bach-Gausmot T: Signal alterations, artifacts and image distortion induced by a superparamagnetic contrast medium. A phantom study in a 0.3 Tesla MR system. *Acta Radiol* 1990;31:213–216.
5. Zygmunt S, Säveland H, Brattström H, et al: Reduction of rheumatoid periodontoid pannus following posterior occipito-cervical fusion visualised by magnetic resonance imaging. *Br J Neurosurg* 1988;2:315–320.

PART III

The Spine

Posttherapeutic Neurodiagnostic Imaging,
edited by J.R. Jinkins,
Lippincott-Raven Publishers, New York © 1997.

CHAPTER IIIA

The Posttherapeutic Cervicothoracic Spine

Jill Thompson, Michelle Smith, Mauricio Castillo, and Suresh K. Mukherji

Correct interpretation of images of the postsurgical spine requires knowledge of the underlying pathology and of the surgical procedure performed. Because of differences in embryologic origins and biomechanics, we have divided the cervical spine into two sections: upper (base of the skull to C2) and lower (C3 to C7). Surgical techniques from each section are divided into those performed via anterior and posterior approaches. The indications and hardware utilized are different for each surgical approach. In addition to bony abnormalities, we have included discussions on the posttherapeutic appearance of the spinal cord. There is a relative paucity of literature on this latter subject; therefore, the ideas expressed in these sections are mostly based on our experience.

UPPER CERVICAL SPINE

The craniocervical junction and upper cervical spine (C1 and C2) can be surgically approached either posteriorly or anteriorly. Because of the unique biomechanics of the occipitocervical and atlantoaxial articulations, the techniques for fixation and fusion of the upper cervical spine are different from those employed for the lower cervical spine (C3 to C7). The posterior approach is generally used for fusions and decompressions. It provides access to the foramen magnum, spinous processes, laminae, facets, and spinal cord. The posterior approach is the most frequently used and the safest for fixation of the upper cervical spine. Posterior fixation of the occipitocervical joints may be achieved with occipitocervical plates, Luque rectangles, or wiring techniques. Bone grafts are often added to promote fusion. Multiple techniques have been developed to stabilize the atlantoaxial joint posteriorly using wires, cables, titanium plates, clamps, screws, and bone-grafting materials.

J. Thompson, M. Smith, M. Castillo, and S. K. Mukherji: Section of Neuroradiology, Department of Radiology, University of North Carolina School of Medicine, Chapel Hill, North Carolina 27599.

Anterior Surgical Approaches

Over the past 60 years, different anterior approaches have been developed for surgical access to the upper cervical spine. The three most commonly used anterior approaches include the transoral, anterior retropharyngeal, and anterolateral retropharyngeal approaches (1). Each approach has its own risks and benefits. The transoral approach is the most direct; however, it is transpalatal and carries a postoperative infection rate of up to 50% (1). The other two anterior approaches are extramucosal, have a much lower incidence of infection, and, therefore, are more amenable to bone grafting.

The anterior retropharyngeal approach allows for wide exposure and for bone strut graft placement. Of the three anterior approaches, the anterior retropharyngeal approach provides the least exposure to the basiocciput.

Transoral Approach

The transoral anterior approach is useful in selected patients, particularly those with basilar settling or congenital deformities and those requiring resections of the odontoid, drainage of C1 or C2 abscess, or biopsy of a tumor in the anterior arch of C1 or body of C2 (1). This surgical approach carries risks of infectious complications and of limited exposure (1). The patient is placed in the supine position with the neck slightly extended. The face and oropharynx are prepped. A Dingman retractor is used to provide good visualization of the oral cavity. The uvula and soft palate are retracted superiorly by a rubber catheter passed through the nares. The anterior tubercle of C1 and body of C2 can then be palpated. Fluoroscopy or lateral radiographs can be obtained to better define the bony anatomy. A midline longitudinal incision is made in the posterior pharyngeal wall, through the retropharyngeal tissue, and in the anterior longitudinal ligament from C1 to C3, allowing access to the vertebrae and disk spaces. After completion of the procedure, the pharyngeal incisions are closed in layers.

Patients with rheumatoid arthritis may also develop instability at the atlantoaxial joint, which requires fusion. This disease generally involves the dens, necessitating transoral decompression of the medulla followed by a posterior fusion procedure. If the fusion of C1 to C2 is insufficient or impossible to perform because of basilar settling, the dens may be transorally resected, and posterior fusion performed from the occiput to C2.

Anterior Retropharyngeal Approach

After the patient has been placed in the supine position, a T-shaped incision is made with its upper transverse segment in the right submandibular region. A vertical limb provides for additional exposure. The transverse incision is carried deep to the platysma muscle, and subplatysmal flaps are raised. The exposure is kept deep to the retromandibular vein to prevent injury to the facial nerve. The dissection is continued until the hyoid bone and hypopharynx can be mobilized medially, thus avoiding contamination from the mucosa of the nasopharynx, hypopharynx, and esophagus. The carotid artery, jugular vein, submandibular gland, floor-of-mouth musculature, and lingual, hypoglossal, superior laryngeal, and vagus nerves are carefully identified and isolated. The alar and prevertebral fascias are then divided longitudinally, and the longus colli muscles are exposed. These muscles are dissected subperiosteally, providing access to the anterior tubercle of C1 and the body of C2. This approach is used for lesions extending from the clivus to C3, particularly when use of bone-grafting material is indicated.

Spinal fusion for upper cervical trauma is indicated for unstable injuries, fractures prone to nonunion, and for decompression of the spinal canal (2). The anterior retropharyngeal approach provides greater exposure from the

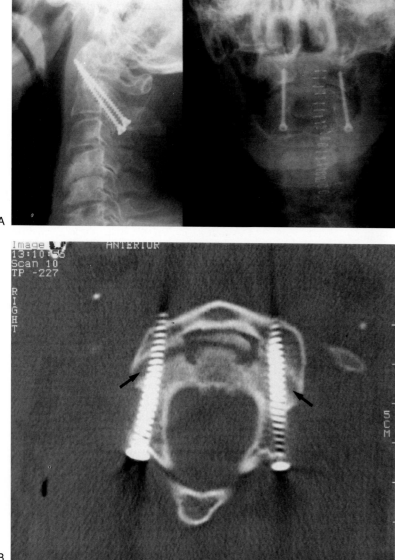

FIG. IIIA-1. Transarticular screws. **A:** Frontal and lateral plain radiographs immediately after procedure show bilateral screws extending from the articular pillars of C2 to the lateral masses of C1. **B:** Oblique coronal CT (bone windows) shows both screws crossing the facet joints (*arrows*) of C1-2.

clivus to C3 and may be used to stabilize fractures from the occiput to C3. Jefferson fractures usually do not require surgical stabilization unless there is 7 mm or more of combined displacement of the lateral masses of C1 on the open-mouth radiograph (2). This is an unstable condition that indicates rupture of the transverse ligament.

Displaced or type II odontoid fractures are frequently associated with nonunion and require fusion (2). Odontoid fractures are typically stabilized by threaded cannulated screws placed via an anterior retropharyngeal approach. If cannulated screws are used, they are advanced over guide pins or wires that have been placed from the inferior C2 body superiorly into the dens, traversing the odontoid fracture. Alternatively, Knoringer screws can be placed primarily across the fracture in a similar trajectory. These screws are threaded at different pitches at both ends and thus achieve compression across the fracture site because of the differential advancement rate of the two ends of the screw. An alternative approach for achieving stability in these patients is transarticular screw fixation of C1 to C2 from a posterior approach (3) (Fig. IIIA-1). This approach tends to be safer but may limit rotational range of motion postoperatively. Some dens fractures heal normally with just external immobilization (Fig. IIIA-2).

Anterolateral Retropharyngeal Approach

The patient is placed in the supine position with the neck extended and head maximally turned. Traction with tongs or a halo device is used. A hockey-stick-shaped incision is made along the anterior border of the sterno-cleidomastoid muscle crossing the base of the temporal bone superiorly. The sternocleidomastoid muscle is mobilized and everted, and the external jugular vein and occipital artery are ligated. Care should be taken to avoid injury to the greater auricular and spinal accessory nerves. Dissection is continued in the retropharyngeal space laterally and posteriorly to the carotid artery sheath. A plane between the alar and prevertebral fascias is created to expose the anterior aspect of the vertebral bodies. The anterior longitudinal ligament is incised in the midline. The proce-

dure is repeated on the opposite side to allow for greater exposure.

The anterolateral approach is used for fusion of C1 to C2 when the posterior ring of C1 is absent or hypoplastic (1). This procedure avoids occiput-to-C2 fusion. The anterolateral retropharyngeal approach tends to have a higher complication rate in patients with rheumatoid arthritis. Alternative approaches should be considered in these patients (1).

Posterior Surgical Approaches

Indications for posterior occipitocervical fusion include instability, intractable neck pain, cervical osteoporosis with loss of bone substance, and severe rheumatoid arthritis that results in spinal cord compression (2). Rarely, occipitocervical fusions are performed in cases of trauma such as those surviving occipitocervical dislocations or in patients with unstable C2 teardrop fractures (4). Stability of the occipitocervical joints can be accomplished with the use of Hartshill–Ransford loops, Luque rectangles, or occipitocervical plates (2,4–6). These devices are placed via posterior approach. If a congenital anomaly with flattening of the occiput or basilar impression exists, the posterior aspect of the foramen magnum can be enlarged for decompression in this region prior to fusion (2).

The contoured occipitocervical loop (Hartshill–Ransford loop) was developed to maintain occipitocervical and atlantoaxial stability and to control progressive vertical migration of the dens (Fig. IIIA-3). The loops were initially used for the treatment of rheumatoid arthritis, but have also been used for patients with congenital malformations, tumors, complicated fractures, degenerative spondylosis, and "bone-softening" conditions such as osteogenesis imperfecta (6). The loops are available in multiple sizes to accommodate pediatric patients and those requiring occipitothoracic fusion. The loop is attached to the occiput with wires and to the posterior elements with sublaminar wires. Bone-grafting material may be placed to facilitate fusion.

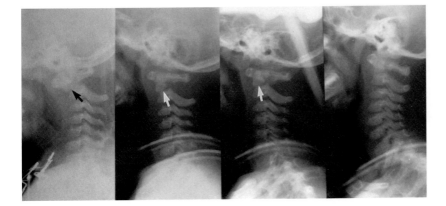

FIG. IIIA-2. External immobilization for dens fracture. Series of lateral radiographs beginning (**left**) immediately after trauma, after initial external immobilization, at 2 weeks, and at 6 weeks after the trauma show adequate healing of type 2 dens fracture (*arrows*) in a child.

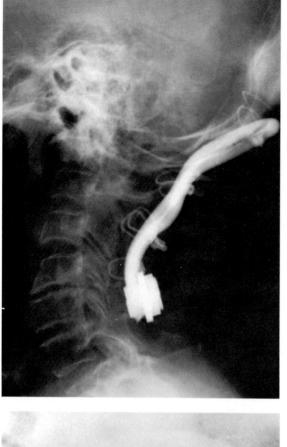

A

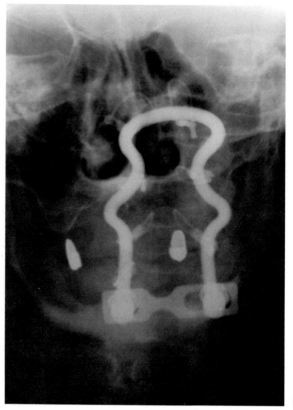

B

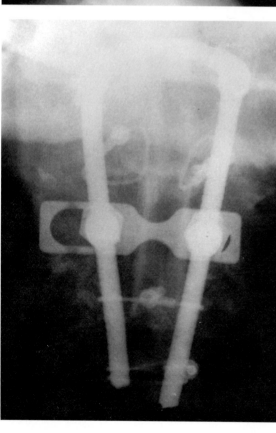

C

FIG. IIIA-3. Hartshill—Ransford loop. **A:** Lateral radiograph shows loop extending from C5-6 to the occiput attached by wires to laminae of several vertebrae and the occipital bone. **B:** Frontal radiograph in same patient shows that the loop has been contoured to fit the patient. The inferior plate holds to loop and prevents it from springing open. **C:** Frontal radiograph from a another patient shows a different contour to this loop.

Luque rectangles are smooth, round rods prebent into a square or shaped as needed to accommodate the occipitocervical junction. The Luque rectangle is fixed to the occiput with wires through the outer table of the calvarium and fixed to the cervical spine with sublaminar wires (Fig. IIIA-4). Occipitocervical plates and Luque rectangles require the placement of bone-graft material to promote fusion.

Occipitocervical plates are special metal plates that are preformed to accommodate the base of the skull. Osteosynthesis with plates attempts to maintain the normal occipitocervical angulation of 105°, giving a normal horizontal direction to the eyes (4). The plates are fixed with 13-mm screws to the occiput superiorly and with screws through the articular masses of C1 or C2 inferiorly. Increased morbidity with this technique results from penetration of the inner table of the calvarium. Occipitocervical plates are currently not FDA-approved for use in the United States.

Basilar impression is an upward movement of the base of the skull in the region of the foramen magnum. It is measured by the intracranial extension of the tip of the odontoid. Patients tend to present in childhood or early adult life with cerebellar and brainstem symptoms occurring from compression by the odontoid (7). Symptoms include extremity weakness with or without spasticity, sensory deficits, cerebellar ataxia, lower cranial nerve dysfunction, and vertebral artery insufficiency. The Arnold–Chiari malformation, syringomyelia, and severe kyphoscoliosis may occur in conjunction with basilar impression (7).

The Arnold–Chiari I malformation consists of displacement of the cerebellar tonsils inferiorly through the foramen magnum into the cervical spinal canal (8). The fourth ventricle remains normally positioned. Reported associations include syringomyelia and anomalies of the occipitocervical junction. Patients may become symptomatic in late childhood or early adulthood. Symptoms include facial pain, deafness, vertigo, paresthesias, and cerebellar signs. The Arnold–Chiari type II malformation consists of displacement of the brainstem and inferior cerebellum into the cervical canal (8). The fourth ventricle is elongated and flattened with no obvious lateral recesses. There may be cervicomedullary kinking and upper cervical cord compression. The bony posterior fossa is small. As in the Chiari I malformation, Chiari II also occurs in combination with other congenital malformations of the upper cervical spine. Patients may present with hydrocephalus, spina bifida, diastematomyelia, or myelomeningocele. The Chiari malformations type I and type II may

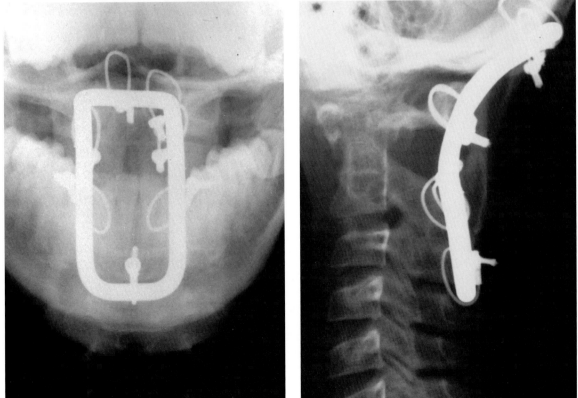

A   B

FIG. IIIA-4. Luque rectangle. **A:** Frontal radiograph shows a Luque rectangle at the posterior craniocervical junction attached to laminae and occiput with Songer cables. **B:** Lateral radiograph in same patient shows rectangle extending from C4 to occipital bones. This patient survived an atlantooccipital dislocation.

require surgical treatment secondary to compression of the medulla and spinal cord. Treatment consists of decompression and fusion and is best accomplished by suboccipital craniectomy and C1 and/or C2 laminectomy followed by fusion (2) (Fig. IIIA-5). Less frequently, compression occurs anteriorly as the odontoid protrudes through the foramen magnum. In these cases, the odontoid can be resected via a transoral approach, and posterior fusion performed for stabilization.

Occipitalization of the atlas is a skeletal abnormality of the upper cervical spine (9). The fusion typically occurs between the anterior ring of C1 and the foramen magnum. A fragment from the posterior arch of C1 may constrict the spinal canal and cause intermittent symptoms depending on head position. Clinically, patients present with symptoms of upper spinal cord compression. The surgical treatment of this condition is essentially the same as that for basilar impression and Chiari malformations and consists of decompression and fixation.

Atlantoaxial instability is defined with reference to measurement of the atlantodens interval, with more than 2.5 mm in the adult and 4.5 to 5.0 mm in children being considered abnormal (10). Indications for atlantoaxial fusion include conditions that produce neck pain and/or instability such as trauma with purely ligamentous injury and/or dens fracture, tumors, congenital anomalies, degenerative arthritis, inflammatory arthritis, infection, and postoperative or rotary instability. In cases of atlantoaxial instability, the patient is placed in the prone position, and a lateral cervical radiograph is obtained. A head–halter halo device may be placed preoperatively if there is instability. A 10-cm midline incision is made from the external occipital protuberance to the spinous process of C3. After placement of self-retaining retractors, dissection is continued in the midline, through the supraspinous ligament, to the spinous process of C2. Ligamentous and muscular attachments are removed, and subperiosteal dissection of C2 is performed to expose the facet joints. Dissection is

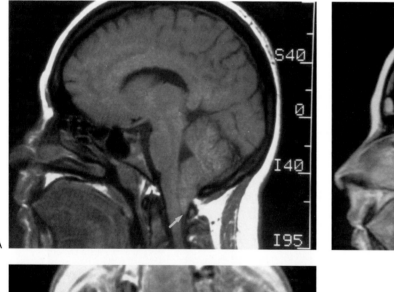

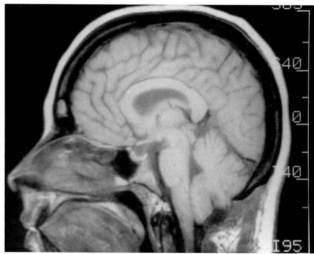

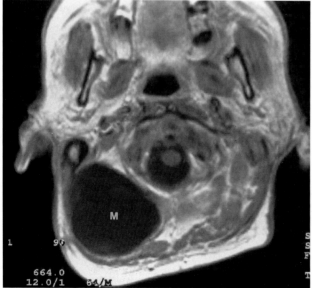

FIG. IIIA-5. Foramen magnum enlargement. **A:** Midsagittal T$_1$-weighted MR image shows typical Chiari type 1 malformation with inferior displacement of the cerebellar tonsils (*arrow*) and a narrowed foramen magnum. **B:** After surgical enlargement of the foramen magnum and lysis of dural bands, the tonsils remain inferiorly placed but with a more normal shape. This patient's symptoms improved after surgery. **C:** Axial T$_1$-weighted MR image in a different patient after decompression of the foramen magnum for Chiari type 1 malformation shows a right-sided postsurgical pseudomeningocele (M).

continued to the base of the occiput and to C1. Dissection at C1 is continued laterally 1.5 cm, with care taken to avoid injury to the vertebral arteries, venous plexuses, and the greater occipital nerves.

Stability of the atlantoaxial joints can be accomplished from a posterior approach with the use of plates, wires, clamps, or screws. Several wiring techniques exist. The technique of C1–C2 fusion is performed by passing stainless steel wire around the posterior arch of C1 and under or through the spinous process of C2 (5). This is referred to as a McLauren fusion. The ends of the wire are twisted together instead of being tied to allow for tension to be adjusted during the procedure. A Brooks fusion uses paired wires or Songer cables that pass under the arch of C1 and around the lamina of C2 (5) (Fig. IIIA-6). Both techniques prevent flexion and, therefore, subluxation of C1 on C2. Bone-grafting material is usually placed between the adjacent laminae or spinous processes to promote fusion. Risks associated with wiring techniques include wire impingement on the underlying cord and wires cutting through weakened bone as they are tightened.

Posterior transarticular screw fixation was introduced by Magerl in 1979 and has become a popular alternative to conventional C1–C2 wiring (3) (Fig. IIIA-7). Transarticular screws pass through the articular pillars of C2 to end in the lateral masses of C1. We perform a preoperative oblique contrast-enhanced axial computed tomography (CT) through the C1–C2 region to evaluate the position of the foramina transversaria and vertebral arteries. The CT illustrates the morphology of this region including bony and arterial anomalies and defines the course of the transarticular screws (11) (Fig. IIIA-1B).

In addition to wiring procedures and transarticular screw placement, laminar (Halifax) clamps may be used for atlantoaxial fixation. Advantages reported with the use of clamps include a reduced risk of dural penetration and neurologic injury (10). Halifax clamps have two C-clamp ends that grip the laminae. Threaded screws hold the C-clamps in place. As the screws are tightened, the C-clamps are drawn together. Often an H-shaped iliac bone graft is placed posteriorly between the adjacent spinous processes to promote fusion. Atlantoaxial fusion is achieved in 12 weeks in 80% of patients using interlaminar clamps (10). Clamp loosening is a potential complication and may result in pseudoarthrosis of the graft.

LOWER CERVICAL SPINE

Anterior Surgical Approaches

The anterior surgical approach was initially described in the 1930s and refined in the 1950s. It offers the most

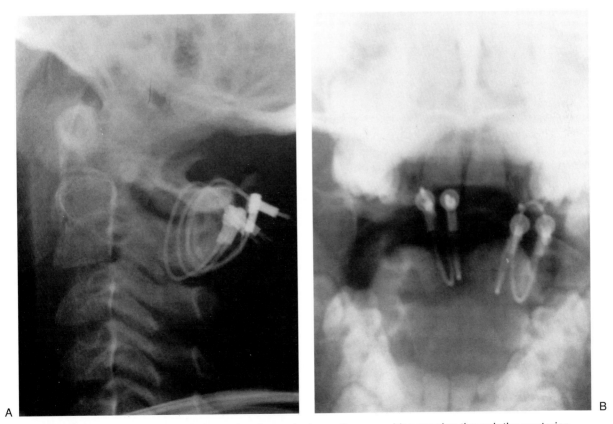

FIG. IIIA-6. Brooks fusion. **A:** Lateral radiograph shows Songer cables passing through the posterior arch of C1 and the laminae of C2. Note normal C1-2 alignment. **B:** Open-mouth frontal radiograph shows both Songer cables in the same patient.

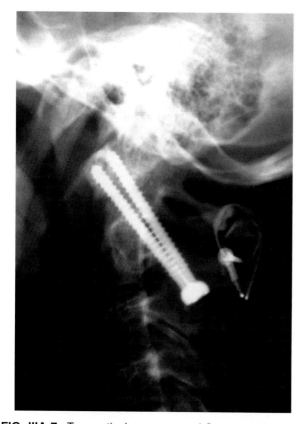

FIG. IIIA-7. Transarticular screws and Songer cables. Lateral radiograph after internal fixation for dens fracture shows Songer cables bridging the posterior arch of C1 to the laminae of C2 and bilateral screws through the C1-2 articulations.

direct method for surgical decompression of the cervical spinal canal. This method is commonly used in the treatment of cervical nerve root or spinal cord compression that results from osteophytes, ossification of the posterior longitudinal ligament (OPLL), congenitally narrowed canal, or herniated disk material. When this surgery is performed exclusively for neck pain, the results are highly variable. According to DePalma et al. (12), good to excellent results were achieved in 63%, and fair results in 29%, of patients in a study of 229 cases treated with an anterior approach for intractable radicular pain. Overall, there is a 60% to 70% improvement rate in neurologic symptoms after anterior cervical procedures (13).

Cervical myelopathy, which is an important indication for anterior canal decompression, is characterized by symptoms of arm pain with paresthesias and weakness, tingling, or numbness in the distal upper extremity, gait disturbance, neck pain, and radicular signs (14). Muscle atrophy and signs of sphincter dysfunction sometimes occur late in the disease. Once the cause for cervical myelopathy has been confirmed, surgical intervention may be indicated. Depending on the extent and size of the

pathology, either a subtotal vertebrectomy and fusion or an anterior diskectomy and fusion will be performed. If the extent of involvement is limited to the intervertebral disk with or without small osteophytes, an anterior diskectomy with fusion may be performed. If the process is more extensive and involves four or more levels, vertebrectomies and long bone strut graft fusion are recommended. Iliac crest grafts are usually used for one-level fusion, and fibular strut grafts are used for fusion of three or more levels. Bone grafts may be obtained from the patient (autologous) or from a graft bank (allografts or homografts). Autologous grafts are preferred by some patients because of the perceived possibility of HIV, hepatitis, and bacterial infection from donor material. However, there is a small risk of infection at the donor site. Pain at the donor site will occur in 15% of patients (13). Rarely, injury to the lateral femoral cutaneous nerve results in myalgic paresthesias. Bone powder and chips are not generally used for anterior spinal fusions. Smaller bone fragments are commonly used for posterior spinal procedures.

Anterior Cervical Diskectomy

Anterior cervical diskectomies and fusion are performed with the patient in head–halter traction or in neutral position via a left-sided neck approach with incision of the prevertebral fascia, exposing the vertebrae and disk spaces. After radiographic confirmation of the desired level(s), all disk material is removed down to the level of the posterior longitudinal ligament and laterally to the uncovertebral joints. Osteophytes are also removed at this time, and if no traction was applied, the vertebrae are then separated from each other with a distractor–spreader. Small inferior and superior posterior lips are left on the vertebral bodies in order to prevent slippage of the subsequent graft material. Likewise, a small anterior lip is left in place to prevent anterior migration. An iliac crest graft is tailored in size and shape, generally that of a plug, and placed within the disk space (Fig. IIIA-8). Decreasing the skeletal traction then locks the graft into place. Anterior fusion with disk removal and placement of a horseshoe-shaped tricortical iliac bone graft is referred to as a Smith–Robinson procedure (14). This procedure has traditionally been the ''gold standard'' for anterior cervical fusions. The Cloward technique entails drilling a hole in the disk space and inserting a prefitted dowel of bone (15). In the Bailey–Badgley procedure, a bone strut graft is utilized (16) (Fig. IIIA-9). After 3 to 5 days of hospitalization, the patient wears a brace for approximately 6 weeks. Six to 12 weeks after surgery, graft incorporation is radiographically evident.

Anterior Cervical Vertebrectomy and Fusion

Anterior vertebrectomies and fusion are performed via a transverse neck incision and mobilization of the deep

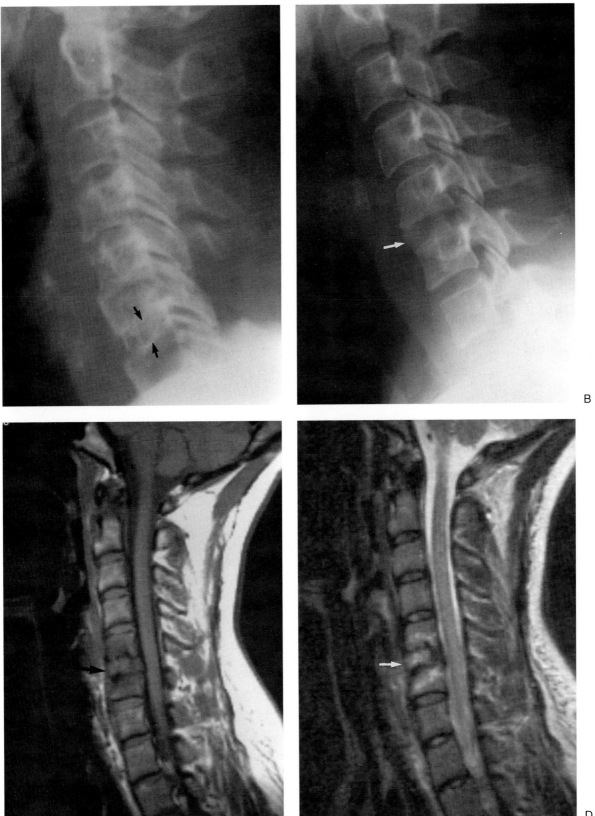

A

B

C

D

FIG. IIIA-8. Bone plug following diskectomy. **A:** Lateral radiograph shows bone plug (*arrows*) at C6-7 secondary to anterior discectomy. There is fusion of C5-6 from prior surgery. **B:** In a different patient, a lateral radiograph shows a bone plug (*arrow*) after a C5-6 diskectomy. **C:** Midsagittal T₁-weighted MR image in same patient shows the bone plug (*arrow*), widening of the disk space, deformity of the adjacent end plates, and signal changes in the bone marrow. **D:** Corresponding T₂-weighted image shows the bone plug (*arrow*) to be bright. The edema of the adjacent end plates is also of increased signal intensity.

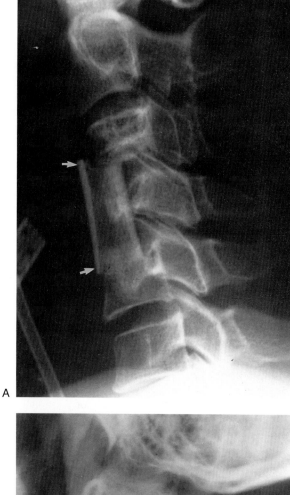

A

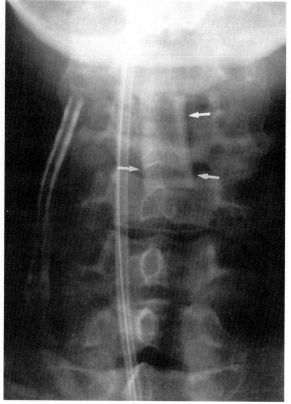

B

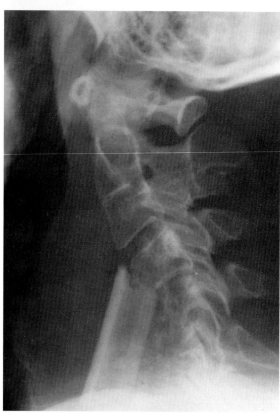

C

FIG. IIIA-9. Bone struts. **A:** Lateral radiograph shows bone strut (*arrows*) extending from C3 to C5 and anterior corpectomy of C4. Note that graft is slightly displaced anteriorly, but this is within acceptable range. **B:** Frontal radiograph in same patient shows graft bone strut (*arrows*). **C:** Lateral radiograph in a different patient following anterior corpectomies of C5 to C7 for osteomyelitis or diskitis shows that the bone strut is markedly displaced anteriorly, and there is exaggerated cervical kyphosis. Note prevertebral soft tissue swelling and congenital fusion of C2-3.

cervical fascia. After diskectomies are performed, the central portions of the vertebral bodies are removed. If the posterior longitudinal ligament is soft, it is removed. After preparation of the end plates and creation of cortical lips (see above), the grafts are locked into the impressions created in the vertebral bodies. Postoperatively, patients are placed in a halo vest for 8 to 12 weeks of immobilization. These patients frequently require postoperative physical therapy and rehabilitation.

Placement of metallic plate and/or screw fixation should be considered following burst fractures, traumatic disk herniation, tumor resection, and grossly unstable injuries (5). Following a corpectomy and removal of disk material below and above the level of corpectomy, a bone graft is placed. Subsequently, a cervical plate is placed anteriorly across the bone graft, and screws are secured to adjacent vertebral bodies, usually two screws above and two screws below. The most commonly used hardware are the Casper and Morscher plates. Caspar plates are trapezoidal in shape, have three rows of holes, and are slightly concave anteriorly to accommodate the vertebral bodies (17) (Fig. IIIA-10). Bicortical (through the anterior and posterior cortices of vertebrae) screws are used for greater stability. Unicortical screws have a smaller incidence of neurologic injury because they do not penetrate the posterior cortex of the vertebral bodies. The Morscher

plate is H-shaped, and its screws are self-locking, preventing them from backing out (18) (Fig. IIIA-11). Some screws have spiral fenestrations that allow the ingrowth of cancellous bone. The initial hollow screw design has been replaced with solid screws because of frequent breakage of the hollow ones. The newer screw system includes lockage by means of an expansion bolt. An additional advantage of titanium hardware is its superior tissue compatibility and increased stealthiness over stainless steel when imaged with CT or MR imaging.

Placement of screws alone is occasionally used as surgical treatment of odontoid fractures, notably types II and III and nonunions. Opinion varies as to which type of screws to use: cortical versus cancellous and cannulated versus noncannulated. Current opinion favors two screws where possible for better rotational stability and the use of safer, cannulated screws. Occasionally, anterior plates and screws are reinforced with posterior plating, thereby producing greater stability.

Intraoperative complications of anterior cervical fusions include arterial (carotid, superior thyroidal, and vertebral) and venous (jugular) laceration, spinal cord injury, esophageal and tracheal injury, and recurrent laryngeal nerve injury (17). Injury to the recurrent laryngeal nerve is the single most common complication of the anterior cervical approach and results in temporary or permanent

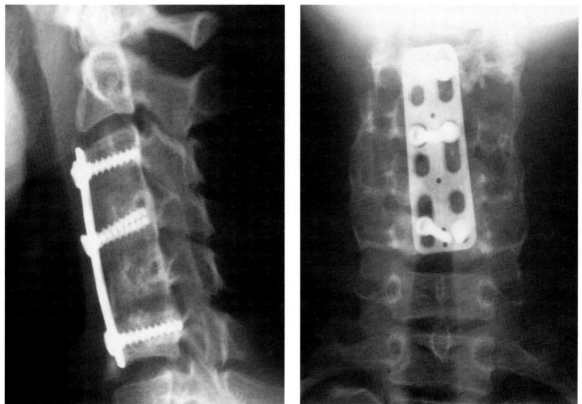

A   B

FIG. IIIA-10. Caspar plate. **A:** Lateral radiograph shows plate extending from C3 to C6 with bicortical screws. Note slight concavity of plate anteriorly to accommodate vertebral bodies. **B:** Frontal radiograph in same patient shows the trapezoidal shape of the Caspar plate.

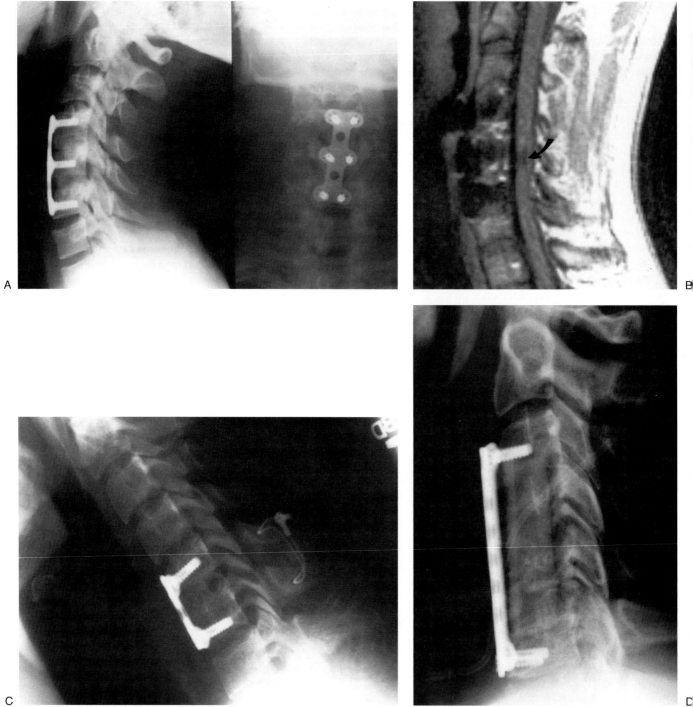

FIG. IIIA-11. Self-locking H-shaped titanium plate (Morscher type). **A:** Lateral and frontal radiographs shows plate extending from C4 to C6 with unicortical screws. Note bone plugs at C4-5 and C5-6 after diskectomies. **B:** Midsagittal T$_1$-weighted MR image in same patient shows only mild artifact from plate; visualization of spinal canal is adequate. The spinal cord shows focal low signal intensity (*arrow*) compatible with myelomalacia. **C:** Short H-shaped plate with unicortical screws at C5-6 with a bone plug at that disk space and Songer cable posteriorly. **D:** Long H-shaped plate extending from C3 to C7 using unicortical screws. There is a bone strut at level of fusion.

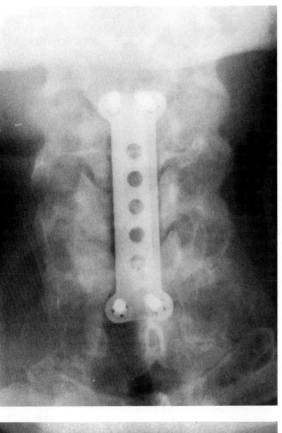

E

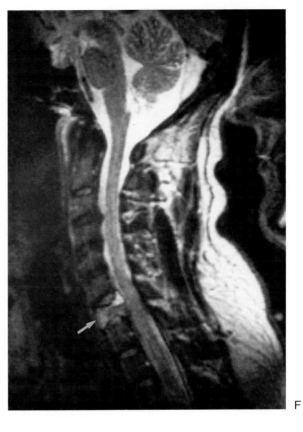

F

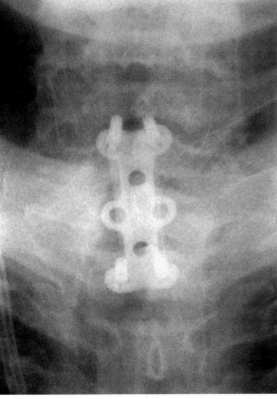

G

FIG. IIIA-11. (*Continued.*) **E:** Frontal radiograph in the same patient shows plate, which obscures the bone strut. **F:** Preoperative mid-sagittal T₂-weighted MR image in a patient with metastatic adeno-carcinoma to C7 (*arrow*). There is compression fracture of the body of C7 and cord compression. **G:** Frontal radiograph in the same patient after C7 corpectomy and placement of H shape.

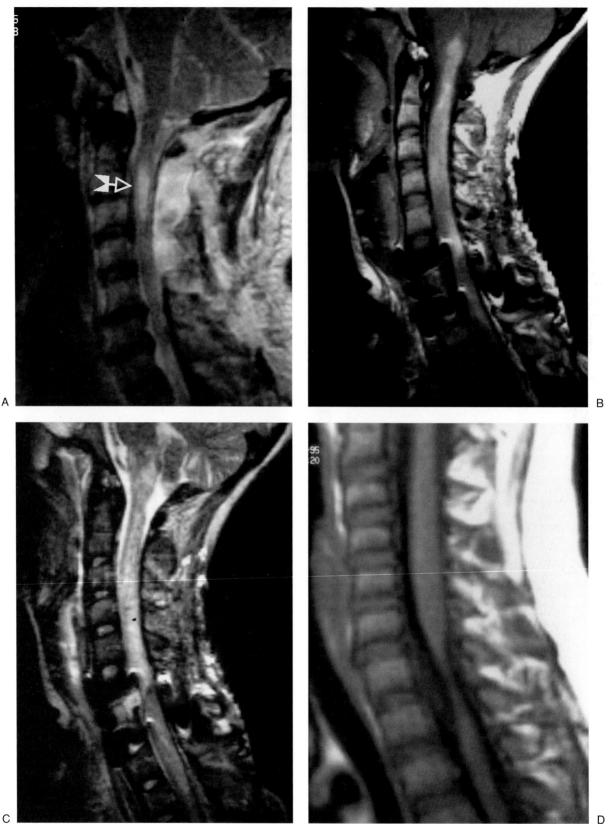

FIG. IIIA-12. Postclosed reduction spinal cord infarction. **A:** Midsagittal T_2-weighted MR image after attempted closed reduction of C2-3 dislocation shows hyperintense zone (*arrow*) in spinal cord, which is also slightly widened in diameter. **B:** Midsagittal T_1-weighted MR image after both closed (initially attempted but failed) and, thereafter, open reduction and fixation of a C6-7 bilateral interfacetal dislocation shows diffuse brightness throughout the cervical spinal cord, which is also expanded. Findings are suggestive of hemorrhagic infarction. **C:** Corresponding T_2-weighted image shows diffuse increased signal intensity in cervical spinal cord extending superiorly to the medulla. Patient expired shortly after this study. **D:** Midsagittal T_1-weighted MR image in a paraplegic child 2 years after cervical spine fracture treated with closed reduction. There is atrophy of the spinal cord suggesting sequelae of infarction.

hoarseness. Right-sided injuries are more common than left-sided ones. Serious injuries to nerve roots and/or the spinal cord occur in 1% to 3% of patients, particularly during closed reduction (Fig. IIIA-12). Computed tomographic myelography or MR is indicated to evaluate for potentially reversible neurologic complications such as acute hematoma. These hematomas acutely appear as an epidural area of medium to low signal intensity on the T_1-weighted images and on T_2-weighted images, reflecting the presence of deoxyhemoglobin. Some hematomas show marginal enhancement after contrast administration. Plain films of the cervical spine should be obtained to evaluate the position of the graft. The bone plug should fit tightly in the intervertebral space. Minimal anterior protrusion is acceptable. Posterior displacement is not normal. Bone struts closely abut the superior and inferior vertebrectomy margins. Ideally, they should not be angled or protrude past a line drawn through the anterior surfaces of the adjacent vertebrae. Persistent CSF leaks will require imaging with plain CT or, preferably, conventional myelography followed by postmyelography CT.

Postoperative infection and abscess formation should be imaged utilizing MR with gadolinium. T_1-weighted contrast-enhanced images will demonstrate an area of thick epidural enhancement with mass effect, posterior displacement of the thecal sac, and occasionally spinal cord compression (Fig. IIIA-13). There may also be enhancement of the underlying disk space. In frank abscesses, the necrotic center does not enhance.

In our experience, most infected disks are hyperintense on T_2-weighted images. After surgery, this sign is not reliable because of the possible presence of blood and/or edema at the disk level.

Within the first few postoperative days, MR imaging reveals discrete rectangular areas of signal abnormality at the superior and inferior corpectomy sites. These vertebral bodies may demonstrate low T_1 and high T_2 signal intensities, consistent with edema. Even after several years, there will continue to be signal intensity abnormalities within the adjacent vertebral bodies, which will vary from iso- to hypointense on T_1-weighted images to iso- or hyperintense on T_2-weighted images. In our experience, unstable graft sites result in prolonged edema in the adjacent vertebrae, whereas stable grafts are characterized by either fatty infiltration or sclerosis at the corpectomy sites. Additionally, the graft itself should continue to be recognized as a rectangular area of variable signal intensity (19). The

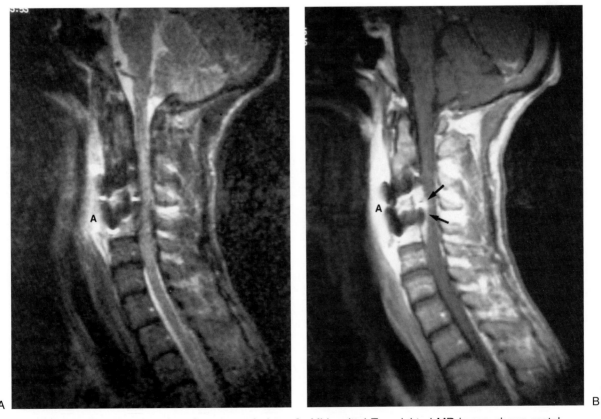

FIG. IIIA-13. Abscess after placement of plate. **A:** Midsagittal T_2-weighted MR image shows metal artifact at C3 to C5 from plate. Note precervical bright abscess (**A**) and compression of spinal cord, which also shows some increased signal intensity (edema?). **B:** Corresponding postcontrast T_1-weighted image shows enhancement of epidural abscess (*arrows*) centered at C4 and enhancement of precervical abscess (A) component.

signal intensity of an autologous bone graft is variable and reflects the state of its marrow (fatty versus cellular). The cortex of autologous bone grafts is always of low T_1 and T_2 signal intensity. Their marrow cavity may be of intermediate signal intensity on T_1- and T_2-weighted images, reflecting cellular marrow, or of high T_1 signal intensity, reflecting a fatty marrow. Bone struts from the graft bank are devoid of bone marrow and freeze-dried. These grafts show low T_1 and T_2 cortical signal intensity as well as absent signal centrally. However, intragraft signal intensity may be variable because of hemorrhage. Marginal and central enhancement may be seen chronically in all types of grafts because of proliferation of granulation tissue and graft incorporation. After successful incorporation, the graft itself should not be clearly definable (19).

Cervical canal stenosis, defined as an anteroposterior canal diameter of less than 1.0 cm, is a significant and abnormal postoperative finding that generally results from hypertrophic bone formation at the levels above and below the surgical decompression site. Degenerative changes of the disk space above and below the graft fusion site occur secondary to increased biomechanical stress at those levels. This new bone is isointense to the vertebral body on T_1-weighted images and may produce a mass effect on the subarachnoid space and spinal cord. On T_2-weighted or gradient-echo images, these osteophytes produce low signal intensity. Occasionally, posterior graft extrusion may cause a functional canal stenosis and cord compression at the corpectomy site (2). In addition, the bone graft material itself may hypertrophy, producing spinal canal stenosis. Delayed graft complications include settling of the graft and telescoping in either caudal or cephalad directions (2). Pseudoarthroses may be seen with long strut grafts and require revision surgery. Pseudoarthroses are directly proportional to the number of levels fused. Therefore, they are more common in multilevel fusions. Approximately 10% to 15% of patients with single-level fusions will eventually develop a pseudoarthrosis at the surgery site; MR or CT myelography may be obtained to evaluate for neural compression.

Metallic artifacts that degrade MR image quality may occur even in the absence of plate or screws and in the presence of plain radiographs in which no metal is seen (Fig. IIIA-14). These artifacts are believed to be secondary to microscopic metal fragments shearing off the drill bits during surgery. The appearance of these artifacts "blooms" on gradient echo images because of their in-

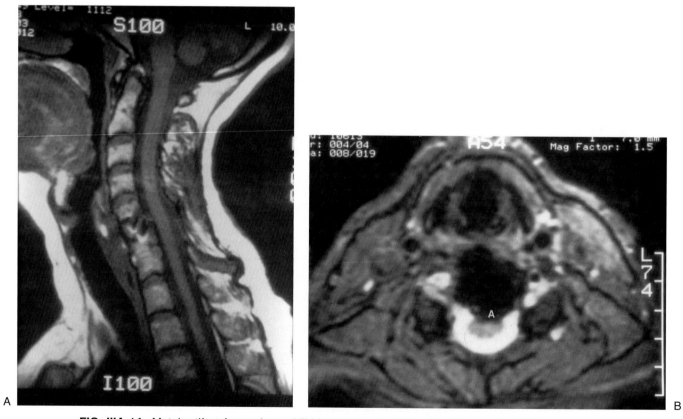

FIG. IIIA-14. Metal artifact from minute drill-bit particles. **A:** Midsagittal T_1-weighted MR image in a patient (same as Fig. IIIA-8) in whom a plain radiograph did not show any metal. Note artifacts presumably arising from microscopic drill-bit particles deposited at diskectomy site. **B:** Axial gradient-echo T_2-weighted image at C5-6 level shows marked susceptibility artifact (A) simulating a large ventral epidural defect.

herent sensitivity to alterations in the magnetic microenvironment (20). For this reason, we routinely image the postoperative cervical spine with sagittal MR fast spin-echo sequences, which are less sensitive to magnetic susceptibility effects. In our experience, it is not possible to estimate the degree of artifact that will be produced by different types of hardware. Because the alternative to MR imaging is generally a myelogram followed by CT scanning, we attempt to image all patients with MR initially.

Posterior Surgical Approaches

The posterior surgical approach is the most commonly performed technique for decompression of the cervical spinal canal and stabilization of the cervical spine. Although the posterior approach offers adequate decompression of the spinal canal, narrowing of the neural foramina cannot be treated with this type of surgery alone unless a concomitant foraminotomy is performed. The posterior approach was developed many years before the anterior cervical approach came into existence. A posterior approach affords considerable access to the posterior elements of the spinal canal, allowing for firm attachment of wires, bone grafts, methylmethacrylate implants, decompressive laminectomies, and fusions. Complications inherent to the anterior approach, including hoarseness, tracheoesophageal tears, tracheal perforation, and carotid artery injury, are avoided with the posterior approach.

In the presence of myelopathic changes and referred pain not responsive to conservative treatment and physical therapy, surgical intervention may be indicated. Three basic posterior approaches for degenerative disease of the cervical spine are available: laminotomy/diskectomy, laminectomy, and laminaplasty (21). Additionally, the wire technique of posterior stabilization may be employed for lower cervical arthrodeses, both with and without plates and screws. The latter is commonly used in the trauma and/or unstable patient.

Posterior laminotomy and diskectomy may be used in the decompression of posterior cervical disk herniations and osteophytes, usually limited to one level (21). Narrowing of a neural foramen by a disk or osteophyte necessitates a foraminotomy. After the patient has been placed in the prone position, appropriate traction is applied. A 3- to 4-cm incision followed by retraction of the paraspinous muscles is performed, exposing the spinous processes. Subsequently, for each level, one or two laminae are either removed or partially drilled, followed by removal of the ligamentum flavum and epidural venous plexus and nerve root retraction to facilitate exposure of the lateral disk space. Following incision of the posterior longitudinal ligament, the extruded disk material and/or osteophytes are removed. Exposure of a neural foramen may necessitate a partial facetectomy. Henderson and associates report satisfactory operative results in 96% of patients in a series of 846 cases using this procedure for posterior disk disease (21). Complications of the posterior approach include wound infection, air embolism, and nerve root compression. Generally, the overall complication rate is comparable to that of the anterior approach (21).

The posterior approach with laminectomy and foraminotomy is favored by some over the anterior approach for the treatment of multilevel spondylitic radiculopathy (22). The patient is placed in the prone position, and a midline incision is made. After adequate exposure of the soft tissues and ligaments, the spinous processes are removed. Multiple laminectomies and foraminotomies are performed, and decompression is carried out to the facets. At this point, consideration to posterior bone fusion should be given. Complications include hematoma, infection, direct cord injury with or without permanent neural deficit, instability, and pseudomeningocele formation (23).

A procedure for increasing the overall canal diameter, a laminaplasty, may be performed in cases of myelopathy secondary to canal stenosis, multilevel spondylosis, and ossification of the posterior longitudinal ligament (OPLL) (21). During this procedure, the spinal processes and laminae are partially resected, a bony gutter is drilled laterally, and the thinned border of the laminae is excised. Subsequently, a second bony gutter is drilled in the contralateral laminae and sutured to prevent this laminar door from closing. The laminae and spinous processes are pushed laterally as in "opening a door," and the bases of all spinous processes are sutured to keep the "door" open (Fig. IIIA-15). The canal diameter may be expanded by approximately 5 mm while its bony architecture is preserved, obviating the need for a posterior stabilization procedure (24). Most complications are secondary to the misplacement of the bony "door" and recurrence of cervical spinal canal narrowing. Transient paresis of the shoulder girdle muscles with severe neck pain may result from a tethering effect on the lower cervical nerve roots immediately postoperatively (24). This complication resolves with conservative treatment in most patients.

Several procedures may be used to stabilize the cervical spine posteriorly. These include (a) interspinous wiring, (b) wraparound interspinous wiring, (c) facet wiring with bone graft, (d) interfacet wiring, and (e) interspinous wiring reinforced with methylmethacrylate. Interspinous wiring, known as the Rogers or modified Rogers technique, is utilized in the lower (C2 to C7) cervical spine. These procedures usually involve fusion of several spinous processes, facets, or laminae with bone-graft placement.

For interspinous wiring, holes are drilled in the outer cortex of the spinous processes near the laminae, and wires are passed through them in adjacent vertebrae. The ends of the wires are then twisted (5). Because the spinal canal is not entered, this is probably the safest posterior spinal procedure. Bone grafts may be secondarily attached

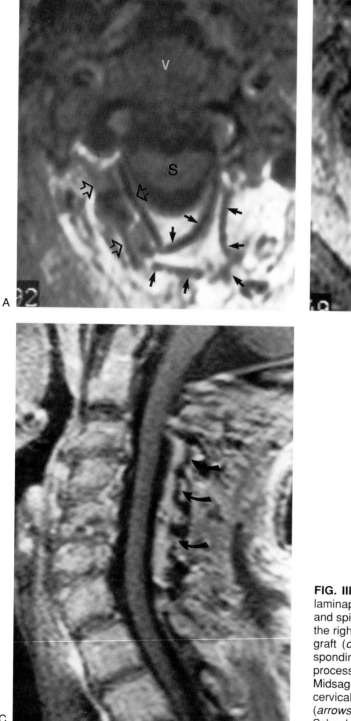

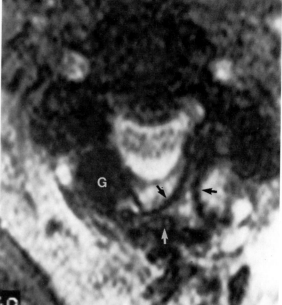

FIG. IIIA-15. Laminoplasty. **A:** Axial T₁-weighted MR image after laminaplasty shows "hinged door" created by rotation of the lamina and spinous process (*small solid arrows*) from right to left. Between the right articular pillar and the rotated lamina, there is a bone strut graft (*open arrows*). S, spinal cord; V, vertebral body. **B:** Corresponding T₂-weighted image shows rotated laminae and spinous process (*arrows*) and blooming artifact from strut bone graft (G). **C:** Midsagittal T₁-weighted image in same patient shows expansion of cervical spinal canal from C3 to C6 created by laminaplasties (*arrows*). (Case courtesy R. M. Quencer, M.D., University of Miami School of Medicine, Miami, Florida.)

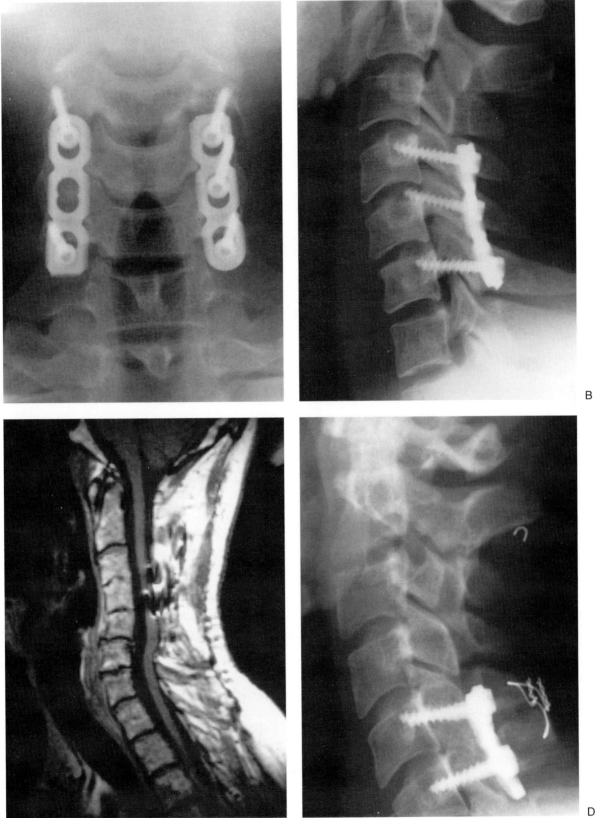

FIG. IIIA-16. Malleable lateral mass plate fixation. **A:** Frontal radiograph shows bilateral metal plates in lateral masses. Note usage of two screws in right side and three screws in left plate. **B:** Lateral view of same patient shows superimposed plates extending from C4 to C6. **C:** Midsagittal T_1-weighted MR image in a different patient with posterior plate fixation at C3-4 shows artifact that partially obscures visualization of the spinal cord, which is atrophic. **D:** Lateral radiograph in a different patient shows lateral mass plates at C5-6 in combination with interspinous wiring at this level. A fragment from a prior broken wire is present superiorly.

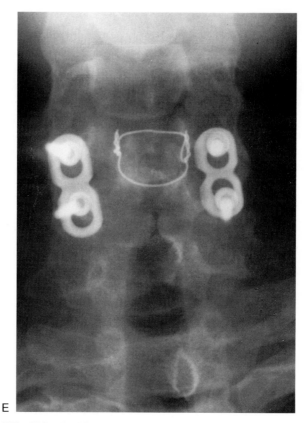

FIG. IIIA-16. (*Continued.*) **E:** Frontal radiograph in the same patient shows short plates and wire.

with wires. Open reduction of cervical spine dislocations and posterior wiring without arthrodesis are not recommended because of the possibility of redislocation.

For facet wiring, holes are drilled in the posterior pillars of the facets, and wires are passed through them. These wires are tied around bone-graft struts. This procedure is fairly safe, as the spinal canal is not entered, and is among the strongest fusions. However, vertebral artery injury is a potentially serious complication.

Sublaminar wiring is favored by many surgeons. This simple procedure involves placement of wire loops around both sides of adjacent laminae. For greater tensile strength, 16 to 18-gauge Luque wires or braided Songer steel cables are employed. At our institution, the latter are preferred for their malleability and snap-lock mechanism. In addition, bone grafts may be placed over the fusion site.

Posterior plating may be used for greater stability. Specially designed posterior cervical plates, Haid plates, are made of titanium and are slightly concave in cross section to accommodate the shape of the spine (5) (Fig. IIIA-16). As with plates in any spinal fixation procedure, titanium plates cause fewer artifacts than stainless steel plates when imaging is done with MR. These plates are attached with screws placed through holes drilled into the articular facets. Malleable plates may be used for areas with un-

usual contours (5). Hook plates or laminar clamps (Halifax clamps) can also be used. The Halifax clamp is a method of posterior stabilization that works by attaching the clamp to adjoining laminae and tightening it until no movement is possible (25). This procedure is commonly utilized for atlantoaxial stabilization and only occasionally used in the lower posterior cervical spine. Often, an H-shaped bone graft is inserted between two spinous processes to encourage bony fusion. Complications unique to plate-and-screw fixations include misplaced screws causing nerve root damage, fracturing or loosening of the devices, bone-graft dislodgement, pseudarthrosis, and instability or failed fusion.

Imaging of the postoperative cervical spine is aimed at identifying potentially reversible complications. These include hematomas, collapse of the vertebral bodies, and extrusion of graft material. Extrusion of graft material occurs most frequently in patients with residual instability (21). The complications can be evaluated by plain films initially and followed by MR imaging and/or CT with or without myelography. Dural tears are typically not identified on imaging studies but may lead to delayed infection, fistulas, or pseudomeningocele. As with any operative procedure, sepsis may occur, and meningitis may result. Delayed postoperative MR imaging of the cervical spine includes evaluation of the bone-graft material and position, nonunion, hypertrophy with canal impingement, resorption of bone around and under implants, degenerative changes above and below the level of the fusion, and recurrent or subsequent herniations. Additionally, because of decreased mobility, patients who have undergone surgery and fixation are prone to adjacent fractures. Complications related to wiring include fractures and loosening of the wires and fractures of the lamina or facets through which the wires were placed.

THORACIC SPINE

Thoracic spine fixation provides stability and restores anatomic alignment in the treatment of fractures, degenerative disease, infection, and tumor. It may also be used to correct congenital deformities such as scoliosis and kyphosis. Internal fixation devices are used to reduce deformities and fractures, to provide spine stability, and to replace vertebrae destroyed by disease. The devices are placed to provide stabilization initially, but most will eventually fail secondary to inadequate strength and prolonged stress. For this reason, these devices are used in conjunction with bone fusion, which maintains long-term position and alignment.

The most common indications for thoracic spinal fixation are scoliosis correction, fracture stabilization, and treatment of degenerative disk disease. Instability occurring as a result of failed surgery is another indication for surgical stabilization of the thoracic spine. Surgical intervention in patients with thoracic trauma is indicated for treatment of instability and spinal canal narrowing. Motor vehicle accidents and falls are the most common causes of fractures of the thoracic spine. Although only a few patients with these injuries have neurologic deficits, spinal fixation may be indicated in these patients to prevent late deformities such as progressive axial vertebral compression and kyphosis.

Scoliosis is another common indication for thoracic spinal fixation. In these patients, surgery is indicated to prevent progressive angulation, pain, and pulmonary and neurologic compromise. Idiopathic scoliosis is a lateral spinal curvature that occurs because of impaired spinal column development. We suggest that patients with idiopathic scoliosis who have other congenital anomalies, unusual curve patterns, and rapidly progressive scoliosis should undergo preoperative MR imaging to define the anatomy of the spinal canal and position of the conus medullaris (to exclude tethering). The MR may be used to detect clinically silent syringomyelia, which has recently been shown to occur in up to 20% of patients with juvenile idiopathic scoliosis (26). The Cobb angle is the internationally accepted method for measuring the magnitude of spinal curvatures in frontal radiographs (27). The degree of scoliosis is measured in the upright position. The first normally angled end plates above and below the curvature

are used as the upper and lower limits of the curve. Curve flexibility on traction radiographs also provides a useful indicator of correctability. Surgery is indicated when the curvature exceeds 45° in a patient with scoliosis (27). Surgical goals are to reduce the curvature to the maximum degree that spinal cord safety permits, restore anteroposterior spinal balance, and fuse as few segments as possible. Surgical revisions may become necessary because of continued growth.

Anterior Approach

The anterior approach to thoracic spinal fixation was first described in 1906 but did not become an accepted procedure until the 1930s, when it was used for the treatment of tuberculosis and spondylolisthesis (28). The anterior approach refers to the placement of instrumentation on the anterior spinal column rather than to the method of surgical exposure. The anterior approach is indicated for the treatment of degenerative disease, failed posterior fusion, high-grade spondylolisthesis, infection, and some vertebral body neoplasms. This approach is also used for anterior decompression in cases of spinal trauma when bone fragments from a vertebral body fracture compress the spinal canal. With this approach, the hardware is usually attached to the lateral aspect of the vertebral bodies. Methylmethacrylate cement and bone grafts are used in conjunction with the rods after corpectomy. Additional stability may be achieved with the use of anterior plates that maintain position but do not correct deformity. Plating is used to treat progressive kyphosis, pseudoarthroses, and failed posterior surgery.

Potential intraoperative complications of the anterior approach include vascular, pleural, and pulmonary injury. Postoperative complications may include ileus, hematoma, and infection. Inaccurate placement of anterior fusion devices may result in impingement on exiting nerves, contact with vascular structures, or penetration of the opposite cortex, which may encroach on the cord (23).

Posterior Approach

This is the most common approach for stabilization of the thoracic spine. A posterior midline incision is made and allows access to the posterior elements, spinal canal, and disk spaces. Laminotomies and/or laminectomies may be performed to provide access for decompression of fractures, diskectomy, and other causes for thoracic spinal canal stenosis. The majority of fixation devices that are used in the thoracic spine are placed from a posterior approach and are secured to the posterior elements. Stability and correction of deformity are achieved in the thoracic spine by the combination of spinal rods and other fixation devices (Fig. IIIA-17). Spinal rods are able to span long segments. The two most commonly used tho-

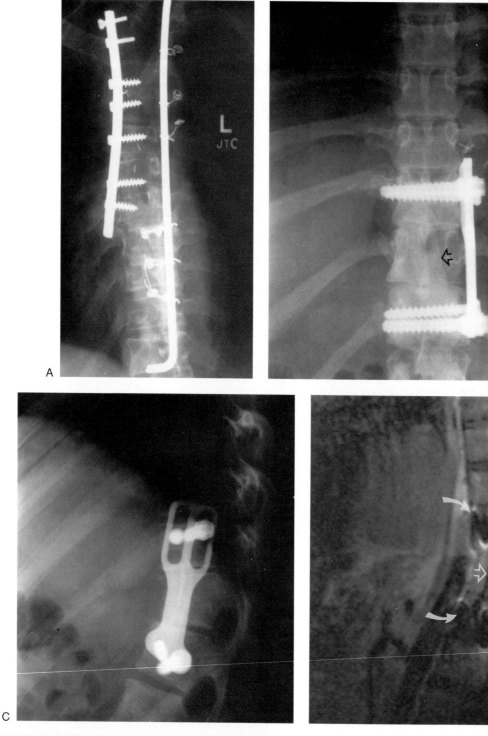

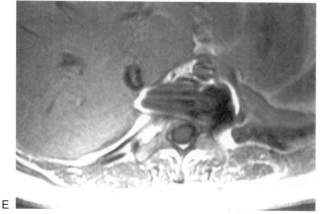

FIG. IIIA-17. Different stabilization devices, thoracic spine. **A:** Frontal view of thoracic spine in a patient with progressive scoliosis after treatment of rib chondrosarcoma. There is a long lateral vertebral plate with unicortical screws and a contralateral Luque rod attached by laminar wires (Luque wires). **B:** Frontal radiograph in a different patient shows lateral vertebral short plate with bicortical screws at T9 and T11. Faintly seen is an anterior fibular bone graft (*arrow*). **C:** Lateral radiograph in the same patient shows the plate, which obscures the fibular bone graft. There is slight anterior wedging of T10. **D:** Midsagittal T₁-weighted MR image in same patient shows fibular bone graft (*open arrow*) and artifact from titanium screws. Note that the spinal canal is well visualized despite the hardware. **E:** Axial T₁-weighted image at T9 level in same patient shows artifact from screws and plate that does not significantly degrade visualization of the spinal canal and spinal cord.

racic rods are Luque and Harrington rods, which are mainly used for correction of scoliosis. These have also been used in the treatment of trauma, tumor, degenerative spondylolisthesis, and disk disease (29). Luque rods are either straight or L-shaped and are attached with wires to the laminae at each level. To facilitate bony fusion, the ligamentum flavum and facet joints are excised prior to wiring. This arrangement distributes the corrective forces over multiple levels. Luque rods can dislodge if not appropriately fixed with a sublaminar wire. Broken wires are a common complication, which may result in neural injury. Harrington rods are smooth, with a collar at one end and ratchets at the other (Fig. IIIA-18). They span at least five vertebral segments. These rods may be bent intraoperatively to conform to a kyphosis or lordosis. Harrington rods correct and stabilize scoliosis by distraction or compression. Harrington rods can fracture with time, especially at the rod–ratchet interface. Other instrumentation includes the Cotrel–Dubousset, Texas Scottish Rite Hospital, and Rogozinski spinal rod systems (30). Occasion-

ally mixed systems of various rods and fixation devices are used.

Three basic types of fixation devices are used in the thoracic spine to secure rods to the posterior elements. These include sublaminar and interspinous wires and cables, laminar and pedicle hooks, and transpedicular screws. Laminar or sublaminar hooks engage the posterior elements inferiorly or superiorly, allowing compression or distraction forces to be applied to the pedicles or laminae (Fig. IIIA-18B). Occasionally, hooks are placed on the transverse processes to provide a more lateral attachment. An up-going and down-going hook at the same level are referred to as a ''claw mechanism.'' This arrangement greatly reduces the risk of rod dislodgement (31). Complications of wire placement and removal include injury to dura, cord, or nerve roots and fracture of the lamina from wire cutting into bone. Hooks rarely fracture but may become detached from a rod and impinge on the cord or nerve roots (29).

A more recently developed technique for attaching fix-

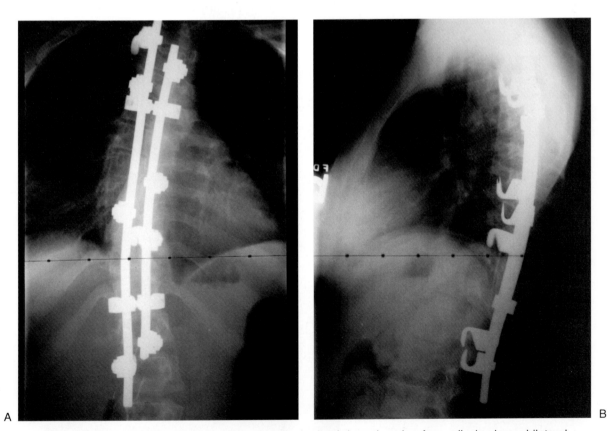

A   B

FIG. IIIA-18. Harrington rods. **A:** Frontal radiograph of thoracic spine for scoliosis shows bilateral Harrington rods. **B:** Lateral radiograph in the same patient shows that both rods are attached to the spine via multiple sublaminar hooks. On the side of the scoliosis apex, the rods are used for compression; therefore, the superior-most hook is supralaminar, and the most inferior one is sublaminar. On the side of concavity, the rods are used for distraction; therefore, the superior-most hook is sublaminar, and the one most inferior is supralaminar.

ation devices is the use of transpedicular screws. The use of these screws was first reported in 1969 by Harrington and Tullos (32). The screws are inserted from a posterior approach and are angled medially as they pass from the pedicle into the vertebral body. When appropriately placed, these screws resist rotation in three dimensions, allowing correction of deformity and stabilization across a point of injury. The pedicular screw strength is decreased if the screws are placed too shallowly or are used in osteopenic bone. Fracture can also occur if the screw diameter is too large. There may be nerve root or cord damage if the medial cortex of the pedicle is violated during screw placement.

A serious complication of spinal surgery and instrumentation is neurologic deterioration, which occurs in 1% of patients (33). The most common causes are malpositioned or migrating hardware and overdistraction. Postoperative neurologic injury may also result from hematoma, cord edema, infection, spinal instability, and disk herniation. Hardware failure may result from migration or fracture of the implant. Common sites of failure include the site of attachment to the spine or the junction between different hardware components. Hardware fracture results from metal fatigue secondary to repeated stress of flexion, extension, and lateral bending. Failed fusion with pseudoarthrosis development is a common end result of implant

or fusion failure. Radiographs in at least two projections are required to evaluate for implant failure, as a complication may not be apparent on only one view.

SPINAL CORD CYST AND MYELOMALACIA

This section deals with the posttreatment MR imaging appearance of nontumoral spinal cord cysts and myelomalacia. The distinction between hydromyelia (dilatation of the central spinal cord canal) and syringomyelia (cyst[s] outside the central canal) is not possible based on MR imaging. The MR is the initial imaging method of choice in patients suspected of harboring a spinal cord cyst, and MR imaging also identifies multicompartamental cysts in which multilevel laminectomies may be needed. The "leading edges" of these fluid-filled spaces are generally of increased signal intensity of T_2-weighted images, probably reflecting softening of the cord at those levels. The term "cyst" is usually applied to an enlarging fluid-filled space, whereas the term "cavity" is used for a static fluid-filled space. Patients with spinal cord cysts commonly present with pain, motor and/or sensory loss, dysesthesias, and hyperhidrosis. Patients who were previously paraplegic or had incomplete paraplegia (generally posttraumatic) may present with worsening symptoms.

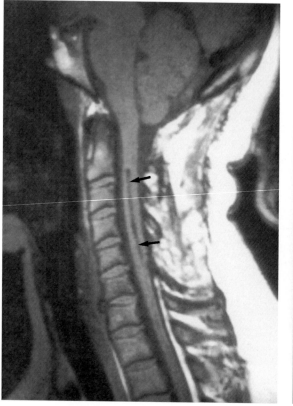

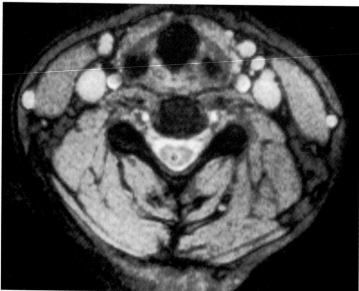

A

B

FIG. IIIA-19. Shunt in spinal cord cyst. **A:** Midsagittal T_1-weighted MR image shows shunt (*arrows*) within a decompressed cyst. **B:** Axial gradient-echo T_2-weighted image in the same patient shows shunt in central position surrounded by high signal intensity (gliosis?).

The differential diagnosis is that of a cord cyst versus progressive myelomalacia. The latter entity is comprised of multiple microcysts in a spinal cord that is scarred and adherent to the dura. By MR imaging, cysts are well defined and have signal intensity similar to CSF in all sequences. Myelomalacia has ill-defined borders and higher signal intensity than CSF on proton-density images. In myelomalacia, the spinal cord is commonly atrophic, but occasionally it may be expanded (progressive myelomalacia). This enlargement is caused by scarring of the pial surface of the cord to the dura in a circumferential fashion that prevents cord collapse.

Once the diagnosis of a spinal cord cyst is suspected, treatment involves decompression of the cyst. Cyst decompression may be accomplished by a myelotomy (syringotomy) with or without placement of a shunt. The shunt not only drains the fluid but serves as a ''wick,'' keeping the myelotomy open. The distal ends of these shunts are commonly placed in the spinal subarachnoid space and peritoneal or pleural cavities. These shunts are radiopaque (barium impregnated) and may be easily seen on plain radiographs of the spine. On MR imaging, they are of very low signal intensity on T_1- and T_2-weighted images (Fig. IIIA-19). Because of their small size, they are not always identified on all MR images. Identification of a cyst, determination of the myelotomy site, and placement of the shunt are greatly aided by the use of intraoperative sonography.

Magnetic resonance imaging and sonography also readily demonstrate tethering of the posterior surface of the spinal cord to dura. In cases of myelomalacia, the lesion is echogenic rather than sonolucent. In cases of progressive myelomalacia, the cord is expanded, echogenic, and in direct continuity with a posterior thickened dura. After shunting, ideally, the cyst should collapse and the spinal cord return to near normal diameter. No change in the size of the cyst (accompanied by no relief of symptoms) is indicative of surgical failure. In cases of progressive myelomalacia, sonography shows the expanded cord returning to a more normal configuration after untethering and duraplasty (which is used to expand the subarachnoid space). In some patients, scarring of the myelotomy and shunt failure may manifest as only mild enlargement of the cyst. This probably occurs because the surrounding spinal cord is gliotic and noncompliant, thus preventing expansion. In these patients, MR evaluation of intracystic fluid motion may help to establish the correct diagnosis.

For these patients, we recommend obtaining two sets of sagittal T_2-weighted images. The first set is a conventional spin-echo (or a fast spin-echo) sagittal T_2-weighted sequence with the motion-compensation gradients turned on. The second set is a conventional spin-echo T_2-

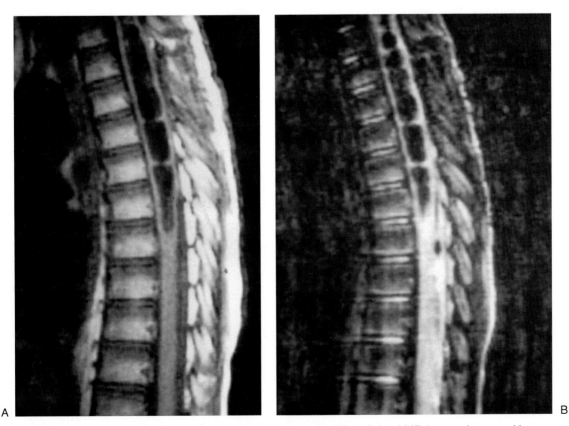

A   B

FIG. IIIA-20. Fluid motion in spinal cord cyst. **A:** Midsagittal T_1-weighted MR image shows multiseptated cyst in upper thoracic cord. **B:** Corresponding spin-echo T_2-weighted image without gradient moment nulling shows intracystic fluid dephasing.

weighted sequence with the motion-compensation gradients turned off. In the latter sequence, because there is no effort to suppress intracystic fluid motion, fluid motion or turbulence may be seen as regions of signal void (Fig. IIIA-20). It is important not to use fast spin-echo sequences for this purpose because, with their long echo train, they have an inherent refocusing effect on fluid motion and turbulence. In addition, the conventional sagittal spin-echo sequence should have only one late echo, as the presence of two symmetric echoes also tends to rephase the effects of constant velocity and makes detection of fluid motion difficult. Sagittal gradient-echo T_2-weighted images may be obtained gated to different portions of the cardiac cycle and displayed in a cine-loop fashion to help identify intracystic fluid motion. The presence of intracystic fluid motion in combination with progressive symptoms in patients known to harbor spinal cord cysts is almost always indicative of myelotomy or shunt failure and may dictate the need for further surgery.

POSTOPERATIVE APPEARANCE OF SPINAL TUMORS AND VASCULAR MALFORMATIONS

Extradural Tumors

Most extradural neoplasias are metastatic in origin, with the primary sites more commonly located in the breast, lung, and prostate. Myeloma, lymphoma, and leukemia may also involve the vertebrae (34). Preoperative embolization reduces blood loss during surgery and may facilitate resectability of the lesions (35). Treatment, aimed at relieving spinal cord compression, is performed by vertebral body resection, placement of banked bone grafts, and anterior plating with or without laminectomies and posterior stabilization devices (34). The appearance of these procedures is described earlier in this chapter.

Intradural and Extramedullary Tumors

Most of these lesions are nerve sheath tumors and meningiomas. Tumors in the neural foramina are commonly removed via an anterior approach. Meningiomas may necessitate anterior or posterior approaches with dural grafting. The site of duraplasty always enhances. This enhancement may be lifelong. Progressive enhancement on serial postoperative studies is suggestive of tumor recurrence. After the resection of nerve sheath tumors, the involved neural foramen may appear widened. There may also be evidence of vertebrectomy with grafting and plating.

Intramedullary Spinal Cord Tumors

In our experience, ependymomas and hemangioblastomas tend to be more commonly operated on than are astrocytomas and metastases, which are treated with irradiation. However, resections of astrocytomas (even holocord ones) are becoming progressively more popular. After surgery, there is always evidence of myelomalacia and blood products. Enhancement may remain for long periods of time and is usually indeterminate in nature. Progressive enhancement is suspicious for a residual enlarging tumor or recurrent tumor (Fig. IIIA-21). Development of cysts is also worrisome for tumors until proven otherwise.

Dural Arteriovenous Fistulas

After successful embolization and/or surgical resections of these malformations, the dilated venous channels on the surface of the spinal cord should almost completely disappear (36). Thrombosis of these vessels may result in high signal intensity within them, resulting from clot-containing methemoglobin. If the spinal cord had high T_2 signal intensity preoperatively (reflecting edema from venous hypertension), after successful surgery, the T_2 signal intensity should return to normal, and there may be slight atrophy (36). The only definite method to prove resolution of these malformations is spinal angiography.

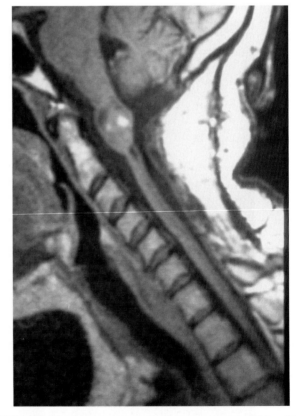

FIG. IIIA-21. Recurrent cervical astrocytoma. Midsagittal postcontrast T_1-weighted MR image shows focal expansion of the cervicomedullary junction, which proved to be recurrent tumor. Note extensive posterior laminectomies.

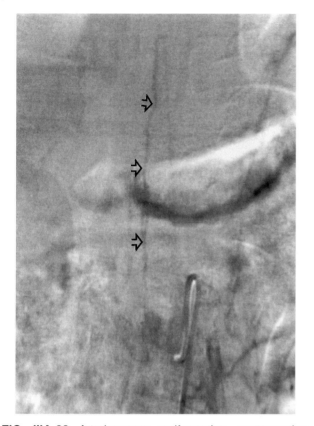

FIG. IIIA-22. Arteriovenous malformation, postresection. Frontal view (subtracted) from a conventional catheter angiogram during infection of left L3 lumbar artery shows opacification of artery of Adamkiewicz that becomes progressively larger distally (*arrows*). This artery was the main supply of a lower thoracic intramedullary AVM. Note that, despite the unusual configuration of this artery, there are no shunting or early draining veins.

Intramedullary Spinal Cord Arteriovenous Malformations

There is no specific appearance following surgery for removal of these malformations. Ideally, the areas of flow–void phenomenon should disappear. Because many of these malformations show some bleeding during surgery, the postoperative MR appearance may be confusing. We have, however, noticed that the spinal cord becomes atrophic and may enhance after contrast administration for prolonged periods of time after surgery. Again, the only definitive method with which to assess the status of a resected malformation is spinal angiography. Spinal angiography may show persistent and somewhat dilated arteries but, after complete resection, may show no arteriovenous shunting (Fig. IIIA-22).

POSTRADIATION THERAPY

Irradiation leads to progressive reduction in hematopoietic bone marrow and its replacement by fat. This is seen as increased signal on T_1-weighted images corresponding to the radiation portal. Immediately after completion of treatment, the vertebral bodies may show increased T_1 signal and enhancement, particularly if fat suppression techniques are used. This is believed to be related to edema and resolves approximately 14 days after completion of therapy. Signal intensity changes reflecting alteration of the hematopoietic marrow may be seen as early as 3 weeks after treatment but at times may develop up to 14 months after completion of treatment. Approximately 50% of irradiated patients show diffuse hyperintensity in the vertebral bodies, and the remaining 50% show hyperintensity centrally with a peripheral band of intermediate signal intensity presumed to represent residual active marrow (37). The latter findings are similar to those seen after bone marrow transplantation.

Irradiation-induced myelitis has two stages. Acutely, edema and transient demyelination may be seen as increased T_2 signal intensity and increased diameter of the spinal cord (Fig. IIIA-23). This occurs 2 to 37 weeks after treatment and tends to resolve spontaneously with the use of steroids. The cord may then become atrophic. Additionally, cord tethering may occur, necessitating surgical untethering and possibly duraplasty. Chronic myelitis develops 3 months to 5 years after completion of therapy. It is characterized by frank necrosis and axonal degeneration (38). There are increased T_2 signal intensity, cord swelling, and postgadolinium enhancement. The abnormality can be placed within the radiation portal.

CONCLUSIONS

In summary, imaging of the posttherapeutic spine requires knowledge of both the specific surgical procedures employed and the imaging features expected after such procedures. In the evaluation of the postsurgical spine, plain radiographs in combination with MR imaging provide the best information. Although most of the surgical hardware now used is considered "MR compatible," it still gives origin to multiple, and at times considerable, artifacts, which may obscure portions of the MR images. Because the degree of artifact the hardware will produce is not known beforehand, postsurgical patients should be given the benefit of MR imaging. Plain radiographs continue to be the ideal method with which to visualize the position of bone grafts and metallic hardware. Patients in whom the therapeutic intervention has been guided toward the soft tissues, such as the treatment of diskitis/osteomyelitis and intramedullary tumors, are better evaluated with contrast-enhanced MR imaging. Postirradiation changes involving the vertebrae and the spinal cord are optimally visualized with MR imaging. Evaluation of vascular malformations after treatment requires both x-ray angiography and MR imaging.

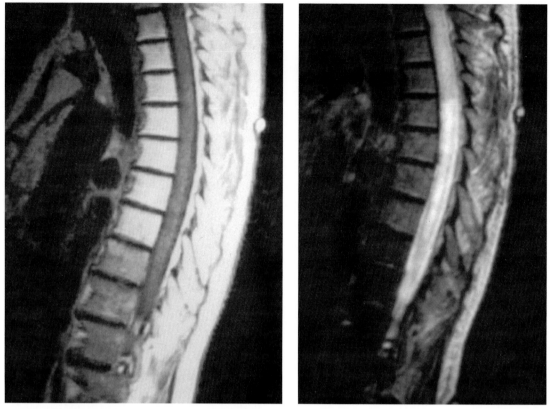

FIG. IIIA-23. Postirradiation changes and myelopathy. **A:** Midsagittal noncontrast T$_1$-weighted MR image shows increased signal intensity in marrow of vertebral bodies corresponding to portal location. **B:** Corresponding T$_2$-weighted image shows increased signal intensity throughout thoracic spinal cord, which, in this symptomatic patient, corresponds to myelopathy.

REFERENCES

1. Richardson WJ, Spinner RJ: Surgical approaches to the cervical spine. In White AH, ed. *Spine Care.* Baltimore: Mosby, 1995:1335–1350.
2. Mike-Mayer H, Cotler HB, Gertzbein SD: Cervical fusions: arthrodesis and osteosynthesis of the cervical spine. In White AH, ed. *Spine Care.* Baltimore: Mosby, 1995:1394–1427.
3. Marcotte P, Dickman CA, Sonntag VKH: Posterior atlantoaxial facet screw fixation. *J Neurosurg* 1993;79:234–237.
4. Roy-Camille R, Saillant G, Mazel C: Internal fixation of unstable cervical spine by a posterior osteosynthesis with plates and screws. In Sherk HH, ed. *The Cervical Spine.* New York: JB Lippincott, 1989:390–403.
5. Slone RM, MacMillan M, Montgomery WJ: Spinal fixation, Part 1. Principles, basic hardware, and fixation techniques for the cervical spine. *Radiographics* 1993;13:341–356.
6. Malcolm GP, Ransford AO, Crockard HA: Treatment of non-rheumatoid occipitocervical instability: Internal fixation with the Hartshill–Ransford loop. *J Bone Joint Surg [Br]* 1994;76-B:357–366.
7. Raynor BB: Congenital malformations of the base of skull: the Arnold–Chiari malformation. In Sherk HH, ed. *The Cervical Spine.* New York: JB Lippincott, 1989:226–235.
8. Ross JS: Cervicomedullary and craniovertebral junctions. In Modic MT, ed. *Magnetic Resonance Imaging of the Spine.* Baltimore: Mosby, 1994:191–215.
9. Hensinger RN: Anomalies of the atlas. In Sherk HH, ed. *The Cervical Spine.* New York: JB Lippincott, 1989:244–247.
10. Moskovich R, Crockard HA: Atlantoaxial arthrodesis using interlaminar clamps: an improved technique. *Spine* 1992;17:261–267.
11. Dull ST, Toselli RM: Preoperative oblique axial computed tomographic imaging for C1-C2 transarticular screw fixation: technical note. *Neurosurgery* 1995;37:150–152.
12. DePalma A, Rothman R, Lewinnek G, et al: Anterior interbody fusion for severe cervical degeneration. *Surg Gynecol Obstet* 1992;134:755–758.
13. Bell GR: The anterior approach to the cervical spine. In: Ross JS, ed. *Neuroimaging Clinics of North America [The Cervical Spine].* Philadelphia: WB Saunders, 1995:465–480.
14. Poletti SC, Handel JA: Degenerative disc disease of the cervical spine: Degenerative cascade and the anterior approach. In: White AH, Schofferman JA, eds. *Spine Care.* Baltimore: Mosby, 1995:1351–1367.
15. Emery SE: Cervical spondylitic radiculopathy and myelopathy: Anterior approach and pathology. In: White AH, Schofferman JA, eds. *Spine Care.* Baltimore: Mosby, 1995:1368–1378.
16. Whitecloud TS: Management of radiculopathy and myelopathy by the anterior approach. In: Sherk HH, ed. *The Cervical Spine.* New York: JB Lippincott, 1989:644–658.
17. Connolly PJ, Yuan HA: Anterior instrumentation of the cervical spine. In: White AH, Schofferman JA, eds. *Spine Care.* Baltimore: Mosby, 1995:1428–1436.
18. Weider A: Anterior plating. In: Sherk HH, ed. *The Cervical Spine.* Philadelphia: JB Lippincott, 1994:151–162.
19. Karasick D: Anterior cervical spine fusion: struts, plugs, and plates. *Skel Radiol* 1993;22:85–94.
20. Tartaglino LM, Flanders AE, Vinitski S, Friedman DP: Metallic artifacts on MR images of the postoperative spine: Reduction with fast spin-echo techniques. *Radiology* 1994;190:565–569.
21. Wetzel FT: Degenerative disc disease of the cervical spine: Posterior approach. In: White AH, Schofferman JA, eds. *Spine Care.* Baltimore: Mosby, 1995:1359–1367.
22. Brower RS, Herkowitz HN: Cervical spondylitic radiculopathy and

myelopathy: Posterior approach. In: White AH, Schofferman JA, eds. *Spine Care*. Baltimore: Mosby, 1995:1379–1393.

23. Slone RM, MacMillan M, Montgomery WJ: Spinal fixation: Part 3. Complications of spinal instrumentation. *Radiographics* 1993; 13:797–816.

24. Hirabayashi K: Expansive open-door laminoplasty. In: Sherk HH, ed. *The Cervical Spine; An Atlas of Surgical Procedures*. Philadelphia: JB Lippincott, 1994:233–250.

25. Maniker AH, Schulder M, Duran HL: Halifax clamps: efficacy and complications in posterior cervical stabilization. *Surg Neurol* 1995; 43(2):140–146.

26. Barnes PD, Brody JD, Jaramillo D, et al: Atypical idiopathic scoliosis: MR imaging evaluation. *Radiology* 1993;186:247.

27. Gaines RW: Spinal deformity in children, adolescents, and young adults. In: White AH, ed. *Spine Care*. Baltimore: Mosby, 1995: 1577–1611.

28. Schlegel J, Yuan HA, Fredricksen B: Anterior intrabody fixation devices. In: Frymoyer JW, Ducker TB, Hadler NM, Kostuik JP, Weinstein JN, Whitecloud TS III, eds. *The Adult Spine: Principles of Practice*. New York: Raven Press, 1991:1947–1959.

29. Krag MH: Spinal fusion: overview of options and posterior internal fixation devices. In: Frymoyer JW, Ducker TB, Hadler NM, Kostuik JP, Weinstein JN, Whitecloud TS III, eds. *The Adult Spine: Principles of Practice*. New York: Raven Press, 1991:1919–1945.

30. Slone RM, MacMillan M, Montgomery WJ, Heare M: Spinal fixation: Part 2. Fixation techniques and hardware for the thoracic and lumbosacral spine. *Radiographics* 1993;13:521–543.

31. Dawson EG, Clader TJ, Bassett LW: A comparison of different methods used to diagnose pseudoarthrosis following posterior spinal fusion for scoliosis. *J Bone Joint Surg [Am]* 1985;67:1153–1159.

32. Yeakley JW, Harris JH Jr: Imaging of spinal fusions. In: Cotler JM, Cotler HB, eds. *Spinal Fusion, Science and Technique*. New York: Springer-Verlag, 1990:335–347.

33. Heller JG, Whitecloud TS III, Butler JC, et al: Complications of spinal surgery. In: Herkowitz HN, Garfin SR, Baldeston RA, Eismont FJ, Bell GR, Wiesel SW, eds. *The Spine*, 3rd ed. Philadelphia: WB Saunders, 1992:1817–1898.

34. Sevick RJ: Cervical spine tumor. In: Ross JS, ed. *Neuroimaging Clinics of North America* [*The Cervical Spine*] Philadelphia: WB Saunders, 1995:385–400.

35. Broaddus WC, Grady MS, Delashaw JB, et al: Preoperative superselective arteriolar embolization: A new approach to enhance resectability of spinal tumors. *Neurosurgery* 1990;27:755.

36. Massaryk TJ: Cystic lesions, vascular disorders, demyelinating disease, and miscellaneous topics. In: Modic MT, Masaryk TJ, Ross JS, eds. *Magnetic Resonance Imaging of the Spine*. St. Louis: Mosby, 1994:388–433.

37. Kricun R, Kricun ME: *MRI and CT of the Spine: Case Study Approach*. New York: Raven Press, 1994.

38. Ross JS: Myelopathy. In: Ross JS, ed. *Neuroimaging Clinics of North America* [*The Cervical Spine*]. Philadelphia: WB Saunders, 1995:367–384.

Posttherapeutic Neurodiagnostic Imaging,
edited by J.R. Jinkins,
Lippincott-Raven Publishers, New York © 1997.

CHAPTER **IIIB**

The Posttherapeutic Lumbosacral Spine

Farid F. Shafaie, Carl V. Bundschuh, and J. Randy Jinkins

It has been estimated that 80% of the population in the United States of America will have back pain at some time in their life (1). In patients between 20 and 50 years old, the evaluation and treatment of low back pain is one of the highest overall costs of health care (2). The incidence of lower extremity pain related to spinal disease is less than that of back pain; however, the prevalence is still quite high. The many mechanisms responsible for back and lower extremity pain include the nonspecific mechanical or chemical irritation of (a) afferent somatic sympathetic neural branches, (b) spinal nerves in the spinal canal or neural foramen, and (c) medial neural branches of the posterior primary spinal rami (3–5). Complicating the diagnosis and treatment of these conditions is the fact that different types of pathology can produce similar clinical syndromes. In addition, the same abnormality may present in typical as well as atypical ways (4).

As a result of conservative treatment failure, there are roughly 200,000 lumbar disk operations performed annually in North America, at an estimated cost of US $1.6 billion (1). International comparisons reveal that the surgery in North America is performed two to four times more frequently than elsewhere and that the rate of failed back surgery is about three times greater than that of some Western European countries (6). In addition, the collected data demonstrate that the number of operations performed for disk excision and spinal fusion is rapidly growing in North America (6).

The likelihood of pain relief through surgical correction has been correlated with several factors. A prospective study showed that such diverse factors as female gender, psychological problems, sick leave from work of more than 3 months' duration, and degenerative radiographic spinal alterations were generally associated with an unsat-

isfactory surgical outcome (7,8). On the other hand, another prospective study identified several clinical variables that were independently predictive of a relatively good outcome from lumbar surgery, including the absence of back pain, the absence of a work-related injury, the presence of a radicular distribution of pain extending to the foot, the presence of leg pain on straight-leg-raising examination, and the presence of lower extremity reflex asymmetry (9). In this latter study, some commonly collected data (e.g., age, motor deficit, and obesity) did not clearly correlate with clinical outcome (9). Indeed, a more recent study has shown that elderly patients (>70 years of age) have had success rates for lumbar surgery comparable to non-age-adjusted patient groups (10).

THE FAILED BACK SURGERY SYNDROME

Despite the loose application of criteria for judging operative success, lumbosacral spinal surgery has been so often unsuccessful (10% to 40%) that failed back surgery is now labeled as a syndrome: the *failed back surgery syndrome* (FBSS) (11). It has been estimated that 20,000 to 50,000 new cases of FBSS occur in the United States every year (12), resulting in an annual cost of US $56 billion in terms of productivity loss, insurance expenses, and employee retraining (13).

The FBSS is characterized by postsurgical intractable pain in the low back and lower extremity(ies) combined with varying degrees of functional incapacitation. The evaluation of this syndrome is a diagnostic challenge because clinical signs and symptoms are often nonspecific. The major identifiable causes of the FBSS include clinically relevant epidural fibrosis, recurrent or residual disk herniation, postoperative spinal infection, sterile arachnoiditis, postsurgical pseudomeningocele formation, and lateral recess, foraminal, or central spinal stenosis that may preexist or follow the spinal surgery (14). Other less common causes of the FBSS include surgery inadvertently performed on the wrong side or at the incorrect level, direct nerve injury at the time of surgery, chronic

F. F. Shafaie: Mallinckrodt Institute of Radiology, St. Louis, Missouri 63110.

C. V. Bundschuh: Department of Radiology, Eastern Virginia Medical School, Norfolk, Virginia 23502.

J. R. Jinkins: Department of Radiology, The University of Texas Health Science Center, San Antonio, Texas 78284.

mechanical spinal pain (e.g., facet joint disease), and fusion failure (14). Still further causes of the FBSS are recurrent or residual symptoms related to anterior spinal disk protrusion, radiculitis (neuritis), herniation at a spinal level other than that operated on, facet joint fracture, and spondylolisthesis (3,15–17). These conditions should be distinguished from acceptable and expected postoperative findings found after successful lumbar surgery.

EXAMINATION TECHNIQUES

Progressive improvements in magnetic resonance (MR) imaging have substantially improved the ability of the medical imaging physician to critically analyze the postoperative lumbosacral spine. Compared to other imaging methods, MR images acquired in multiple planes have superior diagnostic potential, in part because of their greater spatial and contrast resolution characteristics. Nevertheless, the similarity of some postsurgical pathologic processes in regard to MR signal intensity often makes even this imaging technique somewhat difficult to interpret. The development of intravenously administered paramagnetic MR contrast agents (e.g., gadolinium) has materially assisted the diagnostic sensitivity and specificity of MR in the evaluation of the FBSS because of the differential improvement in contrast resolution afforded by these agents.

In general, T_2-weighted fast spin-echo images are superior to conventional spin-echo images in the lumbosacral spine in part because of improved image quality resulting from better spatial resolution and reduced motion artifact (18). Sagittal (with fat suppression) and axial (without fat suppression) fast spin-echo T_2-weighted images are helpful in assessing neural foramen narrowing, central and lateral recess spinal stenosis, hydration status of the intervertebral disk, abnormal signal intensity of the disk and cancellous bone, and signal intensity of abnormal intra- or perispinal soft tissue masses (e.g., disk herniation, epidural scar, epidural abscess, epidural phlegmon). Sagittal and axial T_1-weighted spin-echo images obtained before and immediately after the bolus intravenous injection of a gadolinium product are almost imperative in the evaluation of the postoperative lumbar spine. Fat-suppression techniques can also often be used after intravenous gadolinium administration because they improve relative intensity and homogeneity of contrast enhancement of epidural fibrosis, thereby distinguishing it from recurrent disk herniation (19). However, it makes the critical interpretation of possible abnormal postoperative intrathecal nerve-root enhancement impossible because small degrees of apparently normal nerve root enhancement are not infrequently observed when fat-suppression techniques are used.

The initiation of MR imaging within approximately 2 min of the gadolinium injection is important because some disk herniations can be somewhat vascularized and therefore may enhance relatively early (20). The basis for this imaging strategy is that the vessels in the scar tissue are relatively homoge-

neously distributed, whereas in disk herniation the vessels are quite heterogeneous or centrally absent. Therefore, a markedly heterogeneously or centrally nonenhancing epidural mass would be labeled a partially vascularized disk herniation, but homogeneous enhancement of an epidural process would be termed epidural fibrosis. It should be noted that imaging after 20 to 30 min of contrast agent administration is not helpful because many herniations enhance centrally within this delayed time frame as the gadolinium progressively seeps into the disk.

Overall, intravenously administered gadolinium compounds are an important adjunct to the MR evaluation of the postoperative lumbosacral spine because of their role in the clarification of the probable cause of the postsurgical syndrome. The three major indications for gadolinium utilization in evaluation of postoperative lumbosacral spine are in the elucidation and differentiation of (a) residual or recurrent disk herniation with or without associated scar formation, (b) isolated epidural fibrosis, and (c) spinal, leptomeningeal, and/or neural inflammation (infectious or aseptic) with or without subacute neural degeneration (20–23). The proper differentiation of these pathologic phenomena on MR imaging should allow improved patient triage toward appropriate medical–surgical therapy.

If the patient cannot undergo an MR imaging examination for medical reasons or because of spinal metallic surgical implants, a ''high''-dose (40 to 60g of iodine equivalent) intravenous iodinated contrast-enhanced CT study is recommended after a precontrast survey examination is performed in order to search for the same problems in much the same manner outlined in the foregoing paragraphs. Myelography is helpful for documenting arachnoiditis and its sequelae such as loculations, adhesions, and obstructions but is otherwise not very informative. Computed tomography continues to be the mainstay in evaluating ossific or calcific pathologic changes (e.g., spinal, foraminal, lateral recess stenosis) of the postoperative lumbosacral spine. Kinetic (flexion–extension) MR imaging and flexion–extension conventional radiography both have the potential of depicting postoperative bony instability in the spine.

THE NORMAL POSTOPERATIVE SPINE

The interpretation of images of the lumbar spine acquired in the immediate postoperative period (i.e., initial 6 to 8 weeks) should be undertaken with caution. Normal postoperative changes occur in the bony structures as well as the soft tissues, which vary depending on the time lapsed since the surgical procedure (24,25).

In laminotomy, there is partial resection of the neural arch along with ligamentum flavum removal. Tissue alteration may be minimal if microsurgical techniques have been used. Such changes are usually best appreciated in the axial plane.

In laminectomy, a total resection of the spinal lamina

and associated ligamentum flavum is performed in order to provide a surgical pathway for disk removal or to relieve spinal canal narrowing. On MR, the surgical absence of bone can be best demonstrated on axial T_1-weighted images. There is often an associated asymmetry in the muscle–fat planes posteriorly. The paraspinal musculature may also be temporarily indistinct secondary to edema in the subacute phase after surgery. The posterior border of the dural tube margin may expand posteriorly toward the surgical site and laminectomy defect, reflecting this relative bony insufficiency (Fig. IIIB-1). This is an expected finding and does not represent a pseudomeningocele.

In diskectomy, often performed in association with the postsurgical changes outlined in the foregoing, a partial or complete resection of the degenerated or herniated disk is undertaken. On unenhanced images acquired immediately after surgery, postdiskectomy changes can mimic the preoperative appearance of disk herniation because of annular disk disruption and epidural tissue edema. This renders the outline of the dural sac and intervertebral disk indistinct and may efface the thecal sac. Homogeneous enhancement of this epidural process on MR after intravenous gadolinium administration may be observed. This is caused by granulation tissue and/or fibrosis, and it explains the mild regional epidural mass effect seen commonly in postoperative imaging of successful lumbar discectomy patients (15,20,26).

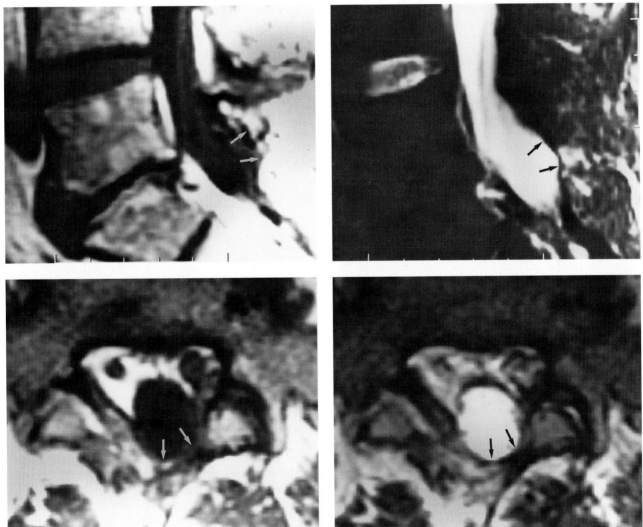

FIG. IIIB-1. Normal postoperative alterations. **A:** Unenhanced sagittal T_1-weighted (550/10) conventional spin-echo image shows focal outward bulging of the thecal sac (*arrows*) at the level of the hemilaminectomy. **B:** Sagittal T_2-weighted (4000/90) fast spin-echo image also shows the focal outpouching of the thecal sac (*arrows*) through the hemilaminectomy defect. **C:** Unenhanced axial T_1-weighted (500/10) conventional spin-echo image shows the outward bulging of the thecal sac (*arrows*) toward the left-sided hemilaminectomy defect. **D:** T_2-weighted (4000/90) fast spin-echo image also shows the left-sided outpouching of the thecal sac into the hemilaminectomy defect (*arrows*).

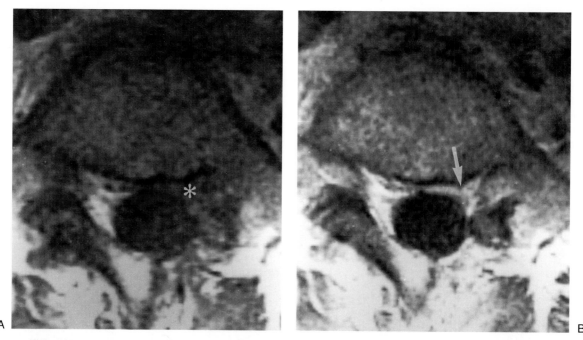

FIG. IIIB-2. Isolated postoperative epidural fibrosis in asymptomatic patient 6 months following successful L5–S1 intervertebral disk surgery. **A:** Precontrast T_1-weighted (600/20) axial image showing obliteration of the epidural fat on the left (*asterisk*). **B:** Gadolinium-DTPA-enhanced T_1-weighted (600/20) axial image demonstrating peripheral epidural enhancement (*arrow*) compatible with epidural fibrosis but absence of detectable enhancement of intrathecal neural tissue.

In one recent study, 100% of asymptomatic patients demonstrated surgical tract subcutaneous soft-tissue enhancement (27). In another study of asymptomatic postoperative patients, 100% of subjects showed evidence of epidural fibrosis (Fig. IIIB-2) (15). In addition, enhancing lumbosacral vertebral end plates have been observed between 6 and 18 months after surgery in 19% of patients (28), and enhancement of the posterior annulus has been reported in the majority of asymptomatic postoperative patients (29).

In surgical *spinal fusion,* placement of a bone graft across the transverse and articular processes for the purpose of spine stabilization is carried out. The MR imaging of the bony fusion tissue usually demonstrates mixed or generally decreased signal intensity on T_2-weighted imaging. Although it is often difficult to determine by MR imaging, a complete fusion may demonstrate a contiguity of the marrow fat across the fused bony elements on T_1-weighted acquisitions. The bone graft itself has a varied MR appearance depending on its site of origin, the extent of trauma to the graft at the time of harvesting, and the degree of vascular infiltration of the graft.

RECURRENT DISK HERNIATION VERSUS EPIDURAL SCARRING

General Considerations Concerning the MR Differentiation of Disk Herniation from Epidural Scar

Magnetic resonance has become the modality of choice for evaluating most spinal syndromes, in part because it is noninvasive and uniquely sensitive to disease. Mass effect, location in relationship to the intervertebral disk, and relative MR signal intensities are all variables that can aid in the differentiation of scar tissue from disk material (30–34). Unfortunately, however, an estimated 30% of anterior epidural or lateral recess scars can be found within close proximity to the disk space, and approximately 30% can demonstrate at least mild degrees of mass effect (32,33,35). For this reason, epidural scarring can be confused with recurrent herniated disk on the basis of unenhanced MR alone. In a study of 20 patients with FBSS, in whom the tissue type was later surgically confirmed, 74% of anterior epidural or lateral recess scar were found to be at least mildly hyperintense relative to the adjacent cancellous bone on T_2-weighted images; however, 69% of disk herniations in this same series were also found to be similarly hyperintense (32). The intensity of disk herniations as noted on T_2-weighted images is in part related to the type of herniation (i.e., contiguous or sequestered) as well as to the length of time from patient symptom onset or exacerbation of symptoms to the time of imaging. This is in part because fresh disk herniations desiccate and shrink at variable rates. As a result of these overlaps in imaging characteristics, unenhanced MR imaging has an accuracy approaching only 85% in the differentiation of epidural scar tissue from herniated disk material (30).

The lack of early central contrast enhancement associated with disk herniations after intravenous gadolinium administration has been claimed to be the major criterion by which recurrent disk herniation can be distinguished from epidural scar (Figs. IIIB-3, IIIB-4, and IIIB-5) (33). However, the occasional generalized enhancement of disk herniations can lead to the erroneous labeling of recurrent herniated disk as epidural scar (Fig. IIIB-6). Early central or homogeneous enhancement of herniated disks is thought to be related to vascular density. The status of the disk matrix itself (i.e., extracellular space) may also be an important factor.

Similarly, the MR imaging characteristics of epidural scar tissue reflect its histologic properties. One reason anterior epidural and lateral recess scar almost always enhances is that fibrosis maintains a fairly large extracellular space. That is also a likely explanation for the lack of significant change in mass effect or T_2 signal intensity of epidural scars older than 2 months (35). Another major

determinant of enhancement grade in epidural scar older than 2 months is the capillary endothelial gap-junction status. If these endothelial junctions are open, the degree of enhancement after gadolinium administration will be greater. In general, the vascular density of scars does not correlate with enhancement grade and, regardless of scar site, appears to remain stable after 2 months of inception (35).

Peridiskal fibrosis is defined as loose, well-vascularized connective tissue (i.e., granulation tissue) that is often found partially or completely surrounding a primary or recurrent disk herniation. It can be seen to be intimately associated with a contiguous disk extrusion or a free fragment and usually has a definable boundary with the disk (Fig. IIIB-3). The basic histologic difference between peridiskal fibrosis and a vas-

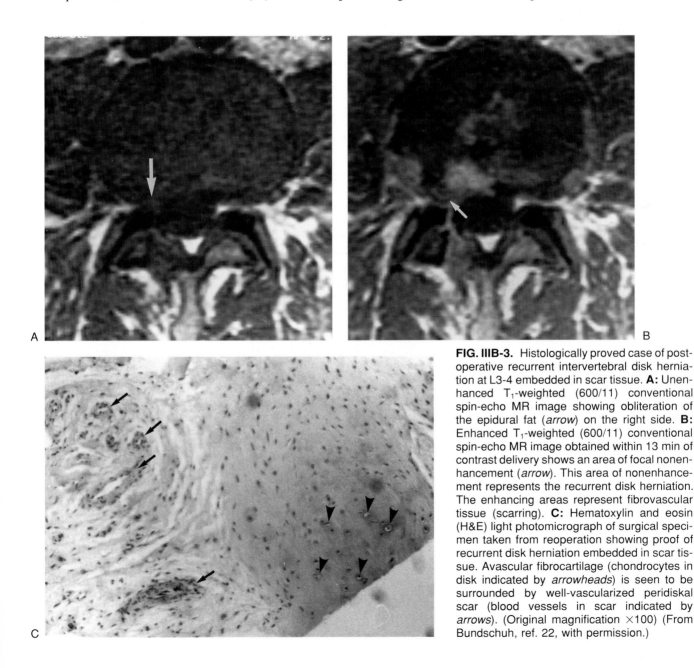

FIG. IIIB-3. Histologically proved case of postoperative recurrent intervertebral disk herniation at L3-4 embedded in scar tissue. **A:** Unenhanced T_1-weighted (600/11) conventional spin-echo MR image showing obliteration of the epidural fat (*arrow*) on the right side. **B:** Enhanced T_1-weighted (600/11) conventional spin-echo MR image obtained within 13 min of contrast delivery shows an area of focal nonenhancement (*arrow*). This area of nonenhancement represents the recurrent disk herniation. The enhancing areas represent fibrovascular tissue (scarring). **C:** Hematoxylin and eosin (H&E) light photomicrograph of surgical specimen taken from reoperation showing proof of recurrent disk herniation embedded in scar tissue. Avascular fibrocartilage (chondrocytes in disk indicated by *arrowheads*) is seen to be surrounded by well-vascularized peridiskal scar (blood vessels in scar indicated by *arrows*). (Original magnification ×100) (From Bundschuh, ref. 22, with permission.)

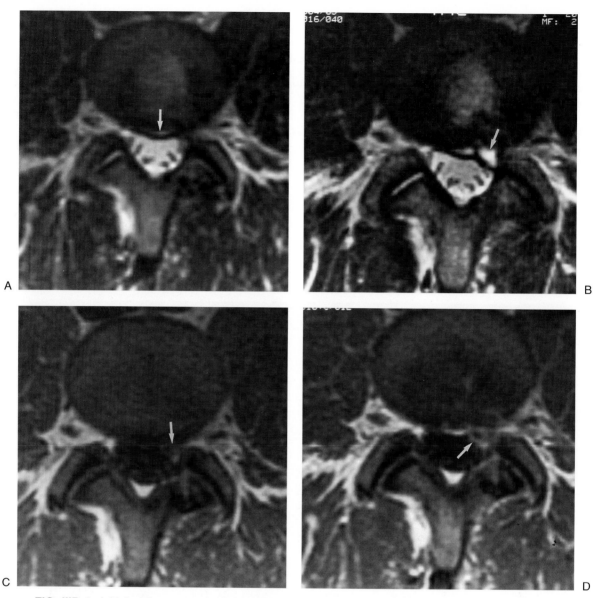

FIG. IIIB-4. Initial and recurrent L4-5 central intervertebral disk herniation with associated L5 lateral recess free disk fragment. **A:** Initial axial T$_2$-weighted (3500/92) fast spin-echo image shows a subtle hyperintense central disk herniation (*arrow*). **B:** Axial T$_2$-weighted (4000/108) fast spin-echo MR image acquired 4 months after diskectomy (**A**) shows the central disk herniation to be larger with the interval appearance of a larger, hyperintense epidural mass (*arrow*) on the left that proved at surgery to be a recurrent disc herniation. **C:** Unenhanced T$_1$-weighted (600/11) conventional spin-echo MR image shows obliteration of the epidural fat (*arrow*) on the left side. **D:** Axial T$_1$-weighted (600/11) spin-echo MR image acquired approximately 8 min after intravenous gadolinium delivery shows that only the periphery of the recurrent disk herniation enhances (*arrow*). Note that **C** and **D** were acquired at the same axial spinal level as B. (From Bundschuh, ref. 22, with permission.)

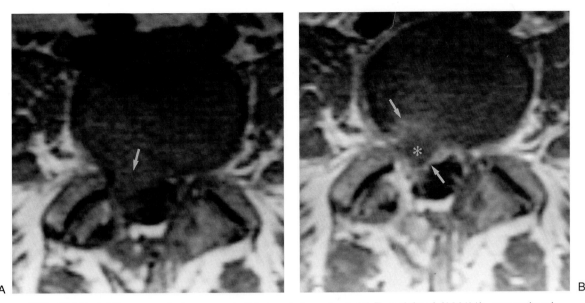

FIG. IIIB-5. L4-5 paracentral recurrent disk herniation. **A:** Axial T_1-weighted (600/11) conventional spin-echo MR image shows a subtle right-sided intraspinal mass (*arrow*). **B:** Enhanced axial T_1-weighted (600/11) conventional spin-echo MR image obtained within 10 min of contrast delivery shows enhancement involving the periphery (*arrows*) of the mass, with relative nonenhancement of the central portion of the disk fragment (*asterisk*).

cularized herniation is that chondrocytes are found only in the herniated disk itself and not typically in scar tissue. Although chondroid metaplasia in scar has been noted, it usually appears in localized congregations and therefore should be readily distinguished from the more uniformly distributed chondrocytes in fibrocartilage (i.e., disk) (36). Aside from the inciting mechanism of the actual trauma of the disk herniation, it is believed that peridiskal fibrosis probably represents a direct response to inflammatory agents released from the herniated disk (e.g., phospholipase A_2 activity) (5,37) as well as a reaction to antigenic material within the intervertebral disk displaced into the epidural space at the time of disk rupture. This process is probably somewhat different from epidural fibrosis secondary to minor hemorrhage associated with bone removal during spinal surgery in the absence of diskectomy. Peridiskal fibrosis appears to result in or contribute to eventual partial resorption of herniated disk material, particularly in cases of noncontained disk fragments. In a recently published report, herniated disk material associated with peridiskal scar in conservatively treated patients was noted to decrease in size over a period of 6 weeks to 6 months (12). It was inferred from this that inflammatory peridiskal granulation tissue may have assisted in the resorption of the herniated disk material.

Vascularized disk herniation, in addition to containing chondrocytes, has a predominantly fibrocartilaginous matrix surrounded by an irregular network of granulation tissue growing into the herniated disk material. The various components are occasionally well intermixed (Fig. IIIB-6). It is likely that a vascularized disk herniation is in a more advanced stage of disk resorption than is a relatively nonvascularized herniated disk surrounded by vascularized peridiskal scar. The distinction with regard to MR imaging is important because a well-vascularized herniation is more likely to be falsely labeled scar on gadolinium-enhanced studies (Fig. IIIB-6). That is, in exceptional cases, a generally vascularized herniation can enhance within minutes of intravenous gadolinium administration. In most cases, however, it appears that the center of the disk herniation will enhance less intensely than the periphery, but only if imaging is completed within 15 to 20 min of contrast agent administration. In a peripherally vascularized disk herniation, the gadolinium gradually seeps into the center of the disk from the surrounding vasculature over time by diffusion, thereby masking its presence on time-delayed imaging (21,27,36). False-negative interpretations on enhanced MR with regard to a diagnosis of disk herniation are in most cases likely attributable to delaying of the scan time to past the immediate postinjection period.

Despite the occasionally confusing patterns of aberrant soft tissue enhancement, it is of paramount importance to recognize that because most scar generally enhances with intravenous contrast material, and most disk herniations do not, the use of intravenous contrast agents is imperative in computed imaging of the postoperative patient in order to differentiate clearly between the two. The quoted accu-

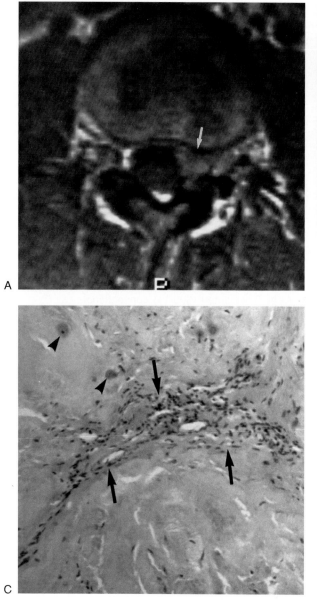

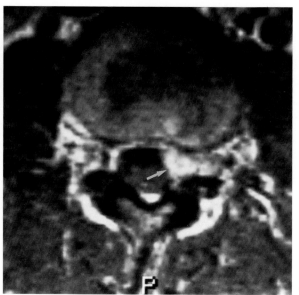

FIG. IIIB-6. Histologically proved case of enhancing L2–L3 free disk fragment. **A:** Unenhanced T_1-weighted (750/35) conventional spin-echo MR image shows an apparent left-sided intraspinal mass (*arrow*). **B:** Enhanced axial T_2-weighted (750/35) conventional spin-echo MR image obtained 10 min after intravenous contrast infusion shows marked, essentially homogeneous enhancement (*arrow*). **C:** Hematoxylin and eosin light photomicrograph of surgical specimen showing fibrocartilage surrounding an island of vascular granulation tissue (*arrows*). Several chondrocytes indicating disk material are seen (*arrowheads*). (Original magnification ×100). (From Shafaie et al., ref. 101, with permission.)

racy of contrast-enhanced MR imaging in the differentiation of herniated disk and epidural scar is 95% to 100% (32,33).

Histopathology of Epidural Scar Tissue

Most of the histologic research on scar tissue has been performed on dermal scars. That research has disclosed striking changes between young scar (i.e., granulation tissue) and mature scar tissue. Capillaries in granulation tissue have scanty micropinocytotic vesicles, a high frequency of luminal occlusion (as low as a 7% patency rate), only a loose network of pericytes, and leaky junctional complexes (38–44). In contrast, mature scar, which can be identified within 5 weeks of tissue injury, has a microvasculature with no evidence of luminal occlusion,

a thin basal lamina, a complete or nearly complete layer of pericytes, and a wealth of micropinocytotic vesicles (41,42,44). The endothelial junction complexes of mature scar tissue are almost certainly less "leaky" than acute or subacute scar (45).

Collagen also undergoes remarkable changes with time following trauma. Within 1 week of injury, a fine meshwork of collagen fibrils restores tissue continuity. In a 3-week-old scar, fibrils are aggregating to form fibers. By 2.5 to 4 months, scar collagen has changed to a mature status, although fiber and fiber-bundle sizes are smaller than those in truly mature scar (46). The water content of scar tissue has also been shown to change with scar age, with young scar containing relatively more water (47).

After 2 months of inception, the vascular density of epidural scar is relatively uniform (35,47). Although the extracellular space in epidural scar is significantly larger during the initial 4 months of growth, after this time it gradually decreases. In a study that concentrated on lateral and posterior epidural scar, the extracellular space of scar tissue less than 4 months old was shown to be 6.65% of the total cross-sectional area, compared with 3.49% for scar tissue older than 4 months (39).

Histopathology and Physiology of Intervertebral Disk Herniation

Until recently, most of the literature concerning the pathophysiology of the intervertebral disk has focused on the nucleus pulposus and inner annulus within the disk space. Less attention has been paid to the biochemistry and histology of the disk once it has ruptured. Some exceptions include work by Eckert and Decker (48), Lindblom and Hultqvist (49), Bobechko and Hirsch (50), Saal et al. (5), and McCarron et al. (51). What is known about the nucleus pulposus and annulus *in situ* must be coupled with these data, and this information must then be extrapolated to the herniated disk in order to begin to understand the pathophysiology involved. Lumbar intervertebral disks are dynamic structures that go through morphologic changes secondary to stress and strain absorbed during daily activities. The intervertebral disk is well vascularized during fetal and newborn life, reflecting the concurrently active metabolic processes present at that time (52,53). Immature disks consist of highly vascularized fibrocartilaginous tissue. As the infant matures and assumes an upright posture, the axial load on the disk increases, with the result that intradiskal hydrostatic pressure exceeds the vascular perfusion pressure. This causes the vessels within the disk to exsanguinate or otherwise occlude, atrophy, and eventually disappear completely (54). The primary means of solute exchange in the intervertebral disk after the newborn period is via diffusion through the vascularized end plates and outer annulus fibrosus (54–56).

Among other things, the adult disk matrix includes proteoglycans, collagen, and water. Chondrocytes, particularly in the outer nucleus and inner annulus, produce specific types of collagen and the building blocks of proteoglycans (Fig. IIIB-7) (57,58). Monomeric proteoglycans are formed when acid mucopolysaccharides are attached to a protein core. A huge multimolecular aggregate results when monomeric proteoglycans are combined with hyaluronic acid and link proteins (36). Aggregated proteoglycans form a cross-linkage with a three-dimensional collagen lattice, with the resultant superstructure directly affecting solute diffusion and probably offering protection against enzymatic degradation (43). Perhaps because of dysfunctional chondrocytes, aging, or other factors, pathologic disks have lower levels of aggregate and total proteoglycans as well as an absolute decrease in water in comparison to healthy disks. It has

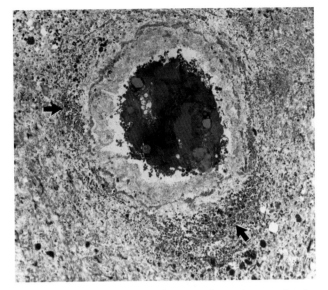

FIG. IIIB-7. Transmission electron photomicrograph of a chondrocyte from a herniated disk specimen (original magnification ×3400). The chondrocyte is the metabolic and matrix-producing workhorse of the intervertebral disk. Numerous chondrocyte processes projecting into the surrounding disk matrix are seen. The matrix at the capsule periphery contains numerous heterogeneously sized elastic fibers (*arrows*). In addition to collagen and elastic fibers, the matrix also contains extracellular (interstitial) fluid, at least two different glycoproteins, noncollagenous proteins, and proteoglycans. (From Bundschuh, ref. 22, with permission.)

been reported that during the first few years of life, the nucleus pulposus and annulus fibrosis contain about 85% and 75% water, respectively, after which time the overall water content decreases to about 70% in adulthood (55). An increase in hyaluronic acid and an increase in collagen content have also been noted with age (36,59,60). These age-related changes correlate with a decrease in signal intensity on T_2-weighted sagittal MR scans (55).

Several of the changes mentioned impact disk nutrition. Because of the body's apparent attempt to aid nutrient and waste disposal, aging intervertebral disks are noted to have a reappearance of blood vessels in the annulus fibrosus and nucleus pulposus as early as the fourth decade; such vessels are present in up to 27% of examined cases by the sixth decade of life (61). This vascular ingrowth can be considered a sign of degeneration of the intervertebral disk. When herniation supervenes, approximately 45% of intervertebral disks show evidence of vascular ingrowth into the disk space (62). Vascular ingrowth also occurs into the disk fragment itself. One study reported blood vessels embedded in the peripheral part of 56.4% of free fragments, in 37.5% of noncontained disk extrusions, and in 11.3% of so-called contained focal disk prolapses (63).

It appears that the vessels associated with disk herniations represent a biological process different from the nutritional and reparative ones described above. The vascularized granulation tissue surrounding and often penetrating disk herniations (i.e., peridiskal scar) in the epidural space seems to represent a resorptive process (48,49). The phospholipase A₂ activity in noncontained herniations (i.e., disk extrusions or free fragments) is approximately 100 times greater than that seen in contained herniations (i.e., disk prolapse). The exposure of noncontained disk herniations to the epidural space may be an important factor in the inflammatory response to phospholipase A₂ and in the consequent resorption of the herniation by peridiskal scar. Sixty-three percent of patients treated conservatively (nonsurgically) demonstrated regression of the size of the disk herniation by an average of 30%, with the largest herniations decreasing to the greatest degree (64). The stimulus for vascular proliferation and inflammation may be the potent inflammatory agents arising from the intervertebral disk at the time of rupture, an autoimmune response to degenerating cartilaginous fractions, or a combination thereof (5,50,51). In laboratory animal models, nonvascularized granulation tissue is noted to surround free disk fragments in the epidural space as early as 5 days after

surgery. At 2 to 3 weeks, prominent vascularity within the granulation tissue response is seen (51). The granulation tissue also contains numerous lymphocytes, plasma cells, and macrophages (51).

Mechanism of Contrast Enhancement of Postoperative Epidural Soft Tissues

Intravascular contrast material (e.g., gadolinium) diffuses through disrupted tight junctions and other areas of endothelial discontinuity into the extracellular space. The rate of delivery of contrast material to a gram of tissue (mmol gadolinium/sec per g tissue) will affect absolute enhancement intensity on the MR image. This rate of delivery depends on vascular density, lumen patency, cardiac output, and intravascular concentration. At 5 min, roughly 20 passes of the contrast agent through a vascular bed can theoretically occur. That allows ample opportunity for the contrast material to accumulate in the extracellular space (65,66), even though a substantial amount of

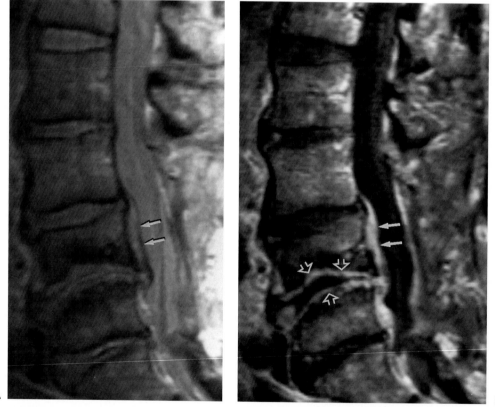

A   B

FIG. IIIB-8. Postoperative L4-5 *Staphylococcus epidermidis* diskitis and osteomyelitis with epidural extension. **A:** Sagittal intermediate-weighted (3000/18) fast spin-echo MR image demonstrates irregularity and volume loss of the L4-5 intervertebral disk and decreased signal intensity of the paradiskal portions of the L4 and L5 vertebrae. There is also an anterior epidural mass extending from L3-4 to L4-5 (*arrows*). **B:** Sagittal T₁-weighted (350/16) conventional spin-echo image obtained 17 min after intravenous gadolinium injection. There is peripheral enhancement surrounding the L4-5 intervertebral disk (*open arrows*). In addition, there is phlegmonous (solid soft tissue) epidural enhancement (*closed arrows*) indicating extension of the disc space infection into the spinal canal. (From Bundschuh, ref. 22, with permission.)

intravascular contrast material normally begins to leave the vascular space by renal excretion and normal extravasation into other tissues within 40 to 60 sec of its administration (67). Although the extracellular space size, vascular density, and endothelial gap junction status are usually the major determinants of contrast enhancement within a given tissue, intravascular gadolinium cannot easily penetrate the normal disk matrix, and, therefore, rates of diffusion and partition coefficients between fluid compartments may also contribute to enhancement grade. In the case of herniated disk, however, vascular density is believed to the most important factor with regard to enhancement characteristics.

Because of the higher rate of luminal occlusion or near occlusion in granulation tissue, the blood flow per gram of tissue (ml/min per g tissue) may be lower than that in mature scar. However, young scar has a greater number of open endothelial junctional complexes relative to older scars. These factors modify the effect of vascular density on contrast enhancement such that there may be no significant relationship between the two in a given tissue.

This has led to the conclusion that the important determinants of contrast enhancement in epidural scar more than 2 months old are the size of the extracellular space and the status of the endothelial gap junction, with vascular density playing a lesser role (35).

POSTOPERATIVE COMPLICATIONS

Postoperative Infection

The onset of progressively severe back pain occurring soon after surgery, especially when accompanied by a persistently elevated erythrocyte sedimentation rate, is suggestive of postoperative infection. T_2-weighted MR imaging is more sensitive early on than combined bone and gallium radionuclide scanning in the diagnosis of postoperative spondylitis and diskitis. However, the specificity of the radionuclide studies is greater than that of MR imaging (100% versus 92%, respectively) (68). The MR manifestations of diskitis include loss of the outline

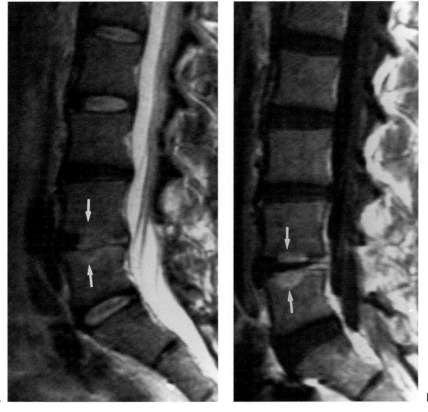

FIG. IIIB-9. Postoperative diskectomy scarring at L4-5 without laboratory evidence of diskitis (including percutaneous biopsy) 3 months following laminectomy, diskectomy, and exuberant disk curettage. **A:** Sagittal T_2-weighted (3000/102) fast spin-echo MR image demonstrates increased signal intensity in the posterior outer annulus, the nucleus pulposus and inner annulus, and the adjacent vertebral bodies at L4-5 (*arrows*). **B:** Sagittal T_1-weighted (300/16) conventional spin-echo MR image obtained 16 min after intravenous gadolinium administration shows that the annulus, vertebral bodies, and end plates enhance (*arrows*), although the central portion of the disk does not. This represents an example of extensive postoperative change in the absence of infection. (From Bundschuh, ref. 22, with permission.)

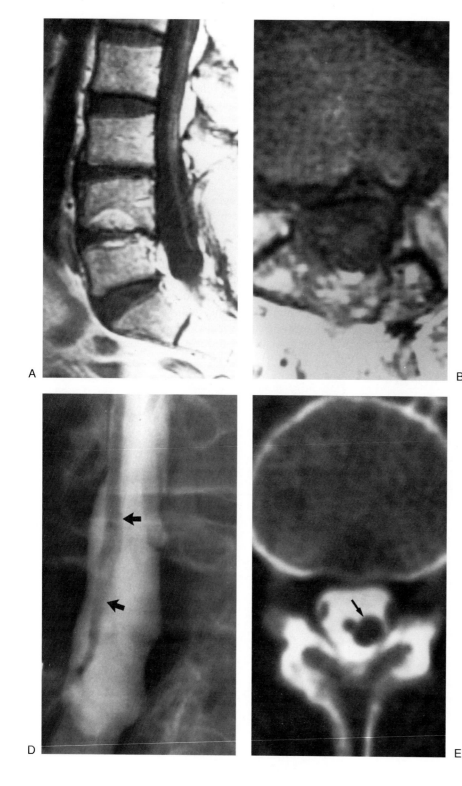

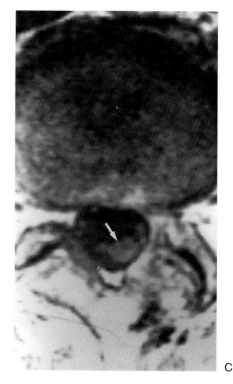

FIG. IIIB-10. Postoperative chronic arachnoiditis. **A:** Sagittal T₁-weighted (600/15) conventional spin-echo image demonstrating narrowing of the L4-5 intervertebral disk space, peridiskal vertebral fatty alteration, and a posterior laminectomy extending from L4 through S1. **B:** Axial T₁-weighted (600/15) conventional spin-echo image at the level of L3 demonstrating the laminectomy without associated abnormality. **C:** Enhanced axial T₁-weighted (600/15) conventional spin-echo image shows enhancement of matted nerve roots forming a thickened cord (*arrow*), indicating the presence of adhesive arachnoiditis. **D:** Oblique conventional radiographs from water-soluble contrast myelogram showing the partially empty sac and the cord-like matting of the nerve roots (*arrows*), proving the presence of arachnoiditis. **E:** Axial CT obtained through L3 showing matting of the nerve roots into a cord-like structure (*arrow*) and peripheral placement of the remaining roots, compatible with adhesive arachnoiditis (compare with **C**). (From Shafaie et al., ref. 101, with permission.)

of the vertebral end plates along with relatively low signal on T_1-weighted images within the peridiskal vertebral body marrow, coupled with high signal intensity on T_2-weighted acquisitions within the abnormal vertebral marrow (Fig. IIIB-8). The combination of extensive disk enhancement, posterior annulus enhancement, and enhancement of the adjacent marrow after gadolinium administration is not typically seen on MR images of asymptomatic postoperative patients in the immediate period after surgery (69). However, it should be noted that limited posterior annulus and peridiskal enhancement is commonly seen in asymptomatic postoperative disks (Fig. IIIB-9) (70).

Unfortunately, degenerative disk disease with fibrovascular alteration of the disk and adjacent vertebral body can also be associated with vertebral marrow enhancement after gadolinium administration, together with MR findings compatible with peridiskal vertebral edema (71). In addition, end-stage degenerative disk disease can on occasion show relatively increased intensity internally within the disk on T_2-weighted images that pathologically represents cystic spaces (72). These factors and possibilities should be taken into account in interpreting postsurgical images of the lumbosacral spine.

Epidural or paravertebral infection may be present postoperatively with or without findings of spondylitis or diskitis. Epidural infection can appear either as a homogeneously or slightly heterogeneously enhancing phlegmonous mass within the spinal canal on intravenous gadolinium enhanced T_1-weighted images, or it may present as a peripherally enhancing mass with a hypointense center representing liquefactive abscess formation. Without coexisting changes of diskitis, separating one type of epidural process from another, either benign or malignant, can be difficult.

Because of the nonspecific appearance of the postoperative spine with regard to spinal infection, correlation of both clinical (e.g., fever, surgical site drainage) and laboratory findings (e.g., blood or cerebrospinal fluid cultures) with the imaging studies is mandatory in such circumstances. The overall appearance on MR of the spinal tissues with or without contrast enhancement after surgical intervention is indeterminate, and percutaneous needle aspiration may be necessary in some cases in order to establish or exclude the presence of active postoperative infection.

Sterile Arachnoiditis

The factors inciting sterile spinal arachnoiditis are much debated but include the surgical procedure itself, the presence of intradural blood, controlled perioperative spinal infection, the previous use of myelographic contrast media (especially oil-based), and the prior intraspinal injection of anesthetic or antiinflammatory agents (e.g.,

steroids) (73,74). Chronically persistent lumbosacral signs and symptoms in 6% to 16% of postsurgical patients may be caused by sterile arachnoiditis (14).

The degree of severity of the imaging findings in a patient with arachnoiditis and the clinical severity do not appear to correlate well with one another (11). The symptoms, when present, are usually polyradicular, with pain and paresthesias extending into both lower extremities. Despite the presence of arachnoiditis, coexisting bony lateral stenosis or recurrent or residual disk herniation should be sought because they may imply a favorable chance of pain relief or diminution with repeat surgery.

Myelography and CT myelography usually clearly depict the changes indicative of arachnoiditis (Fig. IIIB-10) (73,75). However, subtle changes of focal arachnoiditis (i.e., absence of nerve-root sheath filling) may mimic the presence of a herniated disk. The three MR imaging patterns that have been described in adhesive arachnoiditis are (a) matted or clumped nerve roots, (b) an "empty" thecal sac caused by adhesions of the nerve roots to the walls of the thecal sac, and (c) an intrathecal soft tissue mass with a broad dural base that may obstruct the CSF pathways (75–79). These alterations may be either focal or diffuse. Enhancement of the thickened dural scarring on gadolinium-enhanced MR imaging, when present, does not seem to correlate well with actual severity of the arachnoiditis (76). Because pathologic enhancement is not always present in such cases, gadolinium administration does not always aid in its visualization. On the

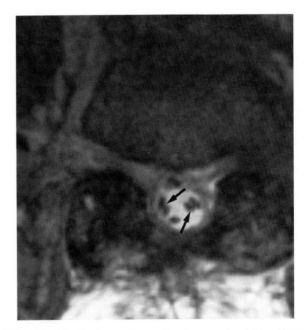

FIG. IIIB-11. Postoperative adhesive arachnoiditis. Unenhanced axial T_2-weighted (4000/108) fast spin-echo image acquired at the L5–S1 level shows matting (*arrows*) of the nerve roots of the cauda equina, indicating chronic adhesive arachnoiditis. (From Shafaie and Bundschuh, ref. 102, with permission.)

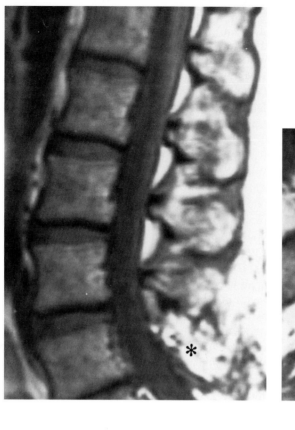

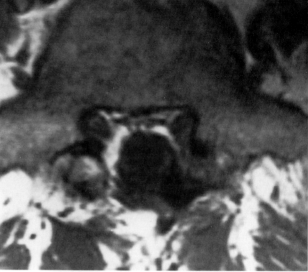

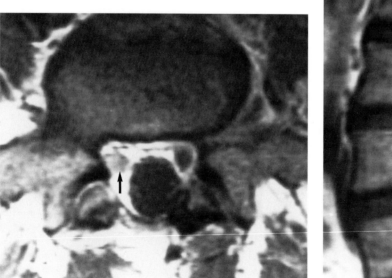

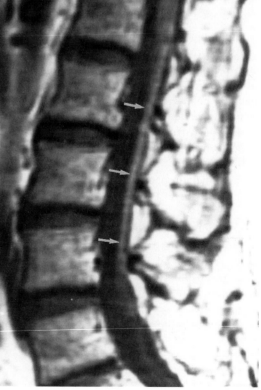

FIG. IIIB-12. Postoperative isolated, sterile radiculitis (neuritis). **A:** Unenhanced sagittal T$_1$-weighted (600/15) conventional spin-echo image demonstrating surgical change posteriorly at the L5 level (*asterisk*) without evidence of associated abnormality. **B:** Unenhanced axial T$_1$-weighted (600/15) conventional spin-echo image demonstrating the bilateral laminectomy without associated abnormality. **C:** Enhanced axial T$_1$-weighted (600/15) conventional spin-echo image shows intense enhancement of the S1 nerve root–sheath complex (*arrow*) without associated abnormalities. **D:** Enhanced sagittal T$_1$-weighted (600/15) conventional spin-echo image shows extensive multilevel enhancement of the S1 nerve root (*arrows*) extending craniad to the level of the conus medullaris of the spinal cord. (From Shafaie et al., ref. 101, with permission.)

other hand, gadolinium may on occasion demonstrate abnormal enhancement of the thickened leptomeninges and matted roots on enhanced MR (Fig. IIIB-10) (32,80,81). Such enhancement may also indicate an underlying element of chronic radiculitis (i.e., nerve root inflammation, see below), giving rise to radicular patient signs and symptoms. At present, the most reliable method of demonstrating the advanced findings of arachnoiditis on MR is the use of unenhanced axial T_2-weighted fast spin-echo acquisitions (Fig. IIIB-11). The classic findings of arachnoiditis identified on MR correlate well with identical findings seen on myelography and postmyelographic CT (74,76). A 92% sensitivity, 100% specificity, and 99% accuracy have been reported in the diagnosis of moderate to severe arachnoiditis by MR imaging (80).

Postoperative Radiculitis

On MR imaging, enhancement of the intrathecal spinal nerve roots of the cauda equina following intravenous gadolinium administration at a conventional dosage of 0.1 mmol/kg is not a normal observation (82). In other

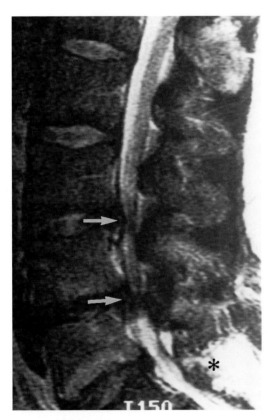

FIG. IIIB-13. Multilevel preexistent central spinal canal stenosis at levels separate from that of previous surgery. Sagittal T_2-weighted (2500/80) conventional spin-echo MR image showing surgical change (laminectomy) at the L5–S1 level (*asterisk*) and severe stenosis of the central spinal canal at the L3-4, and L4-5 levels, craniad to the operated level (*arrows*). (From Shafaie et al., ref. 101, with permission.)

words, spinal nerve roots have a visually intact blood–nerve barrier (BNB) on conventionally enhanced spin-echo MR. On the other hand, the distinction should be noted that there is little or no BNB within the spinal dorsal root ganglia, which explains their intense enhancement pattern after intravenous gadolinium administration (82). With frank compression injury to spinal nerves and nerve roots, however, this otherwise relatively intact BNB may break down (Fig. IIIB-12) (21). The complex and as yet poorly understood sequelae of chronic neural trauma and ischemia are believed to be the cause of the abnormal neurophysiologic changes resulting in clinical radiculopathy that may continue long after the initially offending influence (e.g., disk herniation) has been surgically removed (11,14,61,81,82).

Epidural or perineural fibrosis may cause cerebrospinal fluid nutritional deprivation and a tethering of the nerve root, engendering traction on the nerve during somatic movements. This in turn may induce further aberrant neuroelectrical potentials within the already inflamed, hypermechanosensitive nerve root(s) (15,21,83–86). In addition, actual mechanical circumferential constriction of the underlying nerve root could potentially be amplified by the perineural scar (15,21,87). In some cases, this might constitute a form of the minicompartment syndrome. Quite probably, patient symptoms of a radicular nature reflect the underlying chronic structural and inflammatory–biochemical alterations within the neural tissue (e.g., sodium channel dysfunction, myelinolysis, axonolysis, endoneural fibrosis) and the mechanical effects of the compressive-constrictive changes (e.g., perineural fibrosis, tethering phenomenon) occurring around the spinal nerves and nerve roots (3). The end result is an ectopic discharge within the insulted axon; the clinical manifestation is a radiating radiculopathy, muscular dysfunction, and autonomic derangement (3).

In a recent study of symptomatic postoperative patients, enhancement of spinal nerve roots after gadolinium administration was demonstrated at, and extending away from, the surgical site in the chronic postoperative period (i.e., more than 6 to 8 months after surgery) (Fig. IIIB-12) (15,21). It has been shown in laboratory models that mechanical injury alone is sufficient to cause focal BNB disruption and nerve-root enhancement on MR (88,89). It has also been proven in laboratory models of neural crush that wallerian axon degeneration and regeneration are associated with and may even induce and prolong the BNB breakdown; in fact, BNB disruption is believed to serve as an indicator of such degenerative activity (21,90–92). Almost certainly, the instances of nerve-root enhancement or MR remote to the site of injury (i.e., distant from disk herniation and surgery) are associated with ongoing degenerative and regenerative phenomena within injured nerves.

From a practical standpoint, chronic postoperative nerve root enhancement on MR correlates well with the

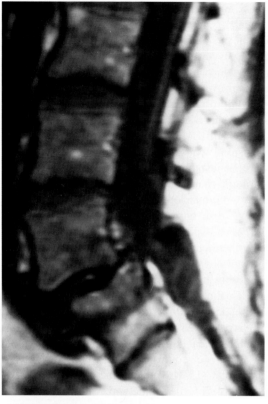

A

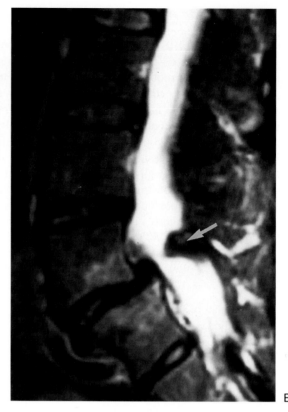

B

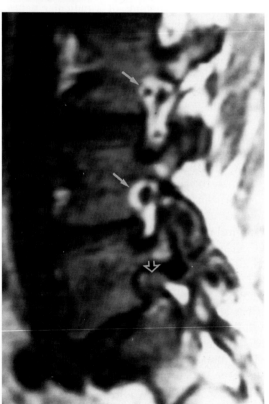

C

FIG. IIIB-14. Postoperative spinal instability resulting in spondylolisthesis and central spinal canal stenosis. **A:** Unenhanced sagittal T$_1$-weighted (600/15) conventional spin-echo MR image demonstrates a postoperative grade I spondylolisthesis at L5–S1. **B:** Sagittal T$_2$-weighted (4000/90) fast spin-echo image again shows the grade I spondylolisthesis. Also noted is surgical change in the posterior soft tissues at the L5–S1 level and severe stenosis of the central spinal canal caused by encroachment of the bony elements of the posterior neural arch (*arrow*). This is a result of the spondylolisthesis occurring in the face of incomplete resection of the posterior neural arch. **C:** Paramedian sagittal T$_1$-weighted (600/15) conventional spin-echo MR image on the patient's left side shows patency of the neural foramina at L3-4 and L4-5 (*closed arrows*) but encroachment on the superior recess of the neural foramen at L5-S1 (*open arrow*), indicating entrapment or impingement of the L5 nerve roots–spinal nerve–dorsal root ganglion. This results from the postoperative spondylolisthesis and may be asymmetric [the patient's right side (not shown) was not involved]. (From Shafaie et al., ref. 101, with permission.)

radicular clinical presentation (15,21). However, a caveat should be noted in that during the first 6 to 8 months after disk surgery, nerve root enhancement can be seen in the asymptomatic patient; this enhancement apparently reflects the nerve root under repair (93). Nevertheless, in the proper clinical setting of the chronic FBSS, nerve root enhancement may be used to confirm the presence of clinically relevant imaging findings in etiologically uncertain cases of postoperative radiculopathy. To reiterate, this is true only in the chronic postoperative period (i.e., more than 6 to 8 months following disk surgery).

Spinal Stenosis

Stenosis of the central spinal canal, the lateral recess of the spinal canal, and the neural foramen may be a cause of the FBSS (14). These forms of spinal stenosis may preexist (Fig. IIIB-13) or follow the spinal surgery (Fig. IIIB-14). Although published studies have methodologic biases and small sample sizes, it appears that the sensitivity and specificity of MR imaging and CT for depicting spinal stenosis are similar to one another (true-positive rate of approximately 90%, false-positive rate of approximately 20%) (93). The appearance of lateral recess spinal stenosis on MR is best depicted utilizing T_2-weighted, fat-suppressed axial fast spin-echo imaging. Central canal stenosis is well seen with T_2-weighted fast spin-echo axial acquisitions. Neural foramen narrowing and dorsal nerve root ganglion deformity are best imaged with direct sagittal T_1-weighted MR imaging (Fig. IIIB-15).

Postoperative Pseudomeningocele

Postlaminectomy pseudomeningocele results either from an inadvertent dural tear or from a persistent opening in the dura following intradural surgery. It is a pseudomeningocele because it is not a true arachnoid-lined sac. This potential cause of FBSS usually presents as a recurrence of low back pain following an asymptomatic interval of several weeks. There may also be radicular signs and symptoms as well (94). Pseudomeningoceles appear as well-defined fluid collections abutting on the surgical site and extending into the posterior paraspinal soft tissues (Fig. IIIB-16) (94–98). Although postoperative pseudomeningoceles usually demonstrate CSF signal intensity on all MR sequences, sometimes fluid–fluid levels or relative differences in MR signal intensity are seen secondary to blood products or internal debris (76,97).

Postoperative Spondylolisthesis and Failed Fusion

Failed operative fusion with resultant spinal instability may reveal a change in bony spinal relationships on MR

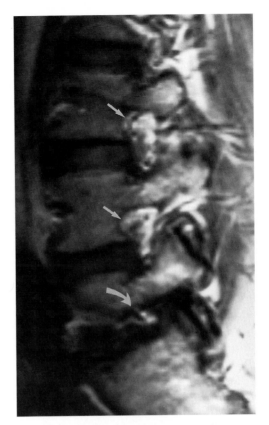

FIG. IIIB-15. Probably preexistent severe right L5 neural foramen stenosis noted in the postoperative period. Unenhanced sagittal T_1-weighted (600/10) conventional spin-echo MR image on the patient's right side shows obliteration of the majority of fat in the L5–S1 neural foramen (*curved arrow*), indicating entrapment of the L5 nerve root–spinal nerve–dorsal root ganglion by the hypertrophied surrounding bony and ligamentous structures. Note the normal neural foramina at L3-4 and L4-5 with hyperintense fat surrounding the L3 and L4 nerve roots (*straight arrows*). (From Bundschuh, ref. 22, with permission.)

imaging. Spondylolisthesis secondary to spinal instability from excessive posterior-element surgical resection or postoperative facet fracture in the absence of a surgical fusion produces similar findings. It is important to note that this spondylolisthesis may be associated with central and foraminal spinal stenosis with entrapment of nerve roots (Fig. IIIB-14) (99,100).

Normally, stable fusions cause a conversion of red marrow to yellow (fatty) marrow secondary to a decrease in biomechanical stresses. This is manifested as a subchondral region paralleling the vertebral end plates demonstrating relative high signal intensity on T_1-weighted images and isointensity or slightly high relative signal intensity on T_2-weighted images. The MR imaging can occasionally depict a failed fusion by demonstrating increased signal intensity in peridiscal regions on T_2-weighted images in the area(s) of bone discontinuity, perhaps representing microfractures and bone edema. It should be noted that a time interval of more than 1 year

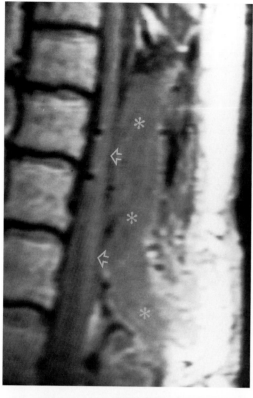

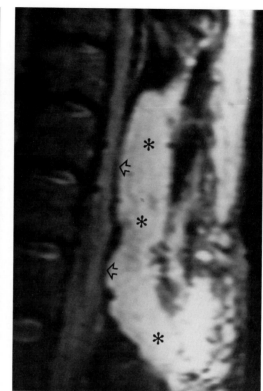

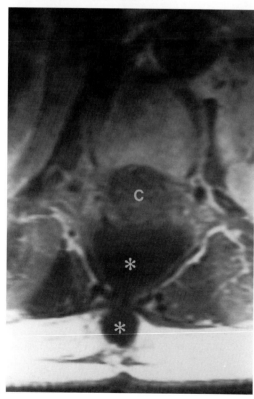

FIG. IIIB-16. Postoperative pseudomeningocele. **A:** Sagittal T$_1$-weighted (600/15) conventional spin-echo MR image showing the extensive lumbar postsurgical change and the large intermediate-intensity abnormality in the posterior spinal soft tissues (*asterisks*) abutting the spinal cord and canal (*open arrows*). **B:** Sagittal T$_2$-weighted (2500/80) conventional spin-echo MR image shows the marked hyperintensity of the CSF collection representing the pseudomeningocele (*asterisks*). The pseudomeningocele can be seen to encroach on the posterior aspect of the spinal cord and canal (*arrowheads*). **C:** Unenhanced axial T$_1$-weighted (600/15) conventional spin-echo MR image shows the spinal canal (C) and the posteriorly located pseudomeningocele (*asterisks*) extending through the posterior paraspinal facia in a dumbbell configuration. (From Shafaie et al., ref. 101, with permission.)

is usually needed between the surgical fusion and the MR examination study in order to fully appreciate and judge these changes. Kinetic flexion–extension MR imaging utilized to judge spinal stability, accomplished with the patient in the lateral decubitus position, may be of use when using MR units that allow such studies to be performed in the lumbosacral region.

CONCLUSIONS

Gadolinium-enhanced MR is at present the single most sensitive and specific imaging modality available to the medical imaging physician for the purpose of evaluation of the postoperative lumbosacral spine in the patient presenting with the FBSS. Unanswered questions remain concerning the elucidation of factors that might more accurately predict surgical success or failure preoperatively and the effective medical approach toward such postoperative findings as arachnoiditis, radiculitis, and fibrosis that as yet do not have clearly defined modes of treatment. The solutions to such clinical problems may enable both medical imaging specialists and clinicians to better understand the origins and means of avoiding the FBSS, to more clearly focus the postoperative imaging evaluation in these patients and to more successfully link the clinical diagnosis and the imaging findings with optimized, effective patient therapy.

ACKNOWLEDGMENT

The authors thank J. Murray for the manuscript preparation and C. Farias for the photographic reproductions.

REFERENCES

1. Rish BL: A critique of the surgical management of lumbar disc disease in a private neurosurgical practice. *Spine* 1984;9:500–504.
2. Ross JS: Magnetic resonance assessment of the postoperative spine: Degenerative disc disease. *Radiol Clin North Am* 1991;29:793–808.
3. Jinkins JR: The pathoanatomic basis of somatic and autonomic syndromes originating in the lumbosacral spine. *Neuroimag Clin North Am* 1993;3:443–463.
4. Kirkaldy-Willis WH, Hill RJ: A more precise diagnosis for low-back pain. *Spine* 1979;4:102–109.
5. Saal JS, Franson RC, Dobrow R, Saal JA, White AH, Goldthwaite N: High levels of inflammatory phospholipase A₂ activity in lumbar disc herniations. *Spine* 1990;15:674–678.
6. McCall IW: Morphology in postdiscectomy problems, importance of magnetic resonance imaging. *Acta Orthop Scand* [*Suppl*] 1993;251:47–48.
7. Weber H: Lumbar disk herniation. A prospective study of prognostic factors including a controlled trial. Part I. *J Oslo City Hosp* 1989;28:33–61.
8. Weber H: Lumbar disk herniation. A prospective study of prognostic factors including a controlled trial. Part II. *J Oslo City Hosp* 1978;28:89–113.
9. Abramovitz JN, Neff SR: Lumbar disc surgery: Results of the prospective lumbar discectomy study of the Joint Section on Disorders of the Spine and Peripheral Nerves of the American Association of Neurological Surgeons and the Congress of Neurological Surgeons. *Neurosurgery* 1991;29:301–308.
10. Quigley MR, Kortyna R, Goodwin C, Maroon JC: Lumbar surgery in the elderly. *Neurosurgery* 1992;30:672–674.
11. Burton CV: Lumbosacral arachnoiditis. *Spine* 1978;3:24–30.
12. Djukic S, Lang P, Morris J, Hoaglund F, Genant HK: The postoperative spine: Magnetic resonance imaging. *Orthop Clin North Am* 1990;21:603–624.
13. Djukic S, Genant H, Helms C, Holt RG: Magnetic resonance imaging of the postoperative lumbar spine. *Radiol Clin North Am* 1990;28:341–360.
14. Burton CV, Kirkaldy-Willis WH, Yong-Hing K, Heithott KB: Causes of failure of surgery on the lumbar spine. *Clin Orthop Rel Res* 1981;157:191–199.
15. Jinkins JR, Osborn AG, Garrett D, Hunt S, Story JL: Spinal nerve enhancement with Gd-DTPA: MR correlation with the postoperative lumbosacral spine. *Am J Neuroradiol* 1993;14:383–394.
16. Ross JS, Modic MT, Masaryk TJ: Tears of the annulus fibrosus: Assessment with Gd-DTPA-enhanced MR imaging. *Am J Neuroradiol* 1989;10:1251–1254.
17. Jinkins JR, Whittemore AR, Bradley WG: The anatomic basis of vertebrogenis pain and the autonomic syndrome associated with lumbar disc extrusion. *Am J Neuroradiol* 1989;10:219–231.
18. Goldwag SS, Frei DF, Gupta KL, et al: Comparison of fast spin-echo and conventional spin-echo MR imaging in the brain, orbit and postoperative spine. Presented at the annual meeting of Roentgen Ray Society, New Orleans, 1994.
19. Mirowitz SA, Shady KL: Gadopentetate dimeglumine-enhanced MR imaging of the postoperative lumbar spine: Comparison of fat-suppressed and conventional T₁-weighted images. *Am J Roentgenol* 1992;159:385–389.
20. Ross JS, Delamarter R, Heuftle MG, et al: Gadolinium-DTPA-enhanced MR imaging of the postoperative lumbar spines: Time course and mechanisms of enhancement. *Am J Roentgenol* 1989;152:825–834.
21. Jinkins JR: Magnetic resonance imaging of benign nerve root enhancement in the unoperated and opostoperative lumbosacral spine. *Neuroimag Clin North Am* 1993;3:525–541.
22. Bundschuh CV: Imaging of the postoperative lumbosacral spine. *Neuroimag Clin North Am* 1993;3:499–516.
23. Bangert BA, Ross JS: Arachnoiditis affecting the lumbosacral spine. *Neuroimag Clin North Am* 1993;3:517–524.
24. Dina TS, Boden SD, Davis DO: Review: Lumbar spine after surgery for herniated disk: Imaging findings in the early postoperative period. *Am J Roentgenol* 1995;164:665.
25. Annertz M, Jonsson B, Stromqvist B, et al: Serial MRI in the early postoperative period after lumbar discectomy. *Neuroradiology* 1955;37:177.
26. Deutsch AL, Howard M, Dawson EG, et al: Lumbar spine following successful surgical discectomy: Magnetic resonance imaging features and implications. *Spine* 1993;18:1054–1060.
27. Van De Kelft EJ, Van Goethem JW, De La Porte C, et al: Early postoperative gadolinium-DTPA-enhanced MR imaging after successful lumbar discectomy. *Br J Neurosurgery* 1996;10:41–49.
28. Grand CM, Bank WO, Baleriaux D, Matos C, Levivier M, Brotchi J: Gadolinium enhancement of vertebral endplates following lumbar disc surgery. *Neuroradiology* 1993;35:503–505.
29. Boden SD, Davis DO, Dinats Sunner JL, Wiesel SW: Postoperative diskitis: Distinguishing early MR imaging findings from normal postoperative disk space changes. *Radiology* 1992;184:765–771.
30. Bundschuh CV, Modic MT, Ross JS, Masaryk TJ, Bohlman H: Epidural fibrosis and recurrent disk herniation in the lumbar spine: MR imaging assessment. *Am J Roentgenol* 1988;150:923–932.
31. Frocrain L, Duvauferrier R, Husson JL, Noel J, Ramee A, Pawlotsky Y: Recurrent postoperative sciatica: Evaluation with MR imaging and enhanced CT. *Radiology* 1989;170:531–533.
32. Hueftle MG, Modic MT, Ross JS, et al: Lumbar spine: Postoperative MR imaging with Gd-DTPA. *Radiology* 1988;167:817–824.
33. Ross JS, Masaryk TJ, Schrader M, Gentili A, Bohlman H, Modic MT: MR imaging of the postoperative lumbar spine: Assessment with gadopentetate dimeglumine. *Am J Roentgenol* 1990;155:867–872.
34. Sotiropoulos S, Chafetz NI, Lang P, et al: Differentiation between

postoperative scar and recurrent disk herniation: Prospective comparison of MR, CT, and contrast-enhanced CT. *Am J Neuroradiol* 1989;10:639–643.

35. Bundschuh CV, Stein L, Slusser JH, Schinco FP, Ladaga LE, Dillon JD: Distinguishing between scar and recurrent herniated disk in postoperative patients: Values of contrast-enhanced CT and MR imaging. *Am J Neuroradiol* 1990;11:949–958.

36. Lipson SJ, Muir H: Proteoglycans in experimental disc degeneration. *Spine* 1981;6:194–210.

37. Naylor A, Happey F, Turner RL, Shentall RD, West DC, Richardson C: Enzymic and immunological activity in the intervertebral disc. *Orthop Clin North Am* 1975;6:51–68.

38. Donoff BR, Burke JF: Abnormality of hypertrophic scar blood vessels. *J Surg Res* 1978;25:251–255.

39. Kischer CW: Fine structure of granulation tissues from deep injury. *J Invest Dermatol* 1979;72:147–152.

40. Kischer CW, Thies AC, Chvapil M: Perivascular myofibroblasts and microvascular occlusion in hypertrophic scars and keloids. *Hum Pathol* 1982;13:819–824.

41. Kischer CW, Shetlar MR: Microvasculature in hypertrophic scars and the effects of pressure. *J Trauma* 1979;19:757–764.

42. Linares HA, Kischer CW, Dobrkovsky M, Larson DL: The histiotypic organization of the hypertrophic scar in humans. *J Invest Dermatol* 1972;59:323–331.

43. Tripathi RC, Tripathi BJ: Functional ultrastructure of endothelium. *Bibl Anat* 1977;16:307–312.

44. Weber K, Braun-Falco O: Ultrastructure of blood vessels in human granulation tissue. *Arch Dermatol Res* 1973;248:29–44.

45. Milici AJ, Furie MB, Carley WW: The formation of fenestrations and channels by capillary endothelium *in vitro*. *Proc Natl Acad Sci USA* 1985;82:6181–6185.

46. Hunter JAA, Finlay JB: Scanning electron microscopy of normal human scar tissues and keloids. *Br J Surg* 1976;63:826–830.

47. Ross JS, Blaser S, Masaryk TJ, et al: Gd-DTPA enhancement of posterior epidural scar: An experimental model. *Am J Neuroradiol* 1989;10:1083–1088.

48. Eckert C, Decker A: Pathological studies of intervertebral discs. *J Bone Joint Surg* 1947;29:447–454.

49. Lindblom K, Hultqvist G: Absorption of protruded disc tissue. *J Bone Joint Surg* 1950;32A:557–560.

50. Bobechko WP, Hirsch C: Auto-immune response to nucleus pulposus in the rabbit. *J Bone Joint Surg* 1965;47B:574–580.

51. McCarron RF, Wimpee MW, Hudkins PG, Iaros GS: The inflammatory effect of nucleus pulposus. A possible element in the pathogenesis of low-back pain. *Spine* 1987;12:760–764.

52. Hassler O: The human intervertebral disc: A microangiographical study on its vascular supply at various ages. *Acta Orthop Scand* 1969;40:765–772.

53. Nguyen CM, Ho K-C, Yu S, Haughton VM, Strandt JA: An experimental model to study contrast enhancement in MR imaging of the intervertebral disk. *Am J Neuroradiol* 1989;10:811–814.

54. Kramer J, Schleberger R, Hedtmann A: *Intervertebral Disc Diseases: Causes, Diagnosis, Treatment and Prophylaxis*, 2nd ed. (Mueller KH, trans). New York: Thieme, 1990.

55. Sether LA, Yu S, Haughton V, Fischer ME: Intervertebral disk: Normal age-related changes in MR signal intensity. *Radiology* 1990;177:385–388.

56. Urban JPG, Holm S, Maroudas A, Nachemson A: Nutrition of the intervertebral disc. An *in vivo* study of solute transport. *Clin Orthop Rel Res* 1977;129:101–114.

57. Higuchi M, Abe K: Ultrastructure of the nucleus pulposus in the intervertebral disc after systemic administration of hydrocortisone in mice. *Spine* 1985;10:638–643.

58. Souter WA, Taylor TKF: Sulfated acid mucopolysaccharide metabolism in the rabbit intervertebral disc. *J Bone Joint Surg* 1970;52(B):371–384.

59. Branemark PI, Ekholm R, Lundskog J: Tissue response to chymopapain in different concentration. Animal investigations on microvascular effects. *Clin Orthop Rel Res* 1969;67:52–67.

60. Mitchell PEG, Hendry NGC, Billewicz WZ: The chemical background of intervertebral disc prolapse. *J Bone Joint Surg* 1961;43(B):141–151.

61. Coventry MB, Ghormley RK, Kernohan JW: The intervertebral disc: Its microscopic anatomy and pathology. Part II: Changes in

the intervertebral disc concomitant with age. *J Bone Joint Surg* 1945;27:233–247.

62. Coventry MB, Ghormley RK, Kernohan JW: The intervertebral disc: Its microscopic anatomy and pathology. Part III: Pathologic changes in the intervertebral disc. *J Bone Joint Surg* 1945;27:460–474.

63. Yasuma T, Arai K, Yamauchi Y: The histology of lumbar intervertebral disc herniation. *Spine* 1993;18:1761–1765.

64. Bozzao A, Gallucci M, Masciocchi C, Aprile I, Barile A, Passariello R: Lumbar disk herniation: MR imaging assessment of natural history in patients treated without surgery. *Radiology* 1992;185:135–141.

65. Kormano MJ, Dean PB: Extravascular contrast material: The major component of contrast enhancement. *Radiology* 1976;121:379–382.

66. Newhouse JH: Fluid compartment distribution of intravenous iothalamate in the dog. *Invest Radiol* 1977;12:364–367.

67. Schmiedl U, Moseley ME, Organ MD, Chew WM, Brasch RC: Comparison of initial biodistribution patterns of Gd-DTPA and albumin-Gd-DTPA using rapid spin echo imaging. *J Comput Assist Tomogr* 1987;11:306–313.

68. Modic MT, Feiglin DH, Pirano DW, et al: Vertebral osteomyelitis: Assessment using MR. *Radiology* 1985;157:156–166.

69. Schultz KP, Assheuer J: Discitis after procedures on the intervertebral disc. *Spine* 1994;19:1172–1177.

70. Boden SD, Davis DO, Dina TS, et al: Postoperative discitis: Distinguishing early MR findings from normal postoperative disc space changes. *Radiology* 1992;184:765–771.

71. Modic MT, Steinberg PM, Ross JS, Masaryk TJ, Carter JR: Degenerative disk disease: Assessment of changes in vertebral body marrow with MR imaging. *Radiology* 1988;166:193–199.

72. Yu S, Haughton VM, Ho PSP, Sether LA, Wagner M, Ho KC: Progressive and regressive changes in the nucleus pulposus. Part II: The adult. *Radiology* 1988;169:93–97.

73. Quencer RM, Tenner M, Rothman L: The postoperative myelogram. Radiographic evaluation of arachnoiditis and dural/arachnoidal tears. *Radiology* 1977;123:667–679.

74. Fitt GJ, Stevens JM: Postoperative arachnoiditis diagnosed by high resolution fast spin-echo MRI of the lumbar spine. *Neuroradiology* 1995;37:139–145.

75. Ruscalleda J: Postoperative spine. *Riv Neuroradiol* 1992;5(S):93–100.

76. Johnson CE, Sze G: Benign lumbar arachnoiditis. MR imaging with gadopentetate dimeglumine. *Am J Neuroradiol* 1990;11:763–790. *Am J Roentgenol* 1990;155:873–880.

77. Castan P, Bourbotte G, Herail JP, Maurel J: Follow-up and postoperative radiculography. *J Neuroradiol* 1977;4:49–93.

78. Meyer JD, Latchaw RE, Roppolo HM, Ghoshkajra K, Deeb ZL: Computed tomography and myelography of the postoperative lumbar spine. *Am J Neuroradiol* 1982;3:223–228.

79. Ross JS, Masaryk TJ, Modic MT, et al: MR imaging of lumbar arachnoiditis. *Am J Roentgenol* 1987;149:1025–1032.

80. Firooznia H, Krischeff II, Rafii M, Golimbu C: Lumbar spine after surgery: Examination with intravenous contrast enhanced CT. *Radiology* 1987;163:221–226.

81. Teplick JG, Haskin MR: Intravenous contrast-enhanced CT of the postoperative lumbar spine: Improved identification of recurrent disc herniation, scar, arachnoiditis, and diskitis. *Am J Roentgenol* 1984;143:845–855.

82. Breger RK, Williams AL, Daniels DL, et al: Contrast enhancement in spinal MR imaging. *Am J Roentgenol* 1989;153:387–391.

83. Charnley J: The imbibition of fluid as a cause of herniation of the nucleus pulposus. *Lancet* 1952;262:124–127.

84. Howe JF, Loeser JD, Calvin WH: Mechanosensitivity of dorsal root ganglia and chronically injured axons: A physiological basis for the radicular pain of nerve root compression. *Pain* 1977;3:25–41.

85. Smyth MJ, Wright V: Sciatica and the intervertebral disc: An experimental study. *J Bone Joint Surg* 1958;40A:1401–1418.

86. Rydevik B, Holm S, Brown MD, Lundborg G: Nuerition of spinal nerve roots: The role of diffusion from the cerebrospinal fluid. *Trans Orthop Res Soc* 1984;9:276.

87. Ransford AO, Harries BJ: Localised arachnoiditis complicating lumbar disc lesions. *J Bone Joint Surg* 1972;54B:656–665.

88. Mackinnon SE, Delton AL, Hudson AR, Hunter DA: Chronic nerve compression: an experimental model in the rat. *Ann Plast Surg* 1984;13:112–120.
89. Kobayashi S, Yoshizawa H, Hachiya Y, Ukai T, Morita T: Vasogenic edema induced by compression injury to the spinal nerve root: Distribution of intravenously injected protein tracers and gadolinium-enhanced magnetic resonance imaging. *Spine* 1993; 18:1410–1424.
90. Sparrow JR, Kiernan JA: Endoneurial vascular permeability in degenerating and regenerating peripheral nerves. *Acta Neuropathol (Berl)* 1981;53:181–188.
91. Weerasuriya A, Rapoport SI, Taylor RE: Perineurial permeability increases during Wallerian degeneration. *Brain Res* 1980;192: 581–585.
92. Boden SD, Davis DO, Dina TS, et al: Contrast-enhanced MR imaging performed after successful lumbar disk surgery: Prospective study. *Radiology* 1992;182:59–64.
93. Kent DL, Haynor DR, Larson EB, Deyo RA: Diagnosis of lumbar spine stenosis in adults: A metaanalysis of the accuracy of CT, MR, and myelography. *Am J Roentgenol* 1992;158:1135–1144.
94. Teplick JG, Peyster RG, Teplick SK, Goodman LR, Haskin ME: CT identification of postlaminectomy pseudomeningocele. *Am J Neuroradiol* 1983;4:179–182.
95. Lee KS, Hardy IM: Postlaminectomy lumbar pseudomeningocele: report of four cases. *Neurosurgery* 1992;30:111–114.
96. Ramsey RG, Penn RD: Computed tomography of a false postoperative meningocele. *Am J Neuroradiol* 1984;5:326–328.
97. Murayama S, Numaguchi Y, Whitecloud TS, Brent CR: Magnetic resonance imaging of post-surgical pseudomeningocele. *Comput Med Imag Graphics* 1989;13:335–339.
98. Barron JT: Lumbar pseudomeningocele. *Orthopedics* 1990;13: 608–609.
99. Jinkins JR, Matthes JC, Sener RN, et al: Spondylolysis, spondylolisthesis, and associated nerve root entrapment in the lumbosacral spine: MR evaluation. *Am J Roentgenol* 1992;159:799–803.
100. Jinkins JR, Rauch RA: Magnetic resonance imaging of entrapment of lumbar nerve roots in spondylolytic spondylolisthesis. *J Bone Joint Surg* 1994;76(A):1643–1648.
101. Shafaie FF, Bundschuh CV, Jinkins JR: Postoperative lumbosacral spine. In: Edelman R, Hesselink J, eds. *Clinical Magnetic Resonance Imaging,* 2nd ed. Philadelphia: WB Saunders, 1996, pp. 1226–1247.
102. Shafaie FF, Bundschuh CV: Spine. In: Deutsch A, Mink J, eds. *MRI of the Musculoskeletal System: A Teaching File,* 2nd ed. New York: Lippincott-Raven, in press.

Posttherapeutic Neurodiagnostic Imaging,
edited by J.R. Jinkins,
Lippincott-Raven Publishers, New York © 1997.

CHAPTER **IIIC**

Principles, Imaging, and Complications of Spinal Instrumentation

Radiologist's Perspective

Richard M. Slone and Kevin W. McEnery

Spinal fusion is often required for the purpose of successful correction or repair of spinal instability or deformity. For certain selected problems, a single-level fusion can be accomplished without the aid of fixation devices. For other pathologies such as spondylolisthesis, it is difficult or impossible to adequately fuse the spine without surgical instrumentation. The likelihood of a successful solid arthrodesis increases when instrumentation is used to span multiple segments (1). Metal wires, plates, screws, and rod instrumentation systems are the most common materials that have been used in the treatment of fractures, degenerative disease, and congenital deformities. The instrumentation is used to provide stability, restore and maintain anatomic alignment, and limit motion as the spine fuses. Although metal instrumentation provides immediate stability, it is subject to fatigue failure, with eventual loosening or fracture from repeated stress if bony fusion does not occur over the involved segment. Providing stability and maintaining alignment during the fusion is the primary purpose of most spinal instrumentation. The success of spinal fusion greatly increases with bone grafting. Such grafts are usually placed in conjunction with the instrumentation to promote a permanent fusion. Exceptions to this rule include patients who have a decreased life expectancy, such as those with metastatic neoplastic spinal disease, who require stabilization but not arthrodesis (2).

The purpose of instrumentation is to provide purchase to an individual level and rigid linkage to other levels. Different instrumentation systems use varying specific approaches to accomplish these two goals. In general, spinal instrumentation using internal stabilization is superior to external immobilization, such as braces and casts, for stabilizing and immobilizing the spine during the fusion process (2).

Spinal elements that are infected, crushed, or involved with tumor often must be removed (corpectomy), leaving a large bony defect and a mechanically unstable spine. Replacement materials such as structural bone grafts, methylmethacrylate, and titanium cages are used to maintain height and restore alignment. Methylmethacrylate is typically used only for the treatment of metastatic tumors to replace vertebral bodies if the life expectancy of the patient is short; it is contraindicated in the treatment of osteomyelitis.

Significant recent changes in spinal fixation have occurred with the development of biocompatible materials that can be left in place permanently and can withstand the repeated stresses of weight bearing, flexion, and extension until arthrodesis occurs. Prior to the development of stainless steel devices in the 1930s, materials used for implants were suboptimal, often requiring removal for failure or because of intervening complications (3).

The first attempts at internal fixation of the spine were undertaken in the late 19th century, and the first successful spinal fusion was reported in 1911 (1,4,5). Graft consisting of autologous iliac bone was first used in the 1930s (6). Facet joint-screw placement for stabilization after

R. M. Slone and K. W. McEnery: Mallinckrodt Institute of Radiology, Washington University School of Medicine, St. Louis, Missouri 63110.

spinal fusion occurred in the 1940s (7). Spinous process plates and distraction rods (Knodt rods) were developed in the 1950s (7,8), rod systems attached to the spine with hooks (Harrington rods) in the early 1960s (9,10), and smooth rods attached with wire (Luque rods) in the 1970s (11,12). The transverse processes were not routinely incorporated into the fusion mass until the late 1960s (13). Although pedicle screws and plates were introduced in the 1960s (13), they did not become popular until the mid- to late 1980s.

The instrumentation is no longer needed once fusion has occurred but is generally left in place indefinitely because of the potential risks associated with repeated surgery. Infection and pain are two indications for removal of the instrumentation following fusion. Fractured and dislodged implants are typical signs of failed fusion and pseudoarthrosis; the instrumentation in such cases is usually removed for the purpose of revision of the fusion. The risk of neurologic injury from migration of the components is low, and instrumentation is rarely removed for this reason. Pressure sores overlying spinal instruments are a potential risk of failure in patients who are neurologically impaired.

INDICATIONS FOR SPINAL SURGERY

Low back pain and radiculopathy are two of the most common medical problems in America. Although conservative treatment provides relief in the majority of cases, some patients require surgical intervention for the treatment of herniated disks, spondylolysis with spondylolisthesis, degenerative spinal disease with instability, scoliosis, or spinal stenosis.

Degenerative Spinal Disease and Instability

Spinal stability is defined as the ability of the spine to resist deformation from physiologic forces. This stability is important because it prevents permanent displacement, deformity, and neurologic compromise. Spinal instability as a result of surgery or degenerative spinal disease is a common indication for spinal fusion requiring instrumentation. Instability of the spine may be chronic or acute, as when it is exposed to sudden external forces. Such acute instability is usually the result of trauma and ligamentous failure or fracture of the vertebral body or facets. Radiologic evidence of acute instability includes subluxation and angulation.

In most cases, spondylolysis, degenerative spondylolisthesis, and scoliosis are all associated with spinal instability, and correction may require surgical instrumentation. However, surgical indications in patients with degenerative disk disease have not been clearly established, and the need for fusion is controversial. A reduction in spinal

stability occurs when the spinal lamina and portions of the posterior elements and facet joints are removed. Significant clinical symptoms can develop if progressive scoliosis or vertebral body slippage occurs. A laminectomy at multiple levels for disk disease or spinal stenosis also may lead to instability requiring posterior fusion and fixation.

Arthrodesis is often the only treatment available in cases of severe degenerative disease and instability (1). Instrumentation is not required for fusion to occur in some cases, such as a single-level fusion after diskectomy. Supplemental bone grafts are usually required for longer fusion segments to promote arthrodesis, and simultaneous spinal instrumentation is needed to provide immediate stability. The extent of surgical decompression and the amount of spinal deformity will determine the nature of the instrumentation and the type of fusion required.

Spinal Scoliosis

Spinal deformities with a component of scoliosis are a common indication for spinal instrumentation and fusion. A great deal of the spinal instrumentation in use today was originally developed for the treatment of scoliosis. A variety of surgical techniques exist, each of which approaches the problem differently. Spinal instrumentation has been used in the treatment of congenital, neuromuscular, degenerative, and idiopathic scoliosis. Surgical indications include marked angulation, pain, progression, pulmonary dysfunction, and neurologic compromise. Congenital scoliosis generally results in short, sharply curved segments and is often treated at an earlier age than scoliosis of other causes. Such early surgical corrections may require later revision because of continued patient growth and progressive deformity. Brace treatment and early recognition to prevent or slow the progression of idiopathic scoliosis have decreased the need for adolescent surgery.

Scoliosis surgery is designed to achieve some correction of the spine in the coronal plane, to preserve the normal sagittal curves, and to fuse as few segments as possible. In principle, it is important that the top and bottom of the spine fusion fall within the stable zone and that the patient be balanced in both the coronal and sagittal plane following surgery. Balance in the coronal plane is defined as the C7 vertebral body falling directly over the midline of the sacrum. Balance in the sagittal plane is defined as the C7 vertebral body falling through or behind the L5–S1 disk.

One of the earliest techniques used to control scoliosis was external bracing, which provided direct pressure at the apex of the scoliotic curve (14). Since that time, it has been found that bracing does not provide permanent correction of scoliosis, but, as noted in the foregoing, it can be useful to prevent progression during the growing years. Early methods of internal fixation, such as Harrington distraction rods, used the concept of distraction. However, the force required for correction of scoliosis increases as the curve angle diminishes, thus limiting the mechanical advantage of the instrumentation and the correction that can be achieved (14). Current improved techniques include paired rod systems such as segmental wiring with Luque rods and Cotrel–Dubousset (CD) instrumentation with pedicle screws and laminar hooks, which provide purchase at multiple spinal levels.

Trauma

Instability that results from fracture or ligament injury and compromise of the spinal canal are indications for surgical instrumentation after spinal trauma. Falls and motor vehicle accidents are the most common causes of acute spinal injuries. Fortunately, only a small percentage of these injuries result in neurologic deficits. Several physical mechanisms may result in spinal injuries, including flexion, extension, rotation, lateral bending, or axial compression. An understanding of the biomechanical stability of fractures can be gained by considering the spine as three anatomic columns. The anterior column consists of the anterior vertebral body, the anterior longitudinal ligament, and the anterior portion of the annulus fibrosus. The middle column consists of the posterior half of the vertebral body, the posterior longitudinal ligament, and the posterior aspect of the annulus fibrosus. The posterior column consists of the posterior elements of the spine, the facet capsules, and the interspinous ligaments (15,16). Disruption of two contiguous columns or of the middle column itself by trauma, congenital disease, or surgery results in an unstable spine.

Four patterns of injury using this three-column concept have been described by Denis (15): (a) compression of the anterior column results in compression fractures, (b) compression of the anterior and middle columns results in burst fractures, (c) distraction of the middle and posterior columns, usually with continuation through the anterior column, causes Chance fractures (i.e., seat belt injuries), and (d) compression of the anterior column with distraction of the middle and posterior columns caused by a rotational shear results in fracture dislocations. The prediction of ligamentous integrity can be accomplished preoperatively by analyzing the fracture pattern and effect of traction on spinal alignment. Spinal stability following trauma can be estimated by evaluating the extent and pattern of injured structures. Inadequate immobilization of an unstable spine, particularly one that is acutely unstable from trauma, can potentially result in progressive pain and neurologic damage.

Apposition of the fracture surfaces and some degree of stabilization are necessary for fracture healing. This often requires the surgical placement of internal or external instrumentation. Instrumentation systems incorporating metallic rods are well suited for the task of reduction. By attaching vertebrae with wire, hooks, or screws to the rod, these vertebrae can be distracted and aligned, and pathologic angular or rotational deformities can be corrected. Bony defects created after removal of the fracture fragments are commonly filled with structural allografts, structural autografts, or titanium cages filled with morselized autograft. Methylmethacrylate is used only infrequently for fracture management and has only a very limited role in spines with advanced pathology, osteoporosis, and osteopenia.

The aim of treatment of spinal trauma is fracture reduction and spinal canal decompression. The purpose of these procedures is the prevention of mechanical damage to nerves and vessels, the restoration of the mechanical integrity of the spine by anatomic reduction and stabilization, the restoration of normal anatomy and function, and the prevention of chronic deformities (18,19). The goals of modern surgical techniques are the reduction and stabilization of fractures with minimal additional injury and risk of subsequent malunion, nonunion, and infection. The nonsurgical treatment of fractures may require months of bed rest. Less spinal immobilization is achieved with external braces (orthoses) than internal fixation, and the former can result in pseudoarthrosis because of continued motion at the fusion level. Unstable fractures of the cervical spine that require distraction to maintain alignment may be treated with external fixation devices such as traction and halo collars. However, early operative intervention with internal fixation and fusion provides rapid correction of the instability and restoration of alignment, allowing early patient rehabilitation. This in turn reduces recovery time and helps prevent disuse osteopenia, stiffness, and loss of motion (20,21).

SPINAL SURGICAL TECHNIQUES

Spinal surgical procedures include anterior (vertebral body), posterior (posterior elements), and sometimes combined fixation techniques to achieve stability. The most common surgical approach is a posterior midline incision that allows access to the posterior elements, spinal canal, and disk space. The term laminotomy refers to removal of only the inferior margin of the lamina and is often used in cases of microdiskectomy. In unilateral laminectomy, the lamina on one side of the spine is removed. A total or bilateral laminectomy involves removal of both laminae and the spinous process. Laminotomies and laminectomies are often performed to improve access for diskectomies and for decompression in cases of trauma and symptomatic stenosis of the central spinal canal. An overzealous laminectomy may contribute to postoperative spinal instability.

Posterior Spinal Fusion

Posterior spinal fusion indicates fusion of the posterior elements and usually includes bone graft material placed bilaterally across the facet joints and laminae. An inter-transverse fusion includes bone graft between the transverse processes. Small H-shaped pieces of bone may be placed between the spinous processes to facilitate union of the posterior elements in the cervical spine. In addition to bone graft placement, the articular cartilage of the facets usually is removed to promote fusion. A dorsal approach is used for posterior spinal fusions performed to correct scoliosis, treat unstable fractures involving the posterior elements, and correct instability created by multilevel laminectomies. Isolated posterior fusion, first reported in the 1940s, has a lower rate of pseudoarthrosis than isolated anterior fusions of the lumbar spine (22).

Anterior Spinal Fusion

Anterior spinal fusion indicates fusion of the vertebral bodies. This procedure was first reported in 1933 (23). Anterior spinal fusions are accomplished through an anterior or posterolateral approach and are performed for post-traumatic decompression when bone fragments or disk material encroach on the anterior aspect of the spinal canal, in degenerative disk disease with spinal instability, and in combination with posterior instrumentation in cases of severe scoliosis. Interbody spinal fusion is accomplished by excising the intervertebral disk or removing a complete vertebral body and replacing it with a piece of bone from elsewhwere, such as rib, iliac crest, fibula, or tibia. Bone graft is occasionally packed into a titanium cage in order to maintain height across the disk and to promote fusion. Anterior fusions may require the addition of posterior surgical fixation to ensure adequate stability.

SPINAL INSTRUMENTATION

Spinal instrumentation includes longitudinal members such as plates and rods attached directly to vertebral bodies or posterior elements using wires, screws, or hooks. Wires and screws can also be used independently as a primary means of fixation. The techniques of fixation differ with their site of attachment to the spine (e.g., lamina, pedicles, or vertebral body), and means of attachment (e.g., screws, wires, or hooks). In addition, instru-

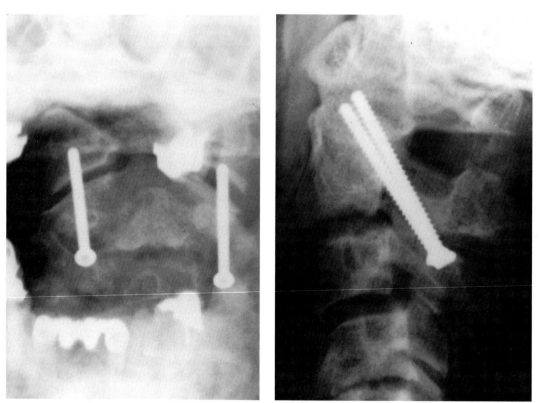

A   B

FIG. IIIC-1. Atlantoaxial fusion with cortical screws. Anteroposterior (**A**) and lateral (**B**) radiographs of the upper cervical spine showing a pair of cortical screws passing through the articular pillars of C2 and into the lateral masses of C1. (From Slone et al., ref. 34, with permission.)

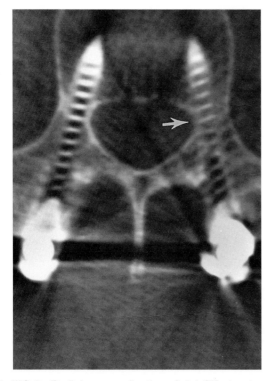

FIG. IIIC-2. Pedicle screw fixation. Axial CT showing optimal placement of the left pedicle screw. The right screw passes very close to the medial cortex (*arrow*). (From Slone et al., ref. 35, with permission.)

mentation used at the cervicooccipital junction, mid- to lower cervical spine, thoracic and lumbar spines, and lumbosacral spine differ significantly. Generally speaking, fixation techniques and fusions may be classified as anterior, posterior, or combined.

Spinal Fusion Screws

Surgical screws are used as a primary means of repair (Fig. IIIC-1) as well as for the attachment of longitudinal instrumentation such as plates and rods. The different types of surgical screws are available in various lengths, pitches, thread diameters, and shank lengths. The shank is the unthreaded portion of the screw. Cortical screws have closely spaced threads designed to gain maximum purchase in cortical bone. These screws are used primarily for the purpose of attaching plates or rods. The bone must be predrilled and tapped (i.e., prethreading of the bone using a special cutting device) before cortical screws can be placed. Plates attached to the vertebral body are often held in place with *bicortical screws*. The term "bicortical" refers to a screw that passed through the entire vertebral body and therefore both cortical layers of bone. *Cancellous screws* have deep threads that are widely spaced to obtain optimal purchase in cancellous bone. They are commonly used as pedicle screws. *Pedicle screws* are placed through a pedicle and into the vertebral body from

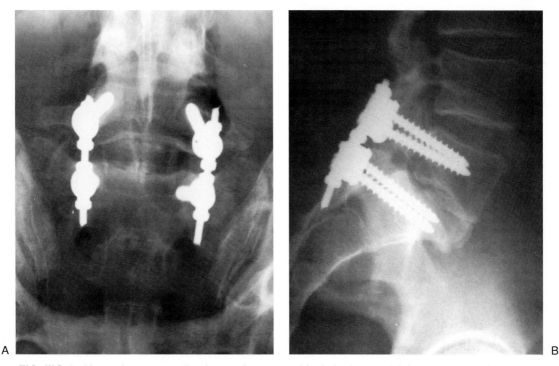

A

B

FIG. IIIC-3. Harms instrumentation in a patient treated for isthmic spondylolisthesis at L5–S1. (**A** and **B**) Placement of bilateral Harms fixation posteriorly, consisting of paired pedicle screws and posterior rods. Iliac bone graft material was placed anteriorly within the disk space to promote fusion. (From Slone et al., ref. 13, with permission.)

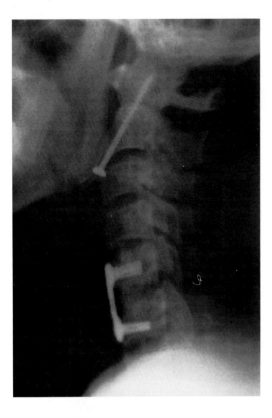

FIG. IIIC-4. Lag screw and Morscher plate in patient with a type II odontoid fracture. Lateral radiograph showing a single partially threaded cancellous screw passing through the body of C2, across the fracture, and into the odontoid. Prior cervical diskectomy with Morscher plate is present at C5–6. (From Slone et al., ref. 13, with permission.)

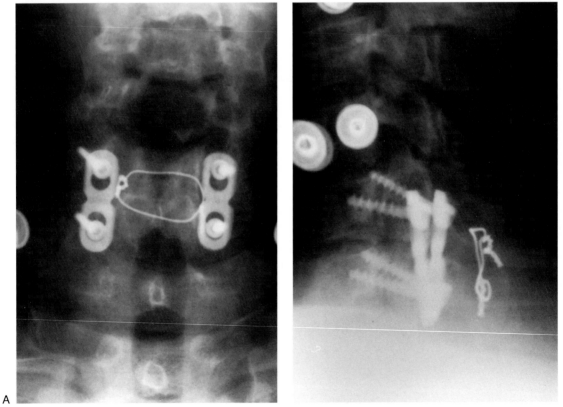

A   B

FIG. IIIC-5. Spinous process wires and cervical reconstruction plates in a patient treated for C5–6 bilateral locked facets. (**A** and **B**) Posterior cervical fusion with short-segment titanium reconstruction plates and paired screws in C5 and C6. A single wire has been placed posteriorly through the spinous processes of C5 and C6 to enhance stability. (From Slone et al., ref. 13, with permission.)

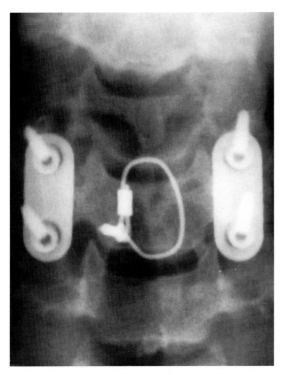

FIG. IIIC-6. Haid plate: AP radiograph showing two Haid plates attached to the articular pillars and a single Songer cable used to attach and stabilize the spinous processes. (From Slone et al., ref. 34, with permission.)

a posterior approach (Fig. IIIC-2). These screws provide excellent purchase of vertebral segments and allow for three-dimensional control when attached to surgical rods (Fig. IIIC-3). Although pedicle screws have been used by spinal surgeons widely since 1985, they still are not approved by the United States FDA. *Cannulated screws* have a hollow center that allows them to be placed over a ''K-wire'' or guide pin for accurate positioning. They are available in both cortical and cancellous thread patterns.

The term *lag screw* refers to the way in which a screw is used rather than to a particular type of screw. Lag screws are used as a primary means of repair and function by pulling two fracture fragments together (Fig. IIIC-4). A screw is considered to function as a lag screw when the threads gain purchase only in the far fragment. The threads in the distal fragment and head of the screw are brought together to achieve compression when the screw is tightened. Partially threaded cancellous screws are typically used as lag screws, although cortical screws can be used if the proximal fragment is overdrilled. Lag screws are oriented perpendicular to the fracture plane.

Spinal Fusion Wires and Cables

Surgical wire can be used as a primary method of fixation such as for attaching two spinous processes together in a posterior cervical fusion (Fig. IIIC-5) or, alterna-

tively, for attaching instrumentation to the spine such as corrective rods. Stainless steel wire is supplied in several diameters; sometimes several strands are used together. The wire ends are usually twisted together, but they may be tied. Cable made of braided strands of titanium or stainless steel wire is much more pliable than wire and less prone to breakage. Songer cables have a loop in one end and a metal collar in the other, which is crimped to secure it in position (Fig. IIIC-6).

Spinal Fusion Plates

Surgical fusion plates can be attached to the vertebral body or posterior elements of the spine with screws. Bolts were used to attach one of the earliest plates to the spinous processes (Fig. IIIC-7). Some of the plates used in the spine, such as tubular plates and malleable reconstruction plates, were originally designed for use in the extremities (Fig. IIIC-8). A number of plates designed specifically for placement on the vertebral body are now available. The *Casper plate* and *Morscher locking plate* are used in the cervical spine (Fig. IIIC-9), and *Armstrong* and *Syracuse plates* in the thoracic and lumbar spines. Specialized plates for use in the posterior spine include *Haid plates*, which are used in the cervical spine, and *Steffee plates*, which are used in the lumbar spine (Fig. IIIC-10). Specialized plates have also been developed for use at the cervicooccipital junction; occasionally, individualized instrumentation must be assembled to allow fusion from the skull base to the thoracic or lumbar spine (Figs. IIIC-11 and IIIC-12).

Spinal Fusion Rods

Surgical rods are used primarily in the thoracic and lumbar spines to provide stability over a long segment. Usually they are paired, although a single rod may be used in special situations. These rods may be connected to the posterior elements with wire, to the lamina and transverse processes with hooks, to the vertebral body posteriorly with pedicle screws or anteriorly with vertebral body screws. Some rods, such as the Luque rods, are smooth and are designed to be attached with wire. Others, such as Harrington distraction rods, are attached to the spine only at the ends with laminar hooks (Fig. IIIC-13). *Knodt rods* are threaded with laminar hooks held in place with nuts. *Harrington compression rods* are also threaded. These rods apply a corrective force primarily at the ends of the rod, where the hooks attach to the lamina. The systems currently in prevalent use include the Cotrel–Dubousset (CD), Texas Scottish Rite Hospital (TSRH), and Isola systems (Figs. IIIC-14–17). These rod systems can be attached to the spine with either hooks, screws, or interspinous or sublaminar wires. These instruments allow

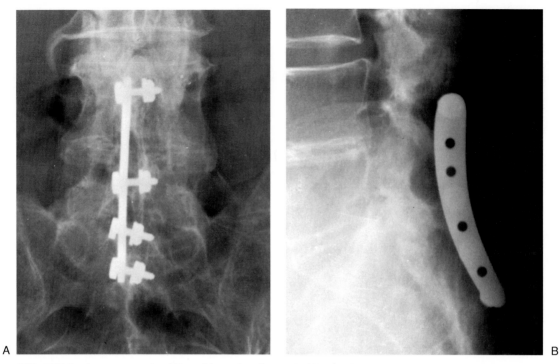

FIG. IIIC-7. Anteroposterior (**A**) and lateral radiograph (**B**) showing a spinous process plate used for a lumbosacral fusion following a multilevel diskectomy. The plate bolts to the spinous processes of the vertebral bodies. (From Slone et al., ref. 35, with permission.)

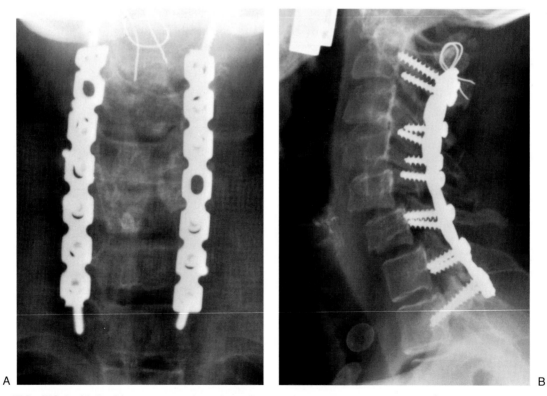

FIG. IIIC-8. Malleable reconstruction plates in a patient with severe rheumatoid arthritis. (**A**) An anteroposterior radiograph shows two malleable reconstruction plates attached to the articular pillars of C2 through T1 for a complete cervical fusion to treat multilevel instability. The broken wire is from a previous C1–C2 fusion. (**B**) Lateral radiograph showing how the plates have been contoured to restore the normal cervical lordotic curvature. (From Slone et al., ref. 34, with permission.)

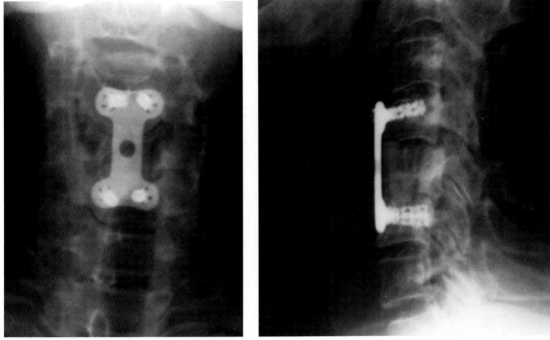

FIG. IIIC-9. Morscher plate. Anteroposterior (**A**) and lateral (**B**) radiographs show a Morscher cervical spine locking plate used for a C4–C5 anterior cervical fusion. The fenestrated screws promote bone ingrowth and further reduce the risk of backing out. A structural allograft was placed anteriorly to maintain the height of the anterior column and promote fusion. (From Slone et al., ref. 34, with permission.)

correction to be achieved through a combination of distraction, compression, translation, and cantilever forces. In addition, the rod may be contoured to accommodate an incompletely correctable curve, and several rod segments may be connected side by side with clamps (*dominoes or double-barreled connectors*) to lengthen the construct. Transverse traction devices are often used to connect paired rods together to improve the rotational stability.

Signal Fusion O-Rings

Occasionally, large metal rings or rectangles called *O-rings* are used in place of a pair of rods or plates (24,25). This type of instrumentation is stiffer than two separate rods and provides more stability. O-rings are attached to the spine with sublaminar wires or cables (Fig. IIIC-18). The closed design of O-rings prevents the wire or cable from slipping off the end as it might with short paired rods.

Methyl Methacrylate for Spinal Fusion

Methyl methacrylate is not an adhesive or glue but rather a space-occupying cement that forms a mechanical interlock with bone. This cement was introduced in the early 1960s and has been used in the spine primarily to replace surgically resected vertebral bodies and to fill in bone defects after corpectomy for tumor. It is contraindicated in spinal infection and usually is not indicated in spinal trauma (26). Although it may be used to strengthen screw sites or to augment other spinal fixation, it is not clearly beneficial when used in these ways. Metal pins or wire mesh are sometimes used to prevent the methylmethacrylate from migrating (Fig. IIIC-19). In patients with a decreased life expectancy, such as those with metastatic neoplastic disease, long-term fusion may be unnecessary, and composite fixation with instrumentation and methylmethacrylate is an acceptable alternative treatment in cases of pathologic spinal collapse (2). Extruded cement or fragments of fractured cement can impinge on spinal nerve roots or the spinal cord and lead to significant complications, particularly when the methyl methacrylate is used posteriorly and placed under tension (27).

Bone Grafts for Spinal Fusion

Surgical bone grafts are commonly placed intraoperatively to promote fusion and increase the size of the bony fusion mass. Homograft or allograft refers to bone taken from a donor or cadaver. Bone harvested from the individual receiving the graft is an autograft. The autografts are

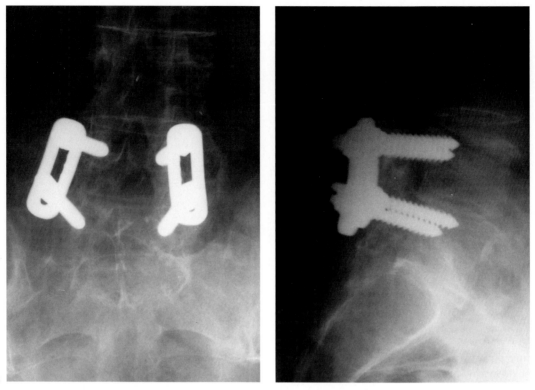

A

B

FIG. IIIC-10. Steffee plates in a 60-year-old patient who developed spondylolisthesis after an L4 laminectomy for degenerative disk disease. Anteroposterior (**A**) and lateral (**B**) radiographs show two Steffee plates and paired pedicle screws placed for stabilization after surgical correction. (From Slone et al., ref. 13, with permission.)

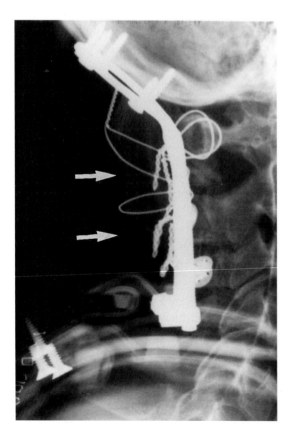

FIG. IIIC-11. Cervicooccipital Cotrel–Dubousset (CD) rod plate system in an 18-year-old patient who was treated for a chordoma of C1 extending into the skull base. Lateral radiograph of the cervical spine shows posterior cervical fusion with occipital cervical plate–rod combination. This is a variation of the standard CD rod system. Sublaminar wires affix the device to C1. Interspinous wires maintain fixation at C2 and C3. Two posterior wires fix faintly visualized (*arrows*) bone graft. (From Slone et al., ref. 13, with permission.)

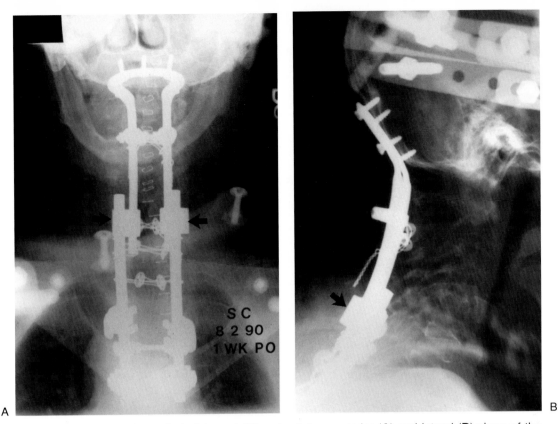

FIG. IIIC-12. Occipital–cervical plate and CD rods. Anteroposterior (**A**) and lateral (**B**) views of the cervical spine showing a cervicooccipital fusion with a CD rod–plate system. Cortical screws fix the device to the occiput. "Dominoes" (*arrows*) at the inferior aspect of the device allow connection to standard CD rods stabilized in the thoracic spine with laminar hooks, pedicle screws, and interspinous wiring. (From Slone et al., ref. 13, with permission.)

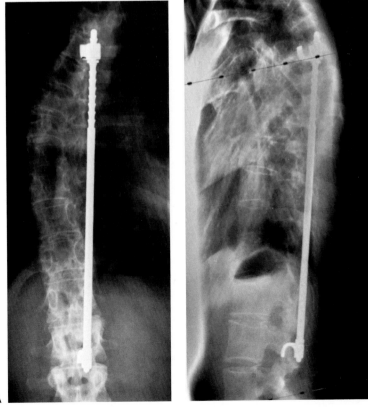

FIG. IIIC-13. Harrington distraction rod for scoliosis treatment. (**A**) Anteroposterior radiograph shows a single Harrington distraction rod placed on the concave side of the scoliosis. Note the extensive bone fusion. (**B**) Lateral radiograph shows a single laminar distraction hook at each end. On the lateral film, note the straightening of the spine with loss of the normal thoracic kyphosis and upper lumbar lordosis. (From Slone et al., ref. 35, with permission.)

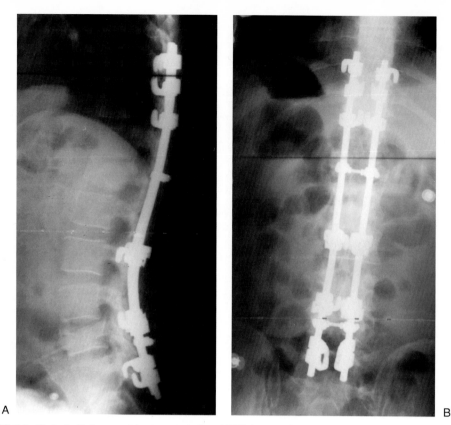

FIG. IIIC-14. Cotrel–Dubousset instrumentation (CDI) in a patient treated for paralysis secondary to fracture dislocation at L1 and burst fracture of L4. (**A**) A CD fixation from T9 to L5 stabilized only with laminar hooks. The rods were contoured to reestablish normal lumbar lordosis. (**B**) On posteroanterior radiograph, note a "CPT claw" configuration at the proximal rod end characterized by nonparallel, paired, distraction, and compression hooks. (From Slone et al., ref. 13, with permission.)

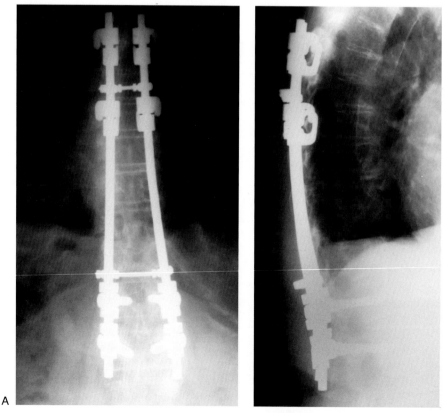

FIG. IIIC-15. Claw mechanism used with CDI in a paraparetic patient with hematogenous vertebral osteomyelitis. Anteroposterior (**A**) and lateral plain (**B**) radiographs of the thoracic spine showing a posterior fusion with CDI. A claw mechanism (paired hooks) has been placed in the thoracic spine and paired pedicle screws in L1 and L2. (From Slone et al., ref. 13, with permission.)

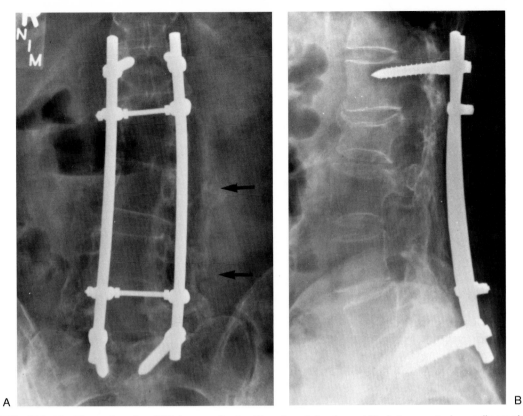

FIG. IIIC-16. Example of a CDI in a patient with a burst fracture. (**A**) Anteroposterior radiograph shows CD rods and pedicle screws spanning L1 to S1 with a posterior fusion for stabilization following a multiple-level laminectomy and L2 burst fracture. Note the extensive bone fusion laterally (*arrows*). (**B**) Lateral radiograph shows the L2 burst fracture and posterior fusion. (From Slone et al., ref. 35, with permission.)

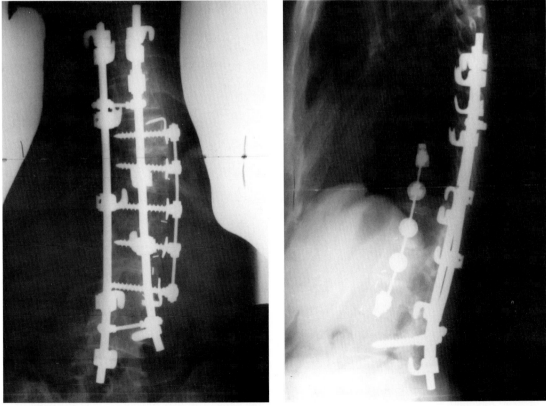

FIG. IIIC-17. Use of CDI and Zielke instrumentation in a patient treated for severe adult thoracolumbar scoliosis. (**A** and **B**) Anterior spinal stabilization with Zielke instrumentation from T11 to L3. Posterior spinal fixation is with CDI from T8 to L3 with interlaminar hooks, including proximal claws, and single distal pedicle screw. (From Slone et al., ref. 13, with permission.)

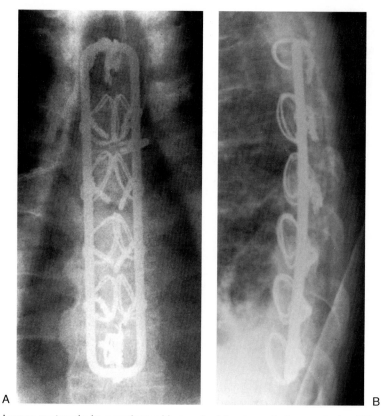

FIG. IIIC-18. Luque rectangle in a patient with a spinal fracture. Anteroposterior (**A**) and lateral (**B**) radiographs show a Luque rectangle and sublaminar wiring used to provide stability for treatment of a thoracic spine fracture. (From Slone et al., ref. 35, with permission.)

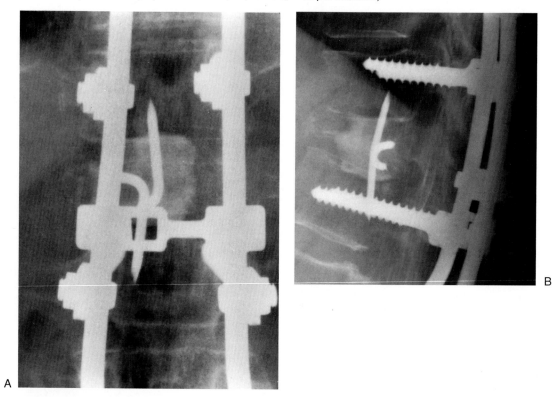

FIG. IIIC-19. Steinman pins. Anteroposterior (**A**) and lateral (**B**) radiographs show methyl methacrylate used to maintain vertebral body height following corpectomy. The two Steinman pins are used to prevent migration of the cement. The spine has been stabilized posteriorly with TSRH hardware and pedicle screws. (From Slone et al., ref. 35, with permission.)

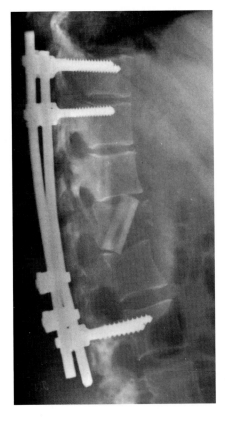

FIG. IIIC-20. Use of TSRH hardware and structural allograft in a patient with a vertebral fracture. Lateral radiograph shows a structural allograft used to treat an L1 compression burst fracture. The TSRH hardware has been used posteriorly to stabilize the spine. Pedicle screws were placed in T10, T11, and L3. (From Slone et al., ref. 35, with permission.)

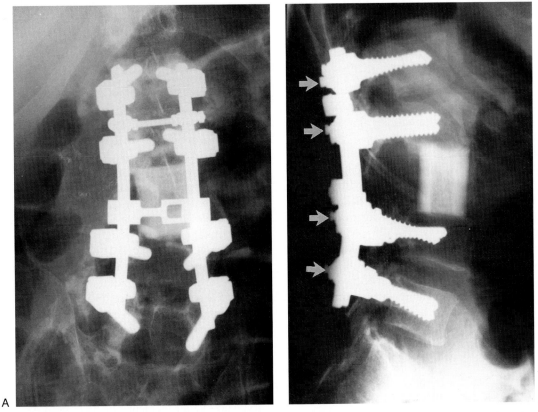

A   B

FIG. IIIC-21. Use of CD instrumentation and anterior allograft in a patient with metastatic colon carcinoma. (**A**) Anteroposterior and (**B**) lateral radiographs show a femoral allograft used for an interbody fusion after an L3 corpectomy for metastatic colon carcinoma. The CD instrumentation is seen posteriorly with paired, top-tightening pedicle screws (*arrows*) within L1, L4, and L5. (From Slone et al., ref. 13, with permission.)

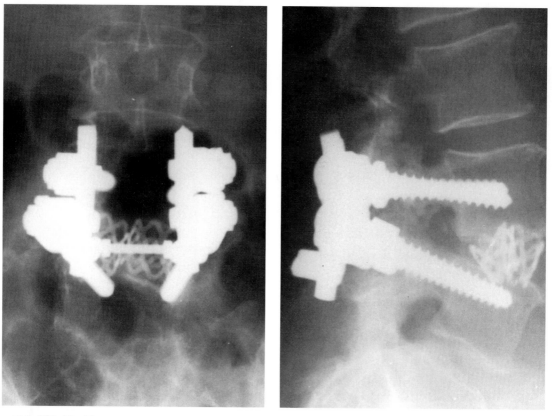

FIG. IIIC-22. Titanium cages and CDI. Anteroposterior (**A**) and lateral (**B**) views of the lumbar spine showing a combined anterior and posterior fusion with CDI and paired variable-angle pedicle screws in L4 and L5. Two titanium cages have been placed in the L4–5 intervertebral disk space. (From Slone et al., ref. 13, with permission.)

commonly surgically removed from the posterior iliac crest during a posterior spinal surgical approach or from the anterior iliac crest during an anterior spinal surgical approach.

The bone graft material is sometimes morselized or cut into small pieces, and placed into the disk space in cases of anterior interbody fusions. Structural allografts or strut autografts are commonly used to restore height to the spinal column following corpectomy or for treatment of traumatic burst fractures (Figs. IIIC-20 and IIIC-21). Structural allografts are usually segments of fibula or tibia from a cadaver. Autografts are sections of rib, ilium, or fibula from the patient. A cadaveric tibial or femoral allograft may also be packed with autologous bone graft material and used as a structural graft element. Following diskectomy or corpectomy, titanium cages can also be used to restore height (Fig. IIIC-22). These cages are usually filled with bone graft material to promote anterior spinal fusion.

COMPLICATIONS OF SPINAL FUSION

Operative complications of spinal surgery include injury to the spinal cord, nerve roots, dura, vessels, and other soft tissues. Postoperative neurologic injury can be the result of direct surgical neural trauma, instrumentation failure, or migration (28). Neurologic injury is an uncommon complication of spinal surgery, occurring in only about 1% of patients (28). Malpositioned instrumentation and overdistraction of bony elements are common causes of surgical fusion failure. Other postoperative complications include hematoma formation, infection, and spinal instability as a result of failure of purchase or failure of accomplishment of rigid linkage. When spinal instrumentation is incorrectly selected or placed, it may contribute to fixation failure. Careful patient, technique, and instrument selection are important factors in determining the success of a particular procedure.

Complications of the bone graft placement include migration of the material with resultant impingement on the spinal canal or neural foramen. Dislodgement of structural allografts may occur if they are not well seated or firmly fixed (Fig. IIIC-23); these grafts are often wired to plates or wedged into the adjacent bone to prevent this possibility. The overall incidence of bone graft extrusion is less than 5%, with most occurring anteriorly (29). Finally, resorption of the graft material may contribute to nonunion.

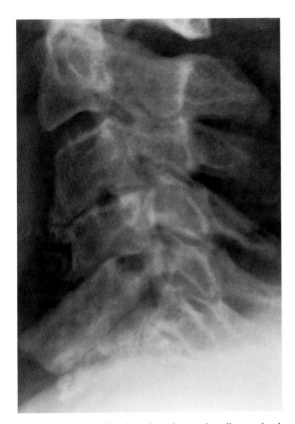

FIG. IIIC-23. Allograft migration. Lateral radiograph shows anterior migration of a structural allograft used for anterior cervical fusion. No metallic fixation was used to secure the graft. (From Slone et al., ref. 36, with permission.)

Instrument Failure

Spinal fusion instrumentation may fail at the site of attachment to the spine (e.g., dislodged hooks, loose screw, broken wire or cable), at the junction of the instrument components (e.g., pedicle screw coming loose from the rod), or along the rigid linkage (e.g., fracture along the midportion of a plate or rod) (Figs. IIIC-24 to IIIC-27). A dislodged or fractured surgical appliance usually indicates instability, clinical failure of the fusion, or both. Fracture of the instrumentation may occur as a result of metal fatigue from the repeated stresses of flexion, extension, and lateral bending. As a result of the loss of stability, these problems can lead to failure of fusion. Redisplacement of the spine can result in neurologic injury. If the fractured appliance is nondisplaced, detection may be difficult.

Failed Spinal Fusion (Pseudoarthrosis)

Typically 6 to 9 months is required for the development of a solid radiographic fusion (20), and 2 years for a solid fusion to completely remodel. Pseudoarthrosis or fibrous

union is a potential complication of spinal fusion. Early recognition and repair of this complication helps prevent surgical implant failure, loss of correction, and pain (30). An increasing risk of pseudoarthrosis is seen with increasing complexity and extent of the spinal surgery and with patient age. Any motion at the intended level of fusion during the healing phase increases the risk of pseudoarthrosis development, and therefore external braces (orthoses) are often worn to minimize motion and maintain stability during healing.

Although perfect surgical technique does not guarantee a successful fusion, the rate of pseudoarthrosis occurrence is decreased by utilizing meticulous surgical technique. Nevertheless, a fibrous union can still sufficiently limit motion to enable a reduction of pain; conversely, a solid bone union does not necessarily ensure a good clinical outcome. Reoperation for surgical repair is necessary only if the patient presents with gross implant failure or pain. In the asymptomatic patient, inter-

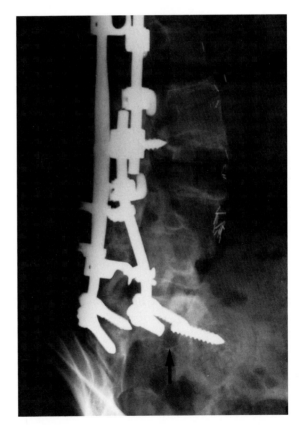

FIG. IIIC-24. Failed pedicle screw fixation and revision with TSRH instrumentation in a patient with spinal fusion for adult scoliosis who noted a several-month history of increasing forward bending and then felt a pop in the lower back and experienced acute back pain. Radiograph shows a fracture through a lower pedicle screw (*arrow*). Note lucency through L5–S1 disk, suggesting lack of fusion at this level. (From Slone et al., ref. 13, with permission.)

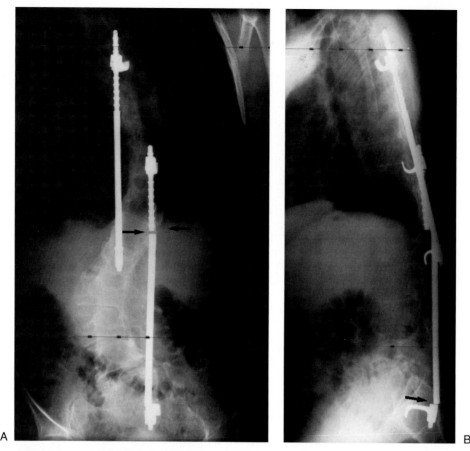

FIG. IIIC-25. Harrington rod failure. (**A**) At superior aspect of rod, lucency at junction of ratchet portion and smooth rod (*arrows*) marks fracture in rod. (**B**) At distal end, displacement of the inferior hook (*arrow*) is present as a result of lower rod fracture. (From Slone et al., ref. 36, with permission.)

vention may be deferred while the patient's condition is followed (31). However, a pseudoarthrosis allows continued stress on the implant, and therefore, instrumentation fracture may follow. Failure of bony fusion may also result from graft fracture or infection in the bony graft site.

Surgical Spinal Instrument Removal

Intact implants generally are left in place for life because of the morbidity associated with repeated surgery. The majority of spinal appliances are placed to provide stability so that bony fusion can take place; their function is complete when this bony fusion has occurred. If successful arthrodesis does not occur, the mechanical devices used in the spine will eventually fail because of continued stresses. Surgical implants that are fractured and dislodged are usually removed because of the need for revision and the risk of migration of the components with subsequent soft-tissue or neural injury. In thin patients, the prominence of the components can cause chronic tissue irritation leading to pain and bursa formation; this

can be an occasional indication for removal (28). Finally, pressure sores developing over appliances occasionally are a problem in neurologically impaired individuals.

Periinstrumental Bone Resorption

Bone resorption can occur around surgical screws and under implants that are in direct contact with bone. Such resorption usually is associated with instrument motion. It may lead to fracture of the weakened bone or detachment of the component with resultant loss of fixation. The pattern of bone resorption occasionally indicates a mechanical etiology such as the arc-like motion of a loose screw about a pivot point. Infection must also be considered when a lucency is seen surrounding an implant (Fig. IIIC-28).

Spinal Trauma and Disk Alterations

In part because of the decreased segmental mobility, patients with spinal fusions are predisposed to traumatic fractures above or below a fused spinal alignment. The

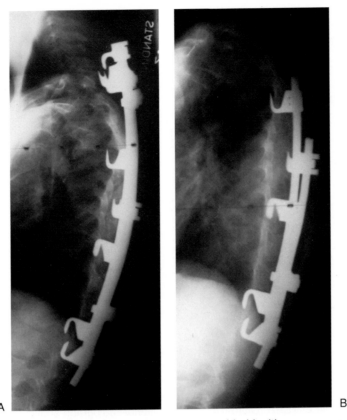

FIG. IIIC-26. Example of TSRH dislodgment in a 10-year-old girl with neuromuscular scoliosis. (**A**) Lateral radiograph shows a posterior thoracic fusion and segmental instrumentation with TSRH hardware. The uppermost thoracic laminar hook has become dislodged and was irritating the overlying soft tissues. (**B**) Lateral radiograph obtained after revision shows the upper hooks removed and the rod shortened. It was determined that the fusion did not need to be as high as originally intended. (From Slone et al., ref. 36, with permission.)

instrumentation or graft itself also may fracture. These patients are somewhat predisposed to premature degenerative changes at the disk levels above and below the fused segment. The development of degenerative spinal changes immediately proximal and distal to a spinal fusion depends on the length of the fusion, the position of the fusion in the coronal and sagittal planes, the normality of the spinal segments above or below the fusion, and the patient's own unique biology and connective tissues.

Complications at Bone Graft Harvesting Site

Complications of bone graft harvesting can include fracture, infection, or hematoma at the graft site or injury to an adjacent nerve (e.g., lateral femoral cutaneous, superior cluneal, and ilioinguinal nerves), the superior gluteal artery, ureter, or sacroiliac joint (32,33). Donor site pain may persist for months after harvesting, and occasionally gait disturbances result (33). These complications can be avoided by using an allograft from a cadaver.

Recurrent Spinal Stenosis

Central stenosis of the spinal canal may occur above or below a fusion as a result of increased stresses and motion immediately proximal and distal to the fused segment(s) that result in hypertrophy of the involved joints and ligaments. This stenosis may require decompression and extension of the fusion. Such stenotic events most commonly occur with long fusions, in fusions that are not well balanced in the sagittal or coronal plane, and in patients with connective tissue problems, who smoke, or who have diabetes. Hypertrophy or overgrowth of the graft material itself does not lead to recurrent stenosis, and stenosis is never encountered in the middle of a segment of spinal fusion.

IMAGING THE POSTOPERATIVE SPINE

The evaluation of spinal fusions can be carried out utilizing conventional radiographs, fluoroscopy, conventional tomography, CT, MR imaging, and nuclear medicine techniques.

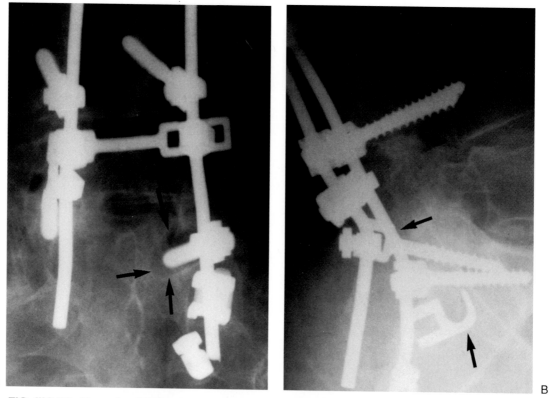

FIG. IIIC-27. Example of TSRH failure. (**A**) Anteroposterior radiograph shows failure of TSRH hardware with disassembly of a lower hook, eyebolt, and pedicle screw. Also note the substantial resorption of bone around the lower screw (*arrows*), indicating loosening. (**B**) Lateral radiograph shows the base of the pedicle screw detached from the rod and eyebolt (*small arrow*) and complete detachment of the lower hook (*large arrow*). (From Slone et al., ref. 36, with permission.)

Proper analysis often requires comparison with previous spinal examinations to facilitate detection of subtle changes that may indicate an impending complication. As is true with any radiologic study, the patient's clinical history, current signs and symptoms, and a knowledge of the prior surgical procedure are very important when evaluating imaging studies. Medical imaging physicians should attempt to familiarize themselves with the procedures and instrumentation devices unique to their institution and discuss equivocal findings with the referring physician.

Conventional Radiography

Conventional radiographs remain the mainstay of implant evaluation. Radiographs demonstrate the position of the spinal elements, the instrumentation, the graft material, and often evidence of complications if present. Orthogonal views of the appliance and spine are necessary because complications are often visible in only one projection. Spinal fusion evaluation usually begins with plain films in the anteroposterior, lateral, and occasionally the oblique projections. Serial radiographs may show subtle changes that become more evident on dynamic lateral flexion and extension films obtained in the erect position. Dynamic radiographs can be helpful in establishing the presence or absence of motion and the integrity of the fusion. Patient splinting during the examination can cause a failed fusion to be missed on flexion views (3).

Fluoroscopy, on the other hand, allows optimal patient positioning, and videotaping allows the examination to be reviewed by others later (3). Conventional x-ray polytomography can be used to determine the extent of bone fusion, the presence of bony overgrowth, fractures, or pseudoarthrosis and can be performed successfully even in the presence of metallic implants. Midline lateral conventional polytomography performed during flexion and extension may increase the detection of subtle motion at the fusion site. This demonstration of motion is helpful in confirming the diagnosis of nonunion or pseudoarthrosis. A fibrous bony union produces a lucent area that is difficult to differentiate from a nonunion on polytomography or conventional radiography, although both are considered failed fusions.

Computed Tomography

Conventional tomography is frequently supplemented by high-resolution, thin-section CT with multiplanar reconstruction, which increases the accuracy of assessing

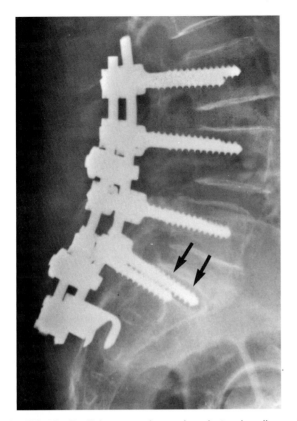

FIG. IIIC-28. Pedicle screw loosening. Lateral radiograph shows a lucent area around a pedicle screw in S1 (*arrows*). This indicates loosening from motion or possibly infection. In this example, TSRH hardware had been used for a lumbosacral fusion with paired pedicle screws in L3 through S1 and sacral foraminal hooks. (From Slone et al., ref. 36, with permission.)

bony spinal fusion. The speed of spiral CT examinations allows reconstructions in the sagittal and coronal planes to be completed quickly. Although metallic implants can generate significant image artifact, adequate information can often be obtained by increasing the radiographic CT technique (e.g., kVp and mA) and oversampling (i.e., obtaining data for more than 360°). Image reformations typically are less affected by beam-hardening artifacts than direct axial images.

Magnetic Resonance Imaging

Imaging in multiple direct planes can be carried out with MR. Magnetic resonance is sensitive for detecting fractures, pseudoarthrosis, and infections. Although the marrow in cancellous bone is well demonstrated, MR imaging provides poor definition of cortical bone because of its solid structure and paucity of mobile water protons. One major drawback is the artifacts that are produced by the ferromagnetic metal implants. This magnetic field distortion can yield im-

ages that are unreadable. More spinal implants are being manufactured using titanium, a metal that produces less image artifact than stainless steel on both CT and MR images.

Radionuclide Imaging

Radionuclide bone scans performed with single-photon emission CT (SPECT) imaging are sensitive to the detection of pseudoarthrosis. Pseudoarthrosis produces focal areas of increased radionuclide activity on images; however, this may be indistinguishable from bony remodeling at the junction of the fusion elements. The reactive changes of the maturing bone graft can also produce areas of increased activity. Finally, the metallic instrumentation itself can attenuate the photons causing cold defects. These factors make image interpretation difficult and limit the utility of radionuclide scans.

CONCLUSIONS

Both CT and MR imaging have provided significant advances in the understanding of spinal disorders and have generally eliminated exploratory spinal surgery (4). Medical imaging physicians can play an important role in accurate diagnosis, preoperative planning, and postoperative evaluation of spinal surgery patients. The many different techniques of spinal fixation vary depending on the patient, type and location of the deformity, the presence of associated injuries or pathology, and the experience of the surgeon. Surgical spinal fixation is a complex issue, and each case is unique. It is not always possible to achieve ideal spinal fixation, and modification of techniques and implants may be needed to accomplish the treatment goals.

Spinal surgical instrumentation is undertaken for the purposes of maintaining the surgical correction and providing stability while bony fusion occurs. The success of intrumentation is dependent on fixation of individual segments to a rigid linkage. A return of signs and symptoms postoperatively may result from an erroneous primary diagnosis, pathology missed during surgery, donor site pain, recurrent disk herniation, infection, hemorrhage, surgical error, graft migration, arachnoiditis, postoperative spinal stenosis, or graft fusion failure with pseudoarthrosis and spinal instability. Postoperative imaging strategies may help in identifying the specific cause of recurrent pain and disability. Conventional radiographs are the mainstay of postoperative evaluation but frequently are supplemented by high-resolution thin-section CT with multiplanar reconstruction. It is important for radiologists to be familiar with the more common surgical spinal fixation devices and understand their intended function in order to properly evaluate the postoperative spine and identify potential complications.

ACKNOWLEDGMENTS

The authors would like to thank Drs. K. H. Bridwell, M. MacMillan, and W. J. Montgomery for their assistance in preparing the material.

REFERENCES

1. Rag MR: Spinal fusion: Overview of options and posterior internal fixation devices. In: Framer JW, Ducker TB, Hadler NM, et al., eds. *The Adult Spine: Principles of Practice.* New York: Raven Press, 1991:1919–1945.
2. An HS, Cotler JM, eds: *Spinal Instrumentation.* Baltimore: Williams & Wilkins, 1992.
3. Yeakley J, Harris JH Jr: Imaging of spinal fusions. In: Cotler JM, Cotler HB, eds. *Spinal Fusion, Science and Technique.* New York: Springer-Verlag, 1990:335–347.
4. Albee FH: Transplantation of a portion of the tibia into the spine for Pott's disease. *JAMA* 1911;57:885–886.
5. Hibbs RA: An operation for progressive spinal deformities. NY Med J 1911;93:1013–1016.
6. Ghormely RK: Low back pain, with special reference to the articular facets with presentation of an operative procedure. *JAMA* 1933; 101:1773–1777.
7. King D: Internal fixation for lumbosacral fusion. *J Bone Joint Surg* [Am] 1948;30:560–565.
8. Knodt H, Larrick RB: Distraction fusion of the lumbar spine. *Ohio State Med J* 1964;12:1140–1142.
9. Harrington PR: The history and development of Harrington instrumentation. *Clin Orthop Rel Res* 1973;93:110–112.
10. Harrington PR: Treatment of scoliosis: Correction and interval fixation by spine instrumentation. *J Bone Joint Surg* [Am] 1962;44:591–610.
11. Luque ER: Interpeduncular segmental fixation. *Clin Orthop Rel Res* 1986;203:54–57.
12. Luque ER: The anatomic basis and development of segmental spinal instrumentation. *Spine* 1982;7:256–259.
13. Slone RM, McEnery KW, Bridwell KH, Montgomery WJ: Principles and imaging of spinal instrumentation. *Radiol Clin North Am* 1995;33(2):189–211.
14. Ogilvie JW: Zielke instrumentation of the spine. In: An HS, Cotler JM, eds. *Spinal Instrumentation.* Baltimore: Williams & Wilkins, 1992:353–358.
15. Denis F: The three column spine and its significance in the classification of acute thoraco-lumbar spinal injuries. *Spine* 1983;8:817–831.
16. Kilcoyne RF, Farrar EL: *Handbook of Orthopedic Terminology.* Boston: CRC Press, 1991.
17. Dickson RA: Thoracolumbar injuries. In: Dickson RA, ed. *Spinal Surgery Science and Practice.* Boston: Butterworth, 1988:307–323.
18. Aebi M, Webb JK: The spine. In: Mueller ME, Allgower M, Schneider R, et al, eds. *Manual of Internal Fixation: Techniques Recom-*

mended by the AO-ASIF Group. New York: Springer-Verlag, 1991: 627–682.
19. Frymoyer JF, Stokes IA: Biomechanics of spinal trauma. In: Dickson RA, ed. *Spinal Surgery Science and Practice.* Boston: Butterworth, 1990:264–271.
20. Foley MJ, Calenoff L, Hendrix RW, et al: Thoracic and lumbar spine fusion. Postoperative radiologic evaluation. *Am J Roentgenol* 1983;141:373–380.
21. Kostuik JP, Huler JR, Esses SI, et al: Thoracolumbar spine fractures. In: Frymoyer JW, Ducker TB, Hadler NM, et al, eds. *The Adult Spine: Principles of Practice.* New York: Raven Press, 1991:1269–1329.
22. Briggs H, Milligan PR: Chip fusion of the low back following exploration of the spinal canal. *J Bone Joint Surg* [Am] 1944;26: 125–130.
23. Burns BH: An operation for spondylolithesis. *Lancet* 1933;1:1233.
24. Dove J: Internal fixation of the lumbar spine: The Hartshill rectangle. *Clin Orthop Rel Res* 1983;203:135–140.
25. Flatley TJ, Devderian H: Closed loop instrumentation of the lumbar spine. *Clin Orthop Rel Res* 1985;196:273–278.
26. Ferguson RL, Allen BL Jr, Tencer AF: Biomechanical principles of spinal correction. In: Cotler JM, Cotler HB, eds. *Spinal Fusion, Science and Technique.* New York: Springer-Verlag, 1990:45–57.
27. McAfee PC, Bohlman HH, Ducker T, et al: Failure of stabilization of the spine with methylmethacrylate: A retrospective analysis of 24 cases. *J Bone Joint Surg* [Am] 1986;68:1145–1157.
28. Heller JG, Whitecloud TS III, Butler JC, et al: Complications of spinal surgery. In: Herkowitz HN, Garfin SR, Balderston RA, et al, eds. *The Spine,* 3rd ed. Philadelphia: WB Saunders, 1992:1817–1898.
29. An HS, Simeone FA: Complications in cervical disc disease surgery. In: Balderston RA, An HS, eds. *Complications in Spinal Surgery.* Philadelphia: WB Saunders, 1991:41–59.
30. Dawson EG, Clader TJ, Bassett LW: A comparison of different methods used to diagnose pseudoarthrosis following posterior spinal fusion for scoliosis. *J Bone Joint Surg* [Am] 1985;67:1153–1159.
31. Schlegel J, Yunan HA, Fredricksen B: Anterior interbody fixation devices. In: Frymoyer JW, Ducker TB, Hadler NM, et al, eds. *The Adult Spine: Principles of Practice.* New York: Raven Press, 1991: 1947–1959.
32. An HS, Balderston RA: Complications in scoliosis, kyphosis, and spondylolisthesis surgery. In: Balderston RA, An HS, eds. *Complications in Spinal Surgery.* Philadelphia: WB Saunders, 1991:5–39.
33. Lane JM, Muschler GF, Kurz LT, et al: Spinal fusion. In: Herkowitz HN, Garfin SR, Balderston RA, et al, eds. *The Spine,* 3rd ed. Philadelphia: WB Saunders, 1992:1739–1776.
34. Slone RM, MacMillan M, Montgomery WJ: Spinal fixation: Part 1: Principles, basic hardware and fixation techniques for the cervical spine. *Radiographics* 1993;13:341–356.
35. Slone RM, Macmillan M, Montgomery WJ, et al: Spinal fixation: Part 2: Fixation techniques and hardware for the thoracic and lumbosacral spine. *Radiographics* 1993;13:521–543.
36. Slone RM, Montgomery WJ, MacMillan M: Spinal fixation: Part 3: Complications of spinal instrumentation. *Radiographics* 1993; 13:797–816.
37. Slone RM, McEnery KW, Bridwell KH, Montgomery WJ: Fixation techniques and instrumentation used in the cervical spine. *Radiol Clin North Am* 1995;33(2):213–232.
38. Slone RM, McEnery KW, Bridwell KH, Montgomery WJ: Fixation techniques and instrumentation used in the thoracic, lumbar, and lumbosacral spine. *Radiol Clin North Am* 1995;33(2):233–265.

Posttherapeutic Neurodiagnostic Imaging,
edited by J.R. Jinkins,
Lippincott-Raven Publishers, New York © 1997.

CHAPTER **IIID**

Principles, Imaging, and Complications of Spinal Instrumentation

Surgeon's Perspective

Denis Laurent Kaech and Guido Meier

Spinal appliances enable stabilization and correction of deformities of the vertebral column. Since Harrington's original publication concerning the management of scoliosis with his system consisting of rods and hooks (1), a number of developments in spinal instrumentation have led to an increase in the surgical treatment of traumatic, degenerative, and neoplastic lesions of the spine. Roy Camille (2) introduced pedicle screw-and-plate fixation in 1963, stimulating further interest in elaborations of posterior devices for spinal stabilization (2–10).

It is impossible to give a comprehensive overview of all the implants (estimated at over 100 total) available today on the market. One cannot expect every radiologist to become familiar with every plate, screw, rod, hook, and intervertebral fusion cage used for spinal fusion, particularly when one is aware of the controversies surrounding which implant is the best for a particular case.

The indications for surgery are based on clinical (e.g., history, neurologic examination) and radiologic (e.g., conventional radiographs, myelography, CT, MR) data (3,5,7,11–17). The choice of the implant and approach depends on the location of the predominant pathology and on the surgeon's preferences and experience. For example, after major trauma or neoplastic vertebral destruction, a combined anterior and posterior procedure may be required. This underlines the importance of a careful preoperative neuroradiologic investigation (15–17).

D. L. Kaech: Department of Neurosurgery, Kantonsspital, CH-7000 Chur, Switzerland.
G. Meier: Department of Orthopedics, Kantonsspital, CH-7000 Chur, Switzerland.

INDICATIONS FOR POSTOPERATIVE IMAGING

Simple postoperative imaging is usually indicated as a routine follow-up in patients who are doing well clinically. However, a more demanding neuroradiologic workup is required for complications and failures of instrumentation placement procedures. In patients doing well postoperatively, CT and MR may also be performed routinely in order to document the success of an operation (i.e., "quality control").

ROUTINE FOLLOW-UP: CONVENTIONAL RADIOGRAPHS

As stated above, the radiologic follow-up after an implant fusion of the spine is routine even in patients who are doing well. In the early postoperative phase, conventional radiographs enable a check of the achieved stabilization, the realignment of the vertebrae, the correct positioning of the implants, the restoration of a physiologic spinal curvature, and the intervertebral disk-space height. In the subacute and in the late phase following surgery (e.g., after 9 to 12 months), radiographs provide the surgeon with relevant information concerning the maintenance of the initial result by comparison with the immediate postoperative films. Bony consolidation can also be assessed, which is essential when removal of the appliance is planned. Dynamic studies (i.e., flexion–extension) can additionally assess the presence or lack of motion across fused segments.

Goals of Instrumentation

The primary goal of spinal instrumentation is to impart sufficient temporary stabilization so that solid bony fusion may occur. Living bone capable of repair and remodeling should permanently replace the temporary function of the instrumentation (except in cases of metastatic disease). Without this fusion, almost all implant constructs will eventually fatigue and fail (3,14,18).

The use of implants is limited by osteoporosis. Major osteoporosis is, for a majority of surgeons, a contraindication for a spondylodesis. Wittenberg et al. (19) have analyzed the importance of bone mineral density in instrumented spinal fusions. Because the screw–cancellous bone interface is the weak link of a rigid-angle stable pedicular system, early screw loosening may be expected when the equivalent mineral density (EMD) of the vertebral cancellous bone is lower than 90 mg/cc, as measured by quantitative CT. Early loosening is less likely when the EMD exceeds 120 mg/cc. However, these measurements are not routinely performed before every fusion procedure in elderly people. In these situations, the surgeon has to decide how much calculated risk he is ready to take when the quality of the patient's bone on gross inspection is less than ideal.

The long-term goal of instrumented surgical spinal fusion is the formation of a solid bony arthrodesis providing permanent stability, thereby preventing pain and neurologic injury under normal loading conditions. On the one hand, the fewest possible motion segments should be lost in order to minimize delayed sequelae of fusion (e.g., chronic pain syndromes and flat back) (14) and to avoid significant additional stress leading to an accelerated decompensation of the adjacent vertebral segments (e.g., secondary instability, disk herniation, stenosis caused by hypertrophic changes) (3,12,15,20,21). On the other hand, adequate decompression of neural elements must be achieved to improve or at least to preserve neurologic function. A wide decompression is permitted when plates and pedicle screws are used for stabilization; there is no need to rely on posterior elements such as laminae for hook fixation (14). Nevertheless, the surgical trauma of a multisegment fusion is considerable, and the "minimally invasive" trend steers the surgeon toward an avoidance of unnecessary damage to otherwise healthy or noninvolved structures (15).

Conventional radiographs and CT are the best imaging modalities for visualizing bone. These two techniques allow the amount of bone removed for decompression and bone grafting for fusion and also the size and position of the metallic implants to be assessed postoperatively.

Investigators checking the fusion status during follow-up should provide radiographic analysis of several factors, including device attachment locations in the spine; presence or absence of fracture of the metallic plates, screws, or bone; evidence of bone resorption; presence or absence of bony callus; endosteal or periosteal new bone deposition; and findings of trabecular bridging or bony remodeling (9).

Description of Fusion Result

Brantigan and Steffee in 1993 and Brantigan in 1994 (22,23) set out several criteria for radiographic fusion, uncertain fusion status, and radiographic pseudarthrosis after posterior lumbar interbody fusion (PLIF) procedures (Table IIID-1). The PLIF consists of either a pedicle screw-and-plate fixation plus ethylene-oxide-sterilized allograft bone (23) or a VSP system (9) of carbon cages filled with autologous bone as anterior column support.

These radiologic findings must be coupled with clinical observations in order to determine their relevance regarding further patient management. For example, pseudarthrosis without collapse of the construct (e.g., loosening, dislocation, or breakage of the hardware, loss of previously achieved correction, recurrence of deformity) is possible, or screw breakage may occur without development of symptomatic pseudarthrosis if the bone graft finally achieves a solid fusion (Fig. IIID-1). Surgeons must treat a symptomatic patient, but they may not necessarily need to correct an unsatisfactory radiologic picture in a satisfied patient (i.e., symptomatic instrumentation failure versus an incidental diagnosis of a broken screw in an asymptomatic patient).

TABLE IIID-1. *Radiographic criteria for success or failure of spinal fusion*

Radiographic criteria of fusion:
- Bone in the fusion area radiographically more dense and more mature than originally achieved immediately after surgery
- No interface lucency between donor bone and vertebral bone (a sclerotic line between the graft and the vertebral bone indicates fusion)
- Mature bony trabeculae bridging the fusion area
- Resorption of anterior vertebral traction spurs [indicating instability, according to MacNab (39), see Fig. IIID-19]
- Anterior extension of the bone graft within the disk space (ossification of the annulus and of the anterior longitudinal ligament)
- Fusion across the facet joints

Radiographic spinal fusion status uncertain:
- Bone graft visible in the fusion area at approximately the density originally achieved surgically, or a small lucency or gap (less than half of the graft area) existing between the graft bone and vertebral bone.

Radiographic criteria of failed fusion:
- pseudoarthritis formation
- Collapse of the construct
- Vertebral slip
- Broken screws
- Resorption of the bone graft
- Major lucency or gap visible in the fusion area (2 mm or more around the entire periphery of the graft or intervertebral fusion cage)

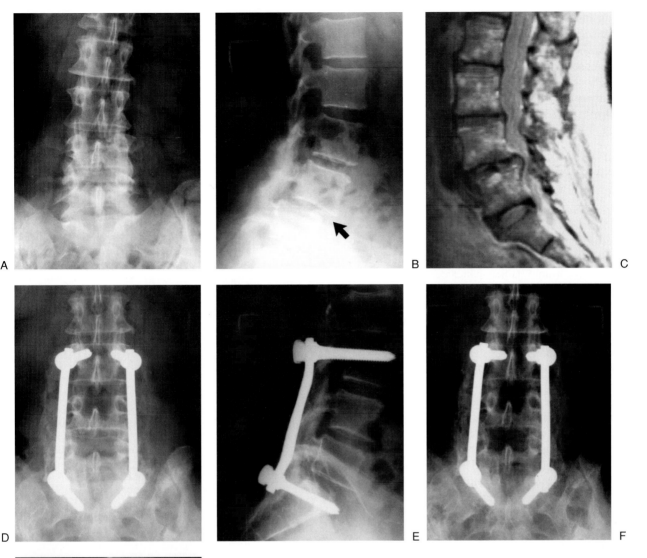

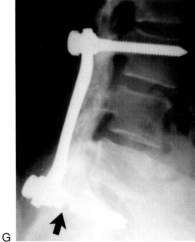

FIG. IIID-1. Degenerative spondylolisthesis L4-5. (**A**) Anteroposterior and (**B**) lateral radiographs demonstrate degenerative spondylolisthesis at L4-5. Note the hypertrophied right L5 transverse process in the anteroposterior image. (**C**) Sagittal intermediate-weighted MR shows the anterolisthesis at L4-5 with marked narrowing of the central spinal canal. (**D**) Anteroposterior and (**E**) lateral radiographs show a distraction spondylodesis of the USS type. The device extends from L3 to S1. There has been a decompression at L4-5 with a reduction of the spondylolisthesis at this level. (**F**) Anteroposterior and (**G**) lateral radiographs at 1 year following surgery shows a breakage of the screw (*arrow*). There is only a minor anterolisthesis of L4 on L5. The intertransversal bone graft bilaterally appears solid on these images. Therefore, even though there has been a breakage of the appliance, the grafted bone provides complete stability.

To check fusion stability, dynamic flexion–extension studies can be performed, generally 3 or 6 months after the surgical procedure. This may indicate that the surgical appliance has performed its intended function. Some appliances are routinely removed after 9 to 12 months; others may or must be left in place (e.g., Morscher's anterior cervical plate) (24) (Table IIID-1).

COMPLICATIONS AND FAILURES OF INSTRUMENTATION PROCEDURES

A more extensive neuroradiologic evaluation will be required in cases of postsurgical complications or in instances of an unsatisfactory clinical course. There are many possible causes for what we could call the "failed spondylodesis syndrome" (FSS), which constitutes a subgroup of the "failed back surgery syndrome" (FBSS) (15,16,20,25,26). The main causes of persistent or recurrent pain after a spinal instrumentation procedure include technical problems occurring during the operation, factors related to surgical trauma, infections, instrumentation failure, new pathology at an adjacent level, and others (Table IIID-2). Postoperative complications and technical errors requiring another surgical procedure must be clarified quickly in the immediate postoperative period or later, when the patient's signs and symptoms begin to progress.

Neural compression and exceptional cases of anterior vascular or visceral injury caused by a malpositioned screw, a large postoperative hematoma, or a major CSF leak after dural tear are some rare indications for emergency reoperation. Neurologic deterioration occurs in only about 1% of spinal fusions (27), mainly because of malpositioned or migrating hardware, and less often because of overdistraction. Arachnoiditis and epidural scars resulting from a previous surgical procedure make nerve roots particularly vulnerable to further manipulations. However, no imaging modality can predict the forces applied on a nerve during a particular procedure or provide a road map for avoiding permanent neurologic deficit postoperatively.

One must be aware of the limitations of postoperative radiologic imaging studies (15,16,28). There are many ultrastructural and microcirculatory changes not detectable by means of neuroimaging. Neurogenic pain related to deafferentation, leading to a vicious circle of overinhibition of central lateral and ventroposterior nuclei by the thalamic reticular nucleus (29), and aberrant and ectopic neurogenic activity related to ultrastructural damage in an injured nerve root, allowing ephaptic transmission and axoaxonal stimulation and associated autonomic dysfunction (30), are some examples of possible mechanisms of symptom production that cannot be imaged.

Nevertheless, it is essential to rule out a "surgical cause" in every case of clinical spinal fusion failure, in part because a neglected "morphologic lesion" will be

TABLE IIID-2. *Factors responsible for the failed spondylodesis syndrome*

Technical complications occurring during surgery:
- Direct injury to thecal sac (e.g., dural tear, CSF leak, pseudomeningocele)
- Malposition of screw (2.6% incidence) (14)
- Iatrogenic traumatic nerve root lesion within the foramen or along the inferomedial surface of the pedicle
- Penetration or fracture of the pedicle wall (i.e., decreased pullout strength)
- Exit of the screw through anterior body cortex (excessive screw length): danger to anterior vascular and visceral structures
- Dislocated bone graft (mainly posterolateral): danger of extraforaminal nerve compression
- Excessive retraction and coagulation of the epidural venous plexus during insertion of intervertebral graft or fusion cages
- Excessive overdistraction: danger of impaired microcirculation of the roots and loss of lumbar lordosis, yielding flat back and causing low back pain
- Excessive bleeding: danger of postoperative hematoma, increased scar formation
- Insufficient decompression (e.g., neglected stenosis or disk herniation)
- Iatrogenic stenosis by sublaminar hooks
- Wrong or insufficient levels fused

Operative trauma:
- Cord/nerve root edema
- Denervation and devascularisation of erector trunci muscle (7,15) (e.g., ischemic back pain, muscle atrophy, and fibrosis)
- Scar tissue formation (e.g., intradural "arachnoiditis," epidural "fibrosis")
- Sympathetic dysfunction, aberrant and ectopic neurogenic activity in damaged nerve (30)
- Reflex sympathetic dystrophy
- Facet fracture
- Pain at the bone donor site (e.g., iliac crest)

Postoperative infections:
- Incidence rate between 1% and 4%
- Independent of instrumentation systems (9,14,47), including cages (45,46)

Instrumentation failure:
- Incidence 4.8% to 16% (10,14,42,47); most frequent cause is insufficient or absent load sharing biomechanical weakness of the anterior column (i.e., 1)
- Screw breakage, pullout, or bending
- Loosening of implants (most likely location the rod–screw interface)
- Migration of hardware
- Resorption of bone graft

Decompensation of an adjacent level:
- Instability
- Facet syndrome
- Spinal stenosis
- Disk degeneration and herniation
- Compression fracture above fusion (e.g., in osteoporosis)

Concomitant diseases, nonfusion-specific causes of failure:
- Neuropathy (e.g., diabetic)
- Radiculitis (e.g., Lyme borreliosis) (28)
- Delayed decompression (insufficient recovery of a radicular deficit, neurogenic pain) (29)
- Tumor remote from operated level (23)
- Major obesity
- Psychosocial problems

an "objective" point against the surgeon in case of litigation. An operation performed at the wrong level or a neglected significant root compression should be identified as a cause of early failure before the patient leaves the hospital (3,7,9,18,23,36).

NEURORADIOLOGIC EVALUATION

The type of surgical spinal implants used will influence or restrict the neuroradiologic evaluation. For example, ferromagnetic appliances produce major artifacts on MR and CT. However, this is not the case with the newer titanium alloys. In cases in which imaging artifact may be a problem, myelography will help to disclose or exclude a major compressive abnormality of nerve roots and thecal sac and to document a gross complication, iatrogenic le-

sion, or new pathology occurring at another level (Figs. IIID-2 through IIID-5).

Magnetic Resonance

In patients with titanium appliances or intervertebral carbon fusion cages and ramps, MR provides the best information concerning the spinal canal and its contents, the nerve roots (especially within the foramen), the paravertebral soft tissues, and the cancellous bone (Figs. IIID-6, IIID-7, and IIID-8). Disk morphology (including herniation), disk space narrowing, and evidence of diskitis are clearly depicted. After removal of ferromagnetic implants, MR can accurately show the traces created by the implantation device (e.g., pedicle screws), enabling

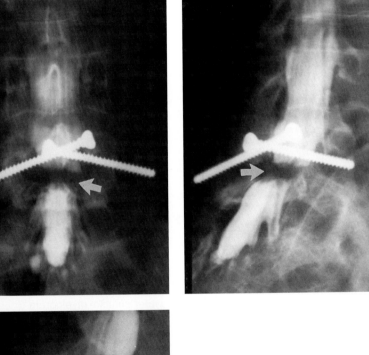

A

B

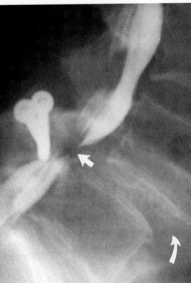

C

FIG. IIID-2. Failed translaminar screw fixation. (**A**) Anteroposterior and (**B**) oblique radiographs following the intrathecal installation of water-soluble contrast medium demonstrates the partial blockage of contrast medium at the L4-5 level (*arrows*). The translaminar screws are identified. (**C**) Lateral radiograph of the myelogram demonstrates the subtotal block to the flow of contrast (*arrow*). The anterolisthesis at L4-5 is also noted (*curved arrow*). In this case, the translaminar screw fixation has failed to halt the anterolysthesis at L4-5.

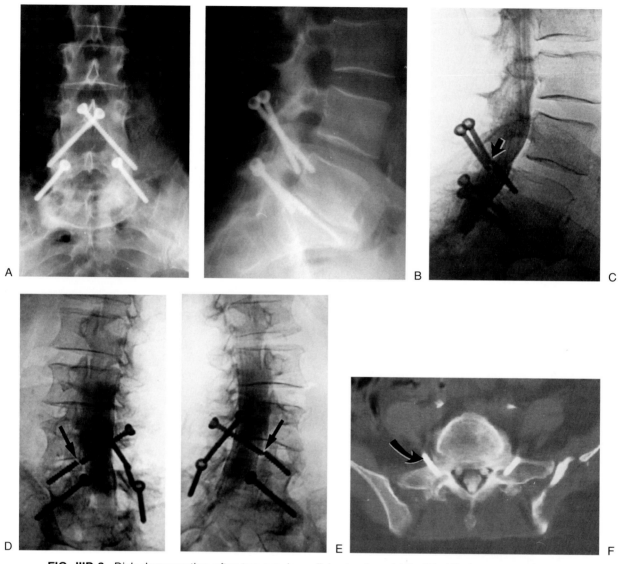

FIG. IIID-3. Disk degeneration after two previous diskectomies at L5–S1. (**A**) Anteroposterior and (**B**) lateral radiographs demonstrate a translaminar screw fixation at L4-5 (8) and a transarticular screw fixation at L5–S1. In addition, there is an intertransversal bone graft predominantly on the left side. (**C**) Lateral, (**D**) left, and (**E**) right oblique negative radiographs from a water-soluble myelogram demonstrate a screw breakage on the right side and mild anterolisthesis at L4-5. The thecal sac is not significantly narrowed at any level. (**F**) Postmyelographic CT at the L5–S1 level demonstrates the suboptimal position of the right transarticular screw, which penetrates laterally from the sacrum into the anterior soft tissues (*arrow*).

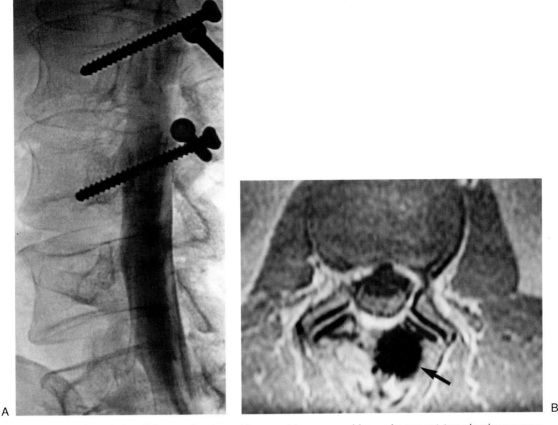

A   B

FIG. IIID-4. Two prior diskectomies in a 40-year-old man requiring subsequent translaminar screw fixation for segmental instability. (**A**) Negative of radiograph from water-soluble myelogram 6 months following translaminar screw fixation shows adequate screw placement without abnormality in the contrast column. (**B**) Axial T$_1$-weighted MR at the L2-3 level shows metallic artifacts (*arrow*) from drill fragments within the soft tissues occurring during the previous surgical procedure.

deductions to be made about former root impingement or compression (Fig. IIID-9) (15–17,20).

Computed Tomography

Computed tomography is best for axial imaging of the bony spinal canal, especially when hypertrophic facet joints and partially calcified ligamenta flava contribute to spinal canal stenosis. The CT gives precise information concerning the cortical bone and the size of the spinal canal and is of paramount importance for the documentation of vertebral fractures. Some illustrative cases (Figs. IIID-10 through IIID-14) document realignment of posteriorly dislocated fragments and bone grafts, which are added to achieve later definitive bony fusion. Using bone window settings on CT acquisitions may minimize metallic artifacts from hardware but may still impede the interpretation, especially when the axial section is placed at a crossing

or connection between vertical rods or plates and horizontal pedicle screws. Computed tomographic myelography may help to better distinguish the dural sac and its contents in a patient with residual mixed lumbar stenosis after fusion (Fig. IIID-15) (12,15,16).

Myelography

Conventional myelography is still indicated to exclude a compression of the thecal sac and nerve root sleeve in patients with ferromagnetic appliances that may interfere with MR (see Fig. IIID-23). Arachnoiditis, pseudomeningocele, and a major CSF fistula.

''Superspecialization'' may influence the priorities different physicians give to the anatomic and functional facts demonstrated on imaging studies. The neurosurgeon will focus on the spinal canal, its content and size; the orthopedic surgeon will look first at the bones, the curvatures, the alignment of the vertebrae,

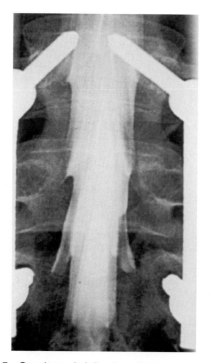

FIG. IIID-5. Good result following diskectomy and distraction spondylodesis for spinal instability. Anteroposterior radiograph of water-soluble myelogram demonstrates the spondylodesis and good filling of the thecal sac and root sleeves.

and at the implanted construct. The rehabilitation specialist will pay attention to the patient's muscles as active stabilizers of the spine, which may be devascularized and denervated by too traumatic and too extensive a surgical procedure. He will care more about socioeconomic and psychological problems of the patient with an operated spine.

Both radiologists and clinicians must, therefore, not forget to examine all clinicoradiologic factors. For example, the erector trunci muscles should not be overlooked on CT and MR (15,16). Kotilainen et al. (31) have confirmed the role of atrophy of these muscles and poor results after disk surgery.

BASIC ANATOMIC AND BIOMECHANICAL CONCEPTS

The Three-Column Spine

According to Louis (32), spinal stability is provided by three columns: one anterior (i.e., suprajacent vertebral body–disk–subjacent vertebral body) and two posterior columns (facet joints on both sides). The weakening of one column may be tolerated, but the weakening of two columns leads to instability.

Another three-column spine concept is presented by Denis (33,34), who describes an anterior, a middle, and

a posterior column. The anterior column consists of the anterior longitudinal ligament, anterior annulus fibrosus, anterior vertebral body, and the anterior two-thirds of the disk. The middle column includes the posterior longitudinal ligament, posterior annulus fibrosus, posterior vertebral body, and posterior disk. The posterior column is made up of the posterior arch and posterior ligamentous complex, including the interspinous ligament, facet capsules, and ligamentum flavum. In acute thoracolumbar spinal injuries, lesions of the middle column are of utmost importance concerning stability. Injuries involving only one column are considered stable, whereas those involving two or three columns are unstable.

Roy Camille (35) prefers to analyze five segments: three vertical and two horizontal. His anterior vertical segment extends more posteriorly than Denis' anterior column. The middle segment includes the posterior wall of the vertebra and disk, the posterior longitudinal ligament, the pedicles, and the facet joints. A lesion of the middle segment elements signifies instability. The posterior segment consists of the spinous and transverse processes and the inter- and supraspinous ligaments.

In the horizontal plane, the mobile segment is located at the level of the intervertebral disk and extends posteriorly through the facet joints to the interspinous ligament, and the immobile segment is at the level of the bony canal (vertebral body–pedicles–lamina). The pedicles and laminae in fact connect the three vertical columns of Louis together.

These variations are interesting but can be confusing when one does not know to which three-column concept an author is referring. In this chapter we use the Louis classification (7,32). A weak anterior column (vertebral body–disk–vertebral body) may lead to a failure of a posterior interbody fusion, as reported in the literature (9,22,36) and illustrated in Figs. IIID-10, IIID-16, and IIID-17.

The Load-Sharing Classification of Spine Fractures

The load-sharing classification (36) is based on the relationship between the amount and characteristics of vertebral injury and the success of posterior short-segment instrumentation (with VSP plates and screws) (9) utilizing intertransverse fusion. The amount of vertebral body comminution, of displacement of fracture fragments, and of correction of kyphotic deformity are analyzed with CT before and with conventional radiographs after the operation, scoring one to three points for each characteristic of the fracture site: (a) the amount of vertebral body actually comminuted by the injury, as best seen on sagittal CT reconstructions of the fracture site (1 point, 30% or less of the vertebral body broken; 2 points, 30% to 60% comminution of the body; 3 points, more than 60% comminution); (b) the amount of apposition or displacement of

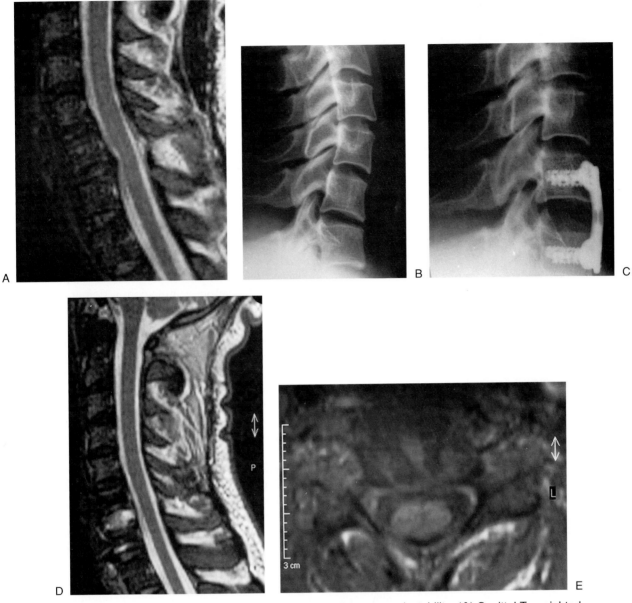

FIG. IIID-6. Traumatic C6-7 disk herniation with diskoligamentary instability. (**A**) Sagittal T$_2$-weighted MR demonstrates the C6-7 focal disk herniation with indentation of the anterior surface of the spinal cord. (**B**) A preoperative lateral radiograph shows a kyphotic deformity C6-7 and enlargement of the interspinous space at this level. (**C**) The postoperative lateral projection radiograph shows that there has been an anterior diskectomy and fusion with Morscher's titanium plate plus a bone autograft (24) taken from the iliac crest. There is a mild overdistraction of the C6-7 intervertebral disk space. (**D**) Postoperative T$_2$-weighted sagittal MR shows that the spinal cord is decompressed and is surrounded adequately by CSF. Only minimal artifacts are seen related to the titanium plate and screws. (**E**) Axial postoperative T$_1$-weighted MR shows that the titanium screws within the vertebral body yield very little MR artifact.

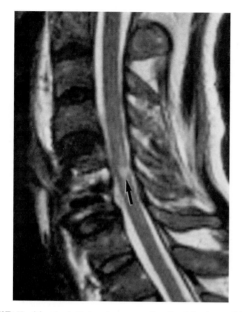

FIG. IIID-7. Ventral diskectomy and spinal fusion with bone graft and Morscher's plate extending from C5 to C6. Postoperative T$_2$-weighted MR in the sagittal plane shows residual abnormal focal hyperintensity (*arrow*) within the spinal cord at the level of C5-6 in this patient with persistent postoperative myelopathy. The metallic artifacts are minimal in this case of titanium screw placement.

fracture fragments, as best seen on axial CT sections through the fracture site (1 point, 0 to 1 mm of displacement; 2 points, at least 2 mm of displacement in less than 50% of the cross-sectional area of the vertebral body; 3 points, 2 mm or greater displacement in over 50% of the cross-sectional area, as viewed on CT); and (c) the amount of correction of kyphotic deformity as best measured by comparing pre- and postoperative conventional radiographs (1 point, 3° or less correction; 2 points, 4° to 9° correction; 3 points, 10° or greater correction).

All three factors describe in different ways the injury to the anterior column. Clearly, vertebral fragments do not transfer load as well as an intact vertebra, and the wider the fracture fragments are displaced, the more poorly they transmit the load. The correction of a kyphotic deformity indicates that there will be a gap in the anterior column when the traumatic kyphosis is corrected. This can be a problem because a major gap eliminates anterior column load sharing and exposes pedicle screw implants to stresses because this configuration generates the highest possible cantilever bending loads.

Spinal fractures can be graded from a minimum total number of 3 to a maximum of 9 points. During the follow-up period (e.g., 3 to 5 years), 10 of 28 patients followed showed evidence of screw breakage. All 10 had point totals of 7 or more; five of the 10 had the maximum of 9 points. There were no screw fractures in cases with point totals of 6 and less. Thus, in the absence of load sharing, hardware failure and nonunion rates greatly increase (36).

The screw–plate (or screw–rod) interface is the most likely location of construct failure because this is the location of the maximum bending moment (i.e., the longest lever arm). A cantilever beam construct with a non-fixed lever arm does not effectively resist axial loads. The application of an axial load may result in screw pullout and/or vertebral body translation as a consequence of toggling of the screw with respect to the plate by such a construct when axial (vertical) stability is not present (12) (Figs. IIID-17 and IIID-18).

Whenever the preoperative CT scan scores 6 points, the surgeon should, in addition to the planned posterior instrumentation, consider reinforcement of the anterior column by transpedicular bone (5) or Bio-Oss (a bovine apatite, see Fig. IIID-14) (48) grafting or, in selected cases, an anterior reconstruction and stabilization.

However, in some trauma cases with late anterior collapse from weakening of the anterior column, the spinal canal and therefore neurologic function are not affected. The posterior wall of the vertebral body heals first, protecting the neural elements. The patients may have some backache and muscular spasm, and the kyphosis on the radiographs may look rather bad, but the neurologic status is intact. Therefore, a second operation is not necessary (see Figs. IIID-10 and IIID-11).

Because of the curved anatomy of the anterior vertebral body cortex, lateral radiographs may be misleading as to the actual depth of penetration pedicle screws. For this reason radiographic penetration of only 75% of the apparent anteroposterior vertebral body diameter can result in actual penetration of the anterior cortex by the screw (37). To avoid anterior cortical perforation with the risk of injury to the perispinous vascular and visceral structures, the screw penetration should not exceed 80% of the apparent vertebral body anteroposterior diameter (14). Divergent insertion of the pedicle screws should especially be avoided in the thoracolumbar spine. It should be noted that some experienced surgeons do not mind minor penetration of the anterior cortex by a pedicle screw, as this increases the stability of the construct (i.e., "penetration" but not "perforation").

The Three-Dimensional Coordinate System

For a standardized description of abnormal increased motion, the tridimensional coordinate system proposed by White and Panjabi (38) can be recommended. Markwalder and Reulen (25) emphasize its use for the analysis of postoperative instability of the lumbar spine. By definition, the X-axis flexion–extension is around the X-axis, and lateral translation to the left or right is along the X-axis. The Y-axis indicates that axial rotation (to the left or right) is around the Y-axis, and axial compression is along the Y-axis. The Z-axis indicates that lateral bending is around the Z-

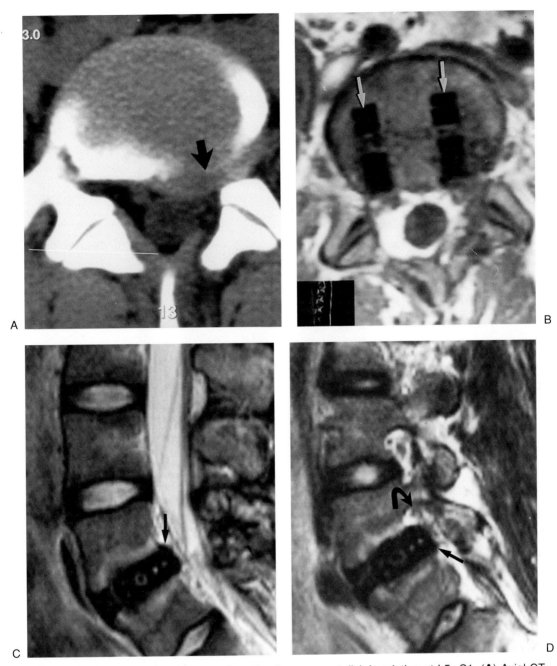

FIG. IIID-8. Intervertebral fusion ramp insertion for recurrent disk herniation at L5–S1. (**A**) Axial CT examination demonstrates a recurrent left-sided disk herniation that extends into the neural foramen (*arrow*). (**B**) Postoperative axial T_1-weighted MR image demonstrates the intervertebral fusion ramps at L5–S1 (*arrows*). Soft tissue seems to surround the left S1 route and sheath complex in the lateral recess and obliterates the fat in this region. (**C**) Sagittal T_2-weighted fast spin-echo MR in the midline shows that the posterior margin of the ramps slightly bulge into the spinal canal (*arrow*). (**D**) A parasagittal view on the right side shows that although the ramp slightly bulges into the inferior neural foramen (*arrow*), the superior recess containing the nerve root remains patent (*curved arrow*).

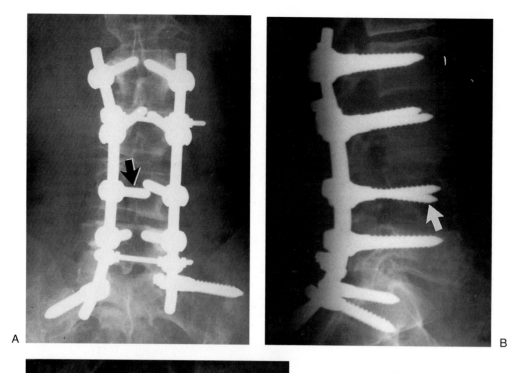

A

B

C

FIG. IIID-9. Cotrel–Dubousset (CD) instrumentation with pedicle screws at multiple levels and vertical rods after L4-5 diskectomy. (**A**) Anteroposterior and (**B**) lateral radiographs show the CD instrumentation placed from L2 through S1 with pedicle screws at each level bilaterally and vertical rods with two cross-connectors at L2-3 and at L5. Note that right L4 pedicle screw crosses the midline and is directed somewhat inferiorly (*arrows*). (**C**) Axial T_1-weighted MR image following removal of the instrumentation at approximately 2 years following the original surgery. Note the track of the right pedicle screw at L4 (*arrows*). The track is too medial, with its tip crossing the midline within the left half of the vertebral body. In fact, the left pedicle screw at L4 went through the medial half of the left L4 pedicle (*curved arrow*).

axis (rotation in the vertical plane with unilateral height loss), and anterior–posterior translation is along the Z-axis (''antero- and retrolisthesis''). Combined abnormally increased rotational–translational motion may occur in an unstable spine.

In Fig. IIID-19, vertical instability after disk herniation is illustrated. Retroposition of the cranial vertebra and the superior facet of the lower vertebra pointing cranially and anteriorly narrows the intervertebral foramen after loss of disk-space height. Finally, traction spurs develop, as

FIG. IIID-10. Burst fracture of T12 with upper end-plate fracture and mild compression of L1. (**A**) Lateral radiograph demonstrates the compression fractures of T12 and L1. (**B**) Axial CT shows the burst fracture of T12 with retropulsion of fragments into the spinal canal (*arrows*). (**C**) Postoperative myelogram shows good alignment of the posterior aspect of the T12 vertebral body with free flow of contrast medium past the fractured vertebral body. The surgical appliance enabled a reposition of the posteriorly displaced fragments in part because the posterior longitudinal ligament was intact. This represents a ''ligamentotactic reduction'' (5,40). (**D**) Immediate postoperative radiographs show parallel implantation of the Schanz screws. Because the anterior column is weakened, this arrangement will not be able to resist the anterior bending forces. (**E**) Lateral radiograph obtained 5 months after **D** shows that the Schanz screws at T11 have eroded almost into the disk space at T10-11. The disk space at T11-12 has become narrowed, and the anterior wedging of T12 has increased since the prior film. (**F**) Lateral radiograph acquired after removal of the spinal appliances at 16 months following surgery shows a marked kyphotic deformity at the thoracolumbar junction and increased collapse of the T12 vertebral body.

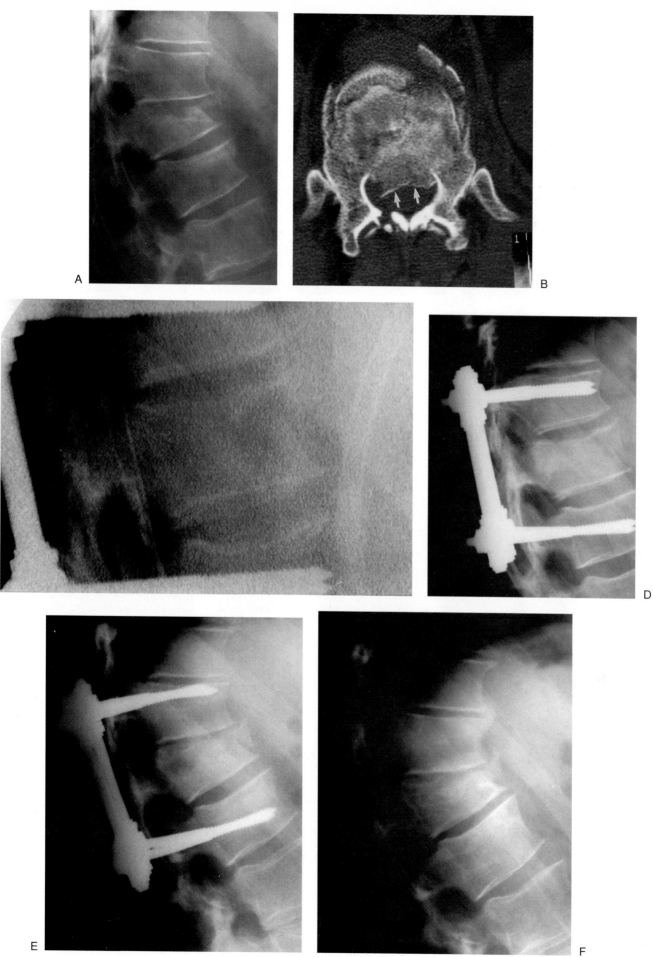

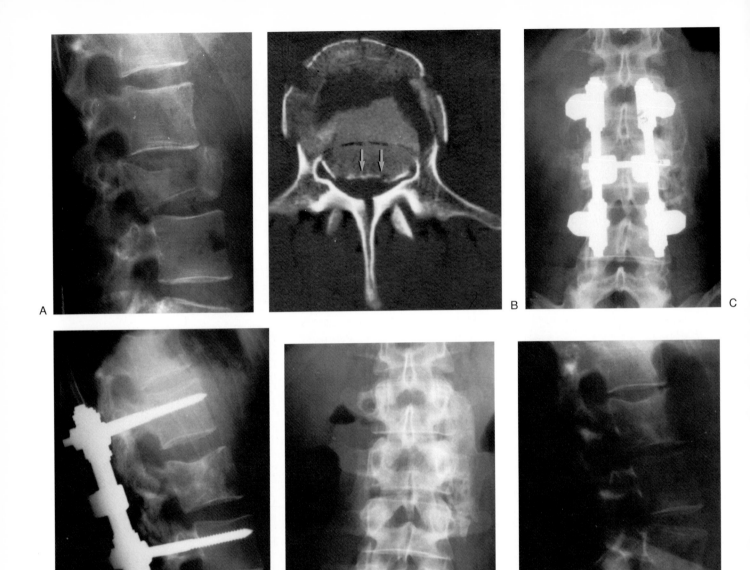

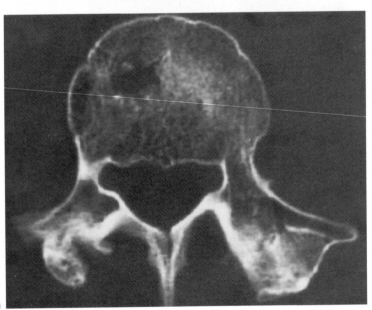

FIG. IIID-11. Burst fracture of L3. (**A**) Lateral conventional radiograph of the lumbar spine shows the burst fracture of L3. (**B**) Computed tomograph through L3 demonstrates a burst fracture of L3 with retropulsion of fragments into the spinal canal. The laminar and spinous process are also fractured. (**C**) Anteroposterior and (**D**) lateral postoperative radiographs after distraction spondylodesis with Dick's internal fixator (5). The device extends from L2 to L4 and contains an additional cross-connector and a predominantly left-sided lateral bone graft extending from L2 to L4. (**E**) Anteroposterior and (**F**) lateral radiographs at 1 year following removal of the internal fixator at 9 months. There is a minimal kyphotic deformity with some straightening of the upper lumbar lordotic curve. The bony fusion predominantly on the left appears continuous. (**G**) Postoperative CT acquired at 9 months following surgery and after removal of the internal fixator shows a normal configuration and size of the spinal canal with realignment of the posterior wall of the L3 vertebral body. The predominantly left-sided bone graft seems to be a solid bone mass (*asterisk*).

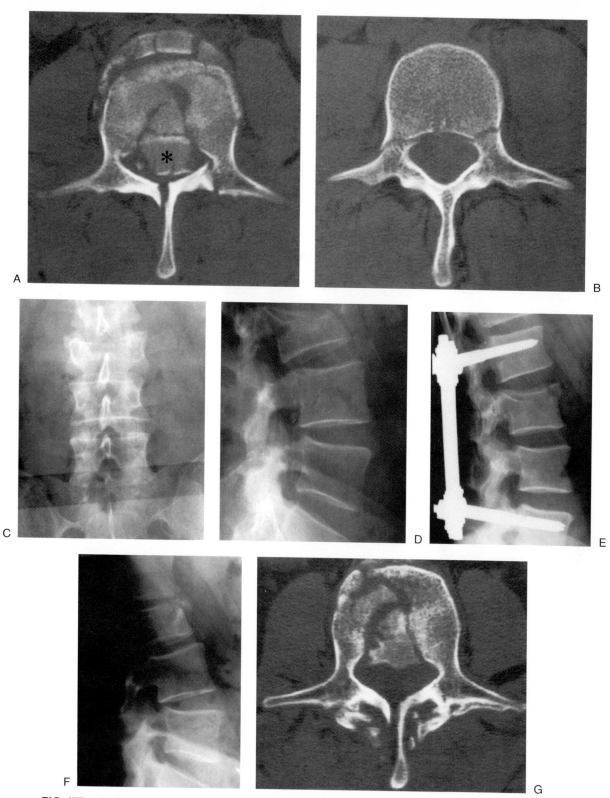

FIG. IIID-12. Burst fracture of L3 with L4 pedicle fracture. (**A**) Axial CT through L3 demonstrates the burst fracture and the marked retropulsion of bone fragments (*asterisk*) into the spinal canal. The central spinal canal is essentially filled with bone fragments. The lamina on the left is also fractured. (**B**) Axial CT through the L4 vertebral body demonstrates bilateral pedicle fractures. (**C**) Anteroposterior and (**D**) lateral radiographs demonstrate the compression burst fracture of L3 and faintly demonstrate the pedicle fractures of L4. (**E**) Lateral radiograph postoperatively following Dick's internal fixator placement. Note that the lordosis in the lumbar region has been reestablished, and the wedging of L3 has been reduced. (**F**) Lateral radiograph of the lumbosacral spine at 1 year following removal of the surgical appliance demonstrates a mild but acceptable kyphosis and only moderate loss of height of the L3 vertebral bodies. The operative appliance was removed in the ninth postoperative month. (**G**) Axial CT obtained during the ninth month after surgery, following surgical appliance removal, demonstrates that the spinal canal is broader in dimension than depicted in **A,** the preoperative CT.

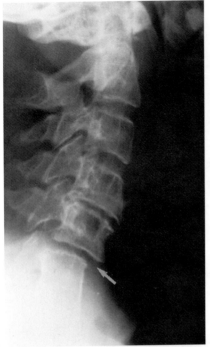

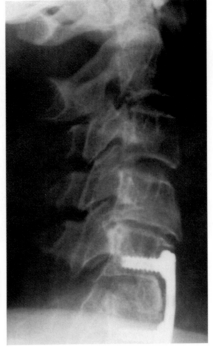

A

B

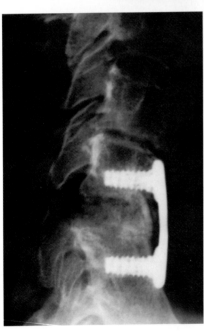

C

FIG. IIID-13. Traumatic subluxation of C5 on C6 following prior C6-7 fusion 10 years earlier. (**A**) Lateral radiograph demonstrates a subluxation of C5 on C6 (*arrow*). Flexion–extension radiograph demonstrated motion and therefore instability at C5-6 (not shown). (**B**) The postoperative lateral radiograph of the cervical spine demonstrates the Morscher's plate and the intervertebral bone graft between C5 and C6. (**C**) Ten weeks following the radiograph in **B,** this lateral radiograph demonstrates that fusion has occurred together with mild kyphotic deformation. There is also an increased gap between the spinous processes of C5 and C6. The inferior articular processes of C5 are almost perched on the tips of the superior articular processes of C6. Because the patient was asymptomatic, no further surgery was carried out.

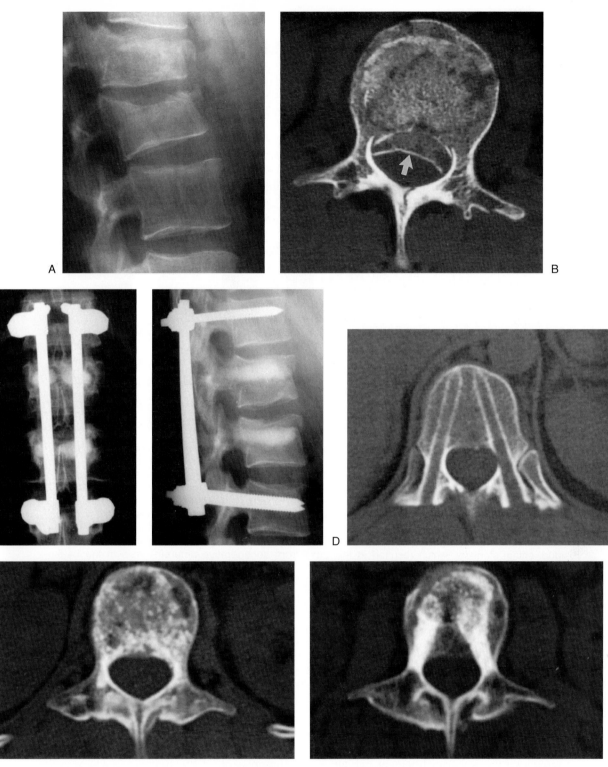

FIG. IIID-14. Burst fracture of L1 and L2. (**A**) A lateral radiograph of the upper lumbar spine shows the burst fractures of L1 and L2 with associated anterior wedging. (**B**) Axial CT through L1 demonstrates the burst fracture with retropulsion of fragments posteriorly into the spinal canal. There is also a fracture extending through the lamina and into the spinal process. (**C**) Anteroposterior and (**D**) lateral radiographs demonstrating treatment with distraction spondylolisthesis with a USS internal fixator and transpedicular grafting of Bio-Oss extending from T12 to L3 (48) in order to reinforce the anterior column. The radiographs demonstrate excellent alignment of the thoracolumbar spine. The previously compressed L1 and L2 vertebral bodies are now of nearly normal height. The hyperdense material identified within the L1 and L2 vertebral bodies is the Bio-Oss. (**E**) The postoperative axial CT after removal of the metallic implants at 9 months following the initial surgery shows the canals of the transpedicular screws bilaterally. Note that the screws were perfectly placed without evidence of penetration into the spinal canal. (**F**) Axial CT through L1 shows a normal size of the spinal canal (compare with **B**). The increased density of the vertebral body results from the placement of Bio-Oss (48). (**G**) Axial CT through L2 showing the marked hyperdensity of the pedicles and the inferior portion of the vertebral body after filling with Bio-Oss (48).

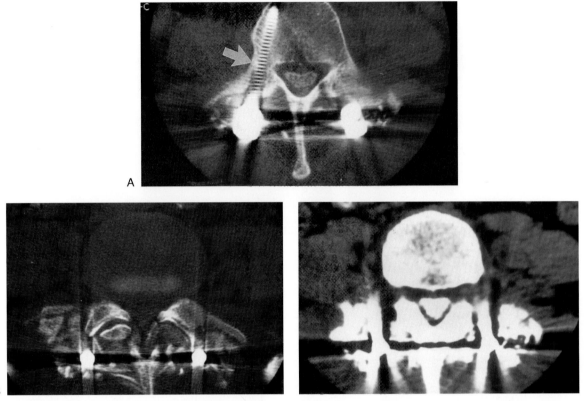

FIG. IIID-15. Residual L4-5 spinal stenosis after USS system L4–S1 spondylodesis. (**A**) This CT following water-soluble myelogram shows contrast medium within the thecal sac at the L4 level. The right-sided pedicle screw is well placed (*arrow*). (**B**) Axial CT through the L4-5 disk level shows almost no contrast within the thecal sac. The intertransversal bone graft is noted bilaterally as well as the metallic artifact from the instrumentation. These do not obscure the spinal canal in this case. (**C**) Above the level of the contrast blockage observed in **B**, the thecal sac is well visualized without compression on this image filmed with soft tissue techniques. Note again that the metallic artifacts do not obscure the spinal canal in this case. In **B**, the obliteration of contrast medium indicates the residual spinal stenosis, which resulted in this case from degenerative anterolisthesis at the L4-5 intervertebral disk level.

described by MacNab (39), indicating degenerative instability (3).

In Fig. IIID-20, rotation–displacement along the *X*-, *Y*-, and *Z*-axes in cases of postoperative instability is illustrated, according to Markwalder and Reulen (25).

In Fig. IIID-21, the principle of "ligamentotactic" reduction by posterior instrumentation is shown. Distraction puts tension on the posterior ligament, which pulls the retropulsed fragment out of the canal (5,40). The same principle applies for bulging ligaments in degenerative stenosis, when a distraction spondylodesis is performed (3) (Figs. IIID-1, IIID-17, IIID-18, and IIID-22).

Figure IIID-23 illustrates the principle of translaminar screw fixation introduced by Magerl (8) and frequently used by Benini (3,11) for degenerative instability and stenosis. In cases of retrolisthesis of the cranial vertebra, distraction will allow a correct re-

alignment, which will be secured by translaminar screws with added posterolateral bone grafts. Failures of this system include screw breakage (see Fig. IIID-3) and fixation of anterolisthesis without repositioning and decompression of central canal stenosis (see Fig. IIID-2). Such cases are better treated with plates and screws or with an internal fixator after prior decompression of the stenosis (3,41).

DISCUSSION OF SPECIFIC IMPLANTS

Hook–Plate Fixation

The hook–plate fixation (6) was designed for posterior stabilization of the cervical spine over one or two motion segments (Fig. IIID-24). Hook plates are available in several sizes. They are inserted with the hook underneath

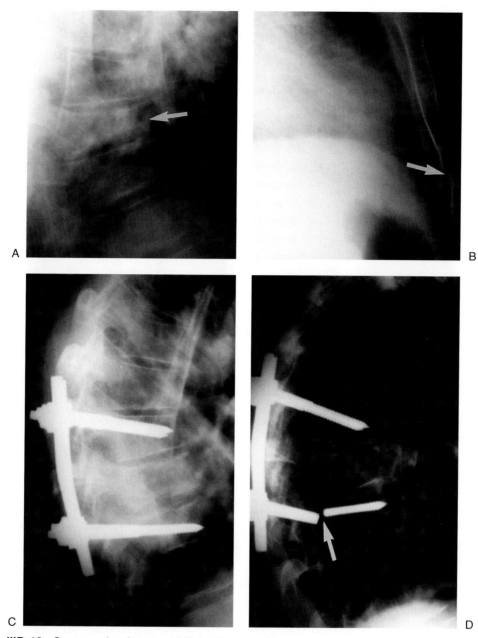

FIG. IIID-16. Compression fracture of T-8 with associated sternal fracture indicating instability. (**A**) Thoracic spine and (**B**) sternal radiographs in the lateral projection show fractures of T-8 and the sternum. (**C**) Schanz screws of the Universal Spine System (USS) internal fixator were, unfortunately, placed in a convergent position. Note that the height of T8 has increased from distraction as compared to the preoperative radiograph. (**D**) A radiograph at a later date demonstrates a fracture of the Schanz screws (*arrow*). This necessitated removal of the implants, and the final result was increased kyphosis (not shown).

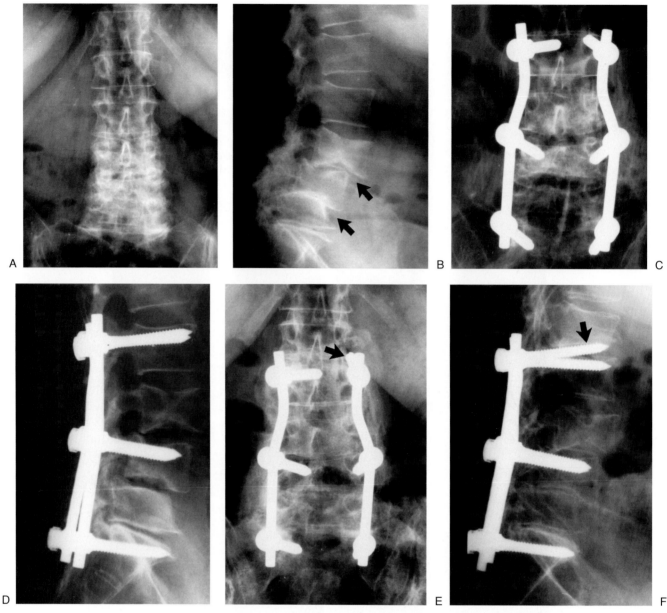

FIG. IIID-17. Degenerative instability in a 73-year-old woman with osteoporosis. (**A**) Anteroposterior and (**B**) lateral radiographs demonstrate marked anterolisthesis of L3 on L4 and L4 on L5 (*arrows*). (**C**) Anteroposterior and (**D**) lateral radiographs show a distraction spondylodesis with the USS internal fixator. Note that there is partial reduction and distraction along the axis of the spine extending from L2 through S1. These films were obtained immediately following the surgical procedure. (**E**) Anteroposterior and (**F**) lateral radiographs obtained at 1 year following the spondylodesis show that the left L2 pedicle screw has migrated out of the pedicle and has been displaced laterally and cranially (*arrows*). There has also been a collapse of the intervertebral spaces at L1-2 and L4-5.

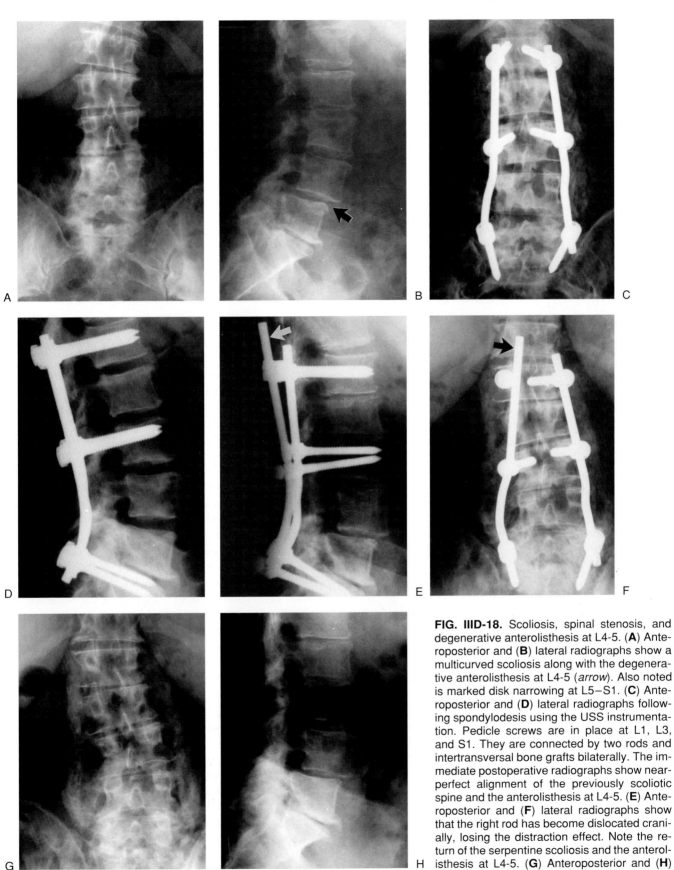

FIG. IIID-18. Scoliosis, spinal stenosis, and degenerative anterolisthesis at L4-5. (**A**) Anteroposterior and (**B**) lateral radiographs show a multicurved scoliosis along with the degenerative anterolisthesis at L4-5 (*arrow*). Also noted is marked disk narrowing at L5–S1. (**C**) Anteroposterior and (**D**) lateral radiographs following spondylodesis using the USS instrumentation. Pedicle screws are in place at L1, L3, and S1. They are connected by two rods and intertransversal bone grafts bilaterally. The immediate postoperative radiographs show near-perfect alignment of the previously scoliotic spine and the anterolisthesis at L4-5. (**E**) Anteroposterior and (**F**) lateral radiographs show that the right rod has become dislocated cranially, losing the distraction effect. Note the return of the serpentine scoliosis and the anterolisthesis at L4-5. (**G**) Anteroposterior and (**H**) lateral radiographs following removal of the surgical implants 1 year later again shows the chronic anterolisthesis at L4-5 and the scoliosis. At surgery, the intertransversal bone grafts were noted to be stable.

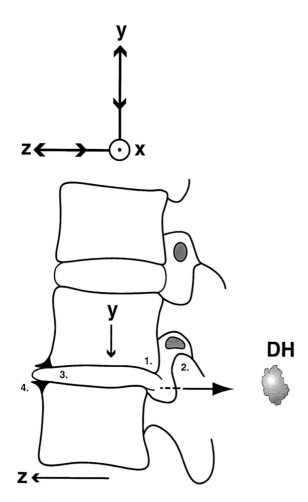

FIG. IIID-19. Features of degenerative spinal instability (3,25). **1:** Retrolisthesis of the craniad vertebral body on the caudal vertebral body; occasionally anterolysthesis occurs. **2:** The superior facet of the caudal vertebral body points craniad and anteriorly and may narrow the intervertebral foramen. **3:** Loss of disk space height. **4:** Anterior traction spurs develop (39). (Note the X-, Y-, and Z-axes of the coordinate system as described by White and Panjabi (38). Following larger disk herniations (DH), the vertical stability and load sharing of the anterior column are diminished.

the lamina of the lower vertebra involved and fixed to the articular process of the upper vertebra by a 3.5-mm AO cortical screw. In very small articular processes, 2.7-mm cortical screws may be used. Tightening the screw creates a posterior axial compressive force and lordosis. To prevent hyperlordosis, a pressure-resistant corticocancellous bone graft is inserted between the two spinous processes. This graft also provides a third bridge together with the two facet joints, creating a three-point fixation. In addition to the corticocancellous bone graft, cancellous graft material is positioned over the articular pillars, laterally and medially to the hook plate. The first or second day after surgery, the patient is placed in a Philadelphia cervical collar for the next 6 to 8 weeks.

Indications for hook–plate fixation are diskoligamentous injuries such as dislocations and subluxations occurring from C2 to C7 with minor damage to the articular processes and vertebral bodies, painful degenerative disease, spondylolisthesis, or anterior postoperative pseudarthrosis of the cervical spine. This fixation can also be used as an adjunct to anterior decompression and fusion in vertebral body fractures, tumor, or infection. The technique is possible only if the lamina of the lower vertebra and the articular pillar of the cephalad vertebra to be fused are preserved.

The main advantage of hook–plate fixation compared with a wiring technique is its better stability. The strength of the hook–plate fixation is attributed to its three-point fixation, which provides stability in all directions (Figs. IIID-24 and IIID-25).

Titanium Hollow-Screw System

Anterior plate fixation of the cervical spine acts as a tension band system in extension and as a buttress plate in flexion. Enhancement of an anterior grafting technique with a plate provides enough primary stability to allow early mobilization without significant external support. This facilitates postoperative nursing and shortens rehabilitation time. Anterior grafting of the cervical spine in combination with anterior plate fixation has proven to be an excellent technique for treating degenerative spine disease and tumors of the cervical spine. This technique is also appropriate for treating most fractures and fracture dislocations, as long as it is possible to obtain reduction through traction maneuvers. It supports the anterior column when instability persists following trauma, diskectomy, or following partial or total vertebrectomy for decompression of the spinal cord.

In such cases, initially the intervertebral disk is removed, or a vertebrectomy and anterior decompression is performed, followed by a bridging graft taken from the anterior iliac crest. A cubic tricortical bone graft is preferred because of its superior mechanical properties. We recommend the use of a slightly wedge-shaped graft, with the higher vertical rim located anteriorly. Through this configuration, the physiologic lordosis of the cervical spine is restored and maintained. When titanium plasma-layered screws are used for this technique, it is not necessary to penetrate the posterior cortex of the vertebral body to gain sufficient stability of the graft–plate construct. In addition to the locking of the screw head into the cylinder of the hollow screw, the angle between plate and screw can be stabilized, and also anterior migration of the screw will be prevented. The titanium plasma spray coating of the screws provides a greater surface area, thus increasing the interlocking between implant and bone interface. Also, the screws are perforated to permit bony ingrowth in order to achieve an increase in pullout strength and a decrease in loosening.

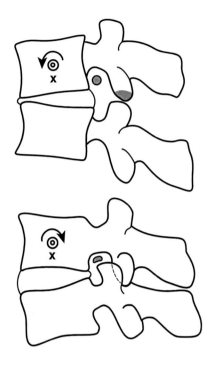

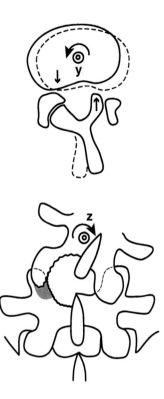

FIG. IIID-20. Rotational displacement along the *X*-, *Y*-, and *Z*-axes in patients with postoperative instability using the three-dimensional coordinate system (16,26,38). (From Kaech, ref. 16, with permission.)

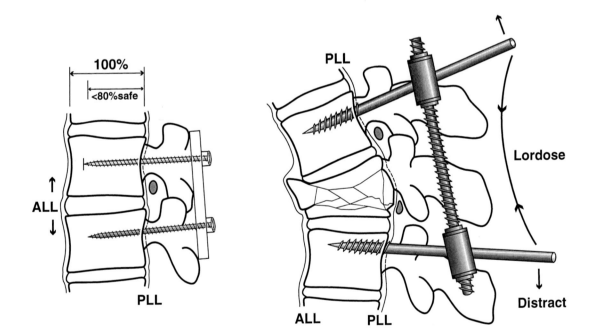

FIG. IIID-21. (**A**) Ligamentotactic reduction by posterior instrumentation (5,40). Lordotic tension puts traction on the posterior longitudinal ligament, which in effect pulls the retropulsed fragments out of the canal and back into line with the posterior aspect of the vertebral bodies on either side of the fractured vertebra. (**B**) In order to avoid cortical bone perforation, the screw penetration should not exceed 80% of the apparent radiographic vertebral body anteroposterior diameter (14,37).

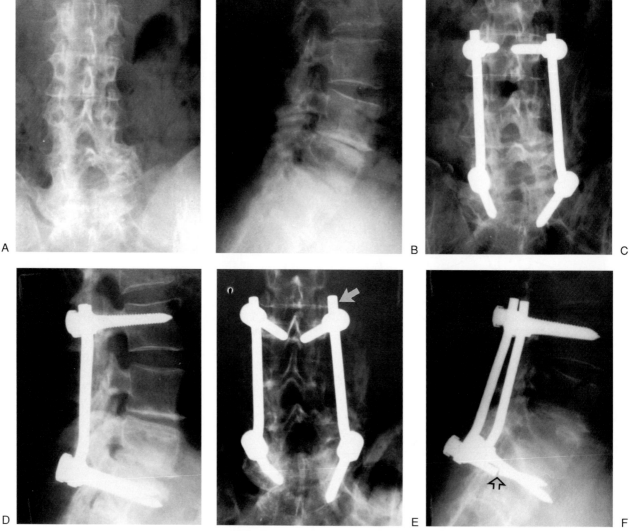

A   B   C
D   E   F

FIG. IIID-22. Patient with past diskectomies at L4-5 and L5–S1 with reoperation for recurrence. (**A**) Anteroposterior and (**B**) lateral radiographs demonstrate marked narrowing of the L4-5 and L5–S1 intervertebral disks. (**C**) Immediate postoperative anteroposterior and (**D**) lateral radiographs show a distraction spondylodesis utilizing the USS internal fixator extending from L3 to S1. The back-opening pedicle screws are connected by rods and locked by locking screws. Note the adequate distraction with an increase in disk height at L4-5 and L5–S1. (**E**) Anteroposterior and (**F**) lateral radiographs performed at 4 months following the surgery show that the L3 locking screw has loosened, resulting in a craniad migration of the left-sided rod (*arrow*). Despite the intertransversal bone graft bilaterally, the overload has caused the right S1 pedicle screw to break (*open arrow*).

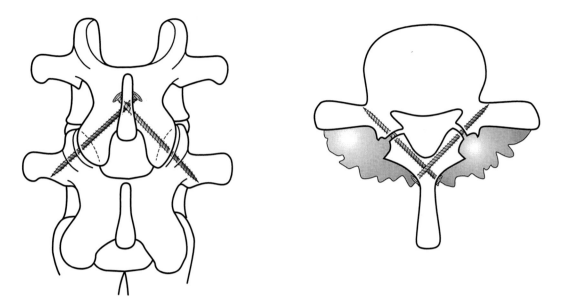

FIG. IIID-23. Translaminar screw fixation of Magerl (8), used also by Benini (3,11), for degenerative spinal instability. In cases of degenerative retrolisthesis, distraction allows a correct realignment, which will be secured by translaminar screws assisted by additional posterolateral intertransversal bone grafts.

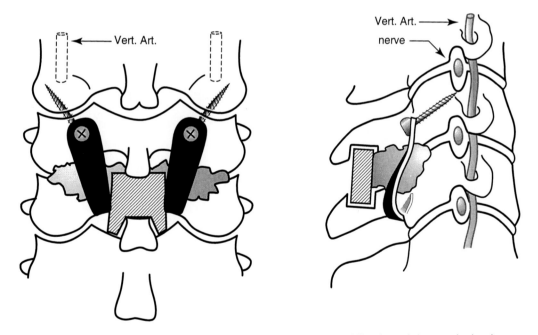

FIG. IIID-24. Hook–plate fixation by Magerl (6) for posterior stabilization of the cervical spine over one or two vertebral segments. A misplaced, excessively long screw may penetrate the bone and injure a nerve root or even the vertebral artery.

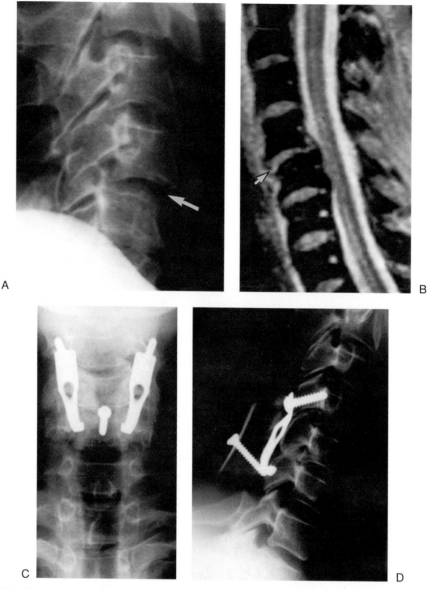

FIG. IIID-25. Fracture subluxation with fusion. (**A**) Lateral radiograph of the cervical spine demonstrates a C4-5 subluxation (*arrow*), a fracture of the right articular process of C5, and a fracture of the lamina of C5 on the left. (**B**) Sagittal T$_2$-weighted MR image demonstrates anterolisthesis of C4 on C5, bulging of the disk posteriorly, and annular rupture anteriorly (*arrow*). (**C**) Anteroposterior and (**D**) lateral postoperative radiographs show a hook–plate spondylodesis extending from C4 through C6. There are screws in the articular process of C4 and a hook extending to the laminae of C6. A posterior bone transplant from the iliac crest is fixed with a screw into the spinous process of C6 [the hook plate is from Grob and Magerl (6), technique modified by G. Meier]. There is correct alignment of the vertebral bodies postoperatively.

The surgical technique for the titanium hollow-screw system is similar to the technique for the anterior standard H plate. To drill the screw holes, a special drill guide is used to prevent overpenetration and damage to the spinal cord. The drill is stopped at a depth of 14 mm. The same principle is applied to the tap sleeve, which also has a stop at 14 mm. The cross-head screwdriver is first inserted into the screwhead before a split sleeve is pushed over the screwhead to hold it in position. A second split sleeve is necessary to prevent the screwhead from expanding on insertion. The screw is driven home until the head of the screw engages at the plate surface. The two split sleeves disengage automatically when the screw is tightened. Finally, the plate is locked into place by insertion of the conical expansion bolt, which expands the head of the larger screw and locks it into the plate.

Anterior plate fixation is also feasible for multisegmental fusion or for single or multiple, subtotal or total vertebrectomy. In such a case, a plate of the appropriate length has to be chosen, and the graft should be fixed to the plate with one to three screws (Figs. IIID-6, IIID-7, IIID-13, and IIID-26).

The AO Internal Fixator

The internal fixator (5) was developed by Dick and has been applied since 1982. The implant is angle stable and is fixed with transpedicular Schanz screws in the vertebral bodies. Therefore, it is not necessary that the dorsal vertebral elements be intact. In contrast to the previously used plates, anchorage in only one vertebra proximally and distally is sufficient. An anchorage in more than two vertebrae is possible. Better stability can be achieved by a cross-link between the two rods.

The pedicle screws will be inserted in a slightly convergent position (10° to 15°). The correct identification of the entry point of the Schanz screws should be checked by fluoroscopy.

The internal fixator can be combined with translaminar screw fixation. Removal of the implants in spinal degenerative cases is not necessary; in cases of spinal fracture, removal is recommended after 9 to 12 months (see Figs. IIID-11, IIID-12, and IIID-21).

Universal Spine System

The SYNTHES Universal Spine System (USS) was developed in 1992 and can be used in the thoracic, lumbar, and sacral spine, either posteriorly or anteriorly. The application of the USS is possible in cases of trauma, infection, tumors, degenerative diseases, and deformities.

The implants of this modular system allow segmental or global three-dimensional correction and a sequential build-up of the construct. In cases of fracture, the implants are Schanz screws of 5- and 6-mm thread diameter, smooth 6-mm rods, clamps with posterior and lateral nuts, and cross-link clamps with 3.5-mm rods.

For degenerative spinal disease and instabilities, back-opening and side-opening pedicle screws are available, in addition to special rod connectors in open and closed versions as well as extension and parallel connectors. Besides the pedicle screws, special pedicle, laminar, and angled laminar hooks are available for the correction of deformities. All implants can be easily manipulated and are easily removable (Figs. IIID-1, IIID-14, IIID-16 through IIID-18, IIID-22, IIID-27, and IIID-28).

The Translaminar Screw Fixation

Immobilization of the facet joints with translaminar 4.5-mm cortex screws as positioning screws provides sufficient stability over one or two segments to secure a bony healing of the spondylodesis. The translaminar screw fixation (8) can be performed from T12 to the sacrum in cases of degenerative spinal disease. The screw fixation fails in the situation of spondylolisthesis secondary to spondylolysis. If significant parts of the facet joint are resected, or if more than two levels have to be fused, a transpedicular implant has to be chosen instead.

For screw fixation, the spinous process, the lamina of the cranial vertebra, the facet joint, and the transverse process of the caudal vertebra should be well visualized. From the opposite side of the spinous process, close underneath the dorsal cortex of the lamina, the drill hole should be made with the 3.2-mm drill bit across the facet joint, directed toward the base of the transverse process. The cartilage of the joint should be removed with a fine curette.

Screw penetration of the dorsal cortex of the lamina is allowed. The length of the screw can be determined with a special length-measuring device. For lumbosacral joints, a direct screw fixation of the joint is preferable. Usually removal of the screws is not necessary. In cases of allergic reactions to standard materials, titanium screws are available for use (see Figs. IIID-2 through IIID-4 and IIID-23).

Intervertebral Fusion Cages

Intervertebral fusion cages or "disk cages" have been tested and developed in the United States since 1989 (22). There are several major types.

Carbon Cages

The first carbon cages created by J. W. Brantigan were implanted after disk removal to support the anterior column and also to prevent screw breakage of a PLIF con-

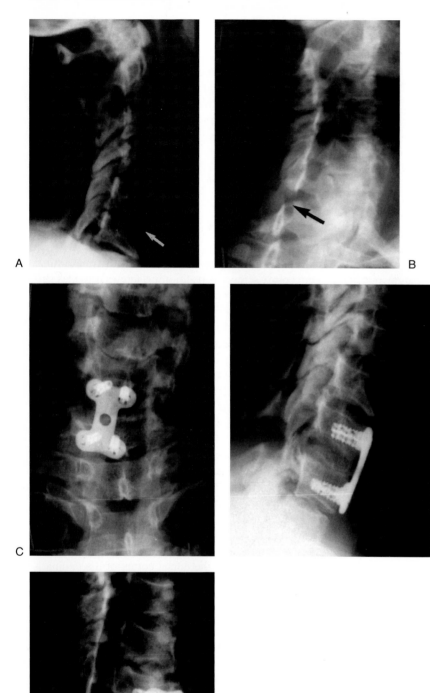

FIG. IIID-26. Traumatic instability at C6-7. (**A**) A lateral cervical spine radiograph demonstrates traumatic instability at C6-C7 (*arrow*). (**B**) The oblique radiograph demonstrates unilateral facet dislocation at C6-7 (*arrow*). (**C**) The postoperative anteroposterior radiograph of the fusion demonstrates Morscher's interlocking plate and a bone graft at C6-7. The plate and screws are not well centered on the cervical spine. (**D**) A lateral radiograph shows the interposed bone graft and the titanium plate and screws. There is a posterior interspinous gap that indicates excessive distraction between the spinous processes of C6-7. (**E**) An oblique radiograph of the cervical spine postoperatively demonstrates the overdistraction, resulting in an enlarged right C6-7 neural foramen (*arrow*). In the absence of neurologic signs and symptoms, no further surgery was carried out.

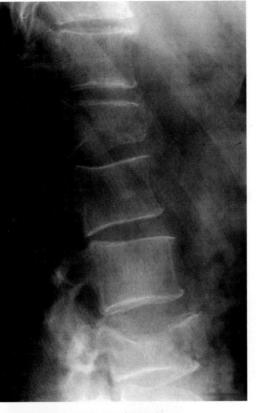

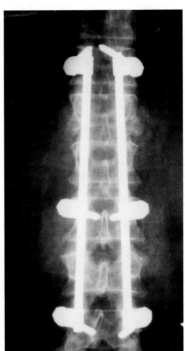

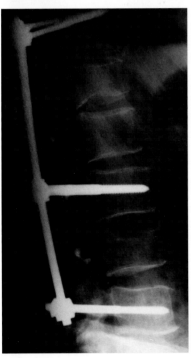

FIG. IIID-27. Burst fractures of the T12 and L3 vertebral bodies. (**A**) A lateral radiograph demonstrates burst fractures of T12 and L3. (**B**) Anteroposterior and (**C**) lateral radiographs demonstrate a distraction spondylodesis extending from T11 through L4 with Schanz screw in T11, L2, and L4 (USS internal fixator). There is a lateral intertransversal bone graft extending from T12 through L1 and L2 through L3. There has been satisfactory realignment with only a minimal kyphosis (i.e., spinal straightening) at L2-3.

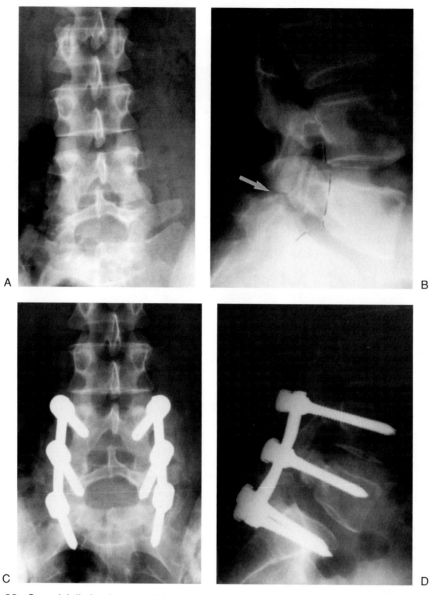

FIG. IIID-28. Spondylolisthesis caused by spondylolysis, associated with degenerative instability at L4-5. (**A**) Anteroposterior and (**B**) lateral radiographs demonstrate the degenerative minor retrolisthesis at L4-5 and the anterolysthesis of L5–S1. The L4-5 abnormalities are degenerative in nature, whereas the L5–S1 spondylolisthesis is caused by spondylolysis (*arrow*). (**C**) Anteroposterior and (**D**) lateral radiographs show a distraction spondylodesis extending from L4 to S1, utilizing the USS internal fixator. There is now good alignment of the vertebral bodies extending from L4 through S1.

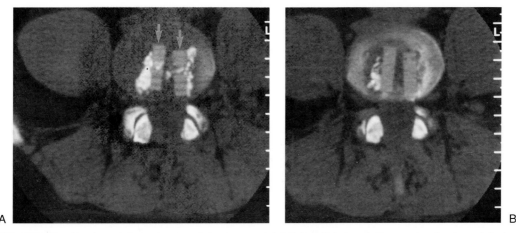

FIG. IIID-29. Previous bilateral microdiskectomy at L4-5 for disk herniation and subsequent fusion with Steffee ramps. **(A)** The postoperative axial CT shows evidence of the radiodense carbon ramps (*arrows*) within the L4-5 disk space. More radiodense bone-graft material is also noted surrounding these ramps. The *posterior erector* trunci muscles appear normal. **(B)** Reevaluation CT at 6 weeks following the surgical procedure demonstrates some increasing sclerosis of the bone surrounding the ramps and bony fusion material.

struct with pedicle screws and plates. The first cages were rectangular with sizes varying between 9 × 9 × 25 mm and 15 × 15 × 25 mm. In order to restore some amount of the physiologic lordosis in the lumbar spine, shaped "wedge cages" were developed, with an anterior height 2 mm more than the posterior height. These cages are filled with autologous bone to allow a solid intervertebral fusion by an additional bony bridge between the end plates. When the posterior structures can be preserved, a fusion without additional pedicular implant may be attempted.

The latest model developed by Steffee is called a "ramp" (Figs. IIID-29, IIID-30, and IIID-31). It is thinner in the transverse plane and requires less removal of bone from laminae and facets for its implantation. In a similar way for cages, the end plates must be cleared of cartilaginous tissue, which would disturb bony fusion. For ramp insertion, the preparation of the intervertebral space does not need to be as exhaustive as for a cage implanta-

tion. This minimizes the risk of additional bony injury. The carbon cages are radiolucent so that only the bone chips within (or beside) the cages appear "hyperdense" on the plain films. The bone graft is placed primarily lateral to the ramps. This radiolucency makes the intraoperative appreciation of insertion depth by lateral fluoroscopy difficult.

Titanium Cages

The Ray Threaded Fusion Cage (42,43) is a titanium cylinder 12, 14, 16, or 18 mm in diameter and 21 or 26 mm in length. These cages are perforated on 70% of their cylindrical wall to allow immediate contact between the graft material inside the cage and the end plates, while the part of the wall facing the disk space is full to prevent soft tissues from invading the bony graft. The cages are easily recognized on x-rays. Evidence of fusion can be

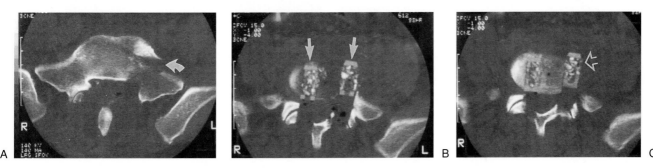

FIG. IIID-30. S1 vertebral body fracture following carbon cage insertion for L5–S1 disk herniation excision. **(A)** Axial CT demonstrates the left S1 fracture (*curved arrow*). **(B)** The CT also visualizes the carbon cages (five filled with bone chips) (*straight arrows*). **(C)** However, an adjacent CT shows that the left-sided carbon cage is too laterally placed and falls within a portion of the left L5–S1 neural foramen and root exit region (*open arrow*).

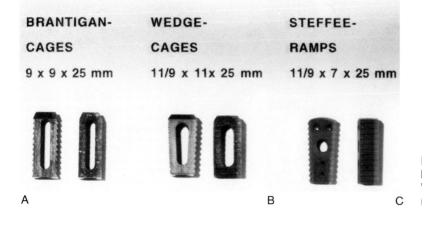

BRANTIGAN-CAGES
9 x 9 x 25 mm

WEDGE-CAGES
11/9 x 11x 25 mm

STEFFEE-RAMPS
11/9 x 7 x 25 mm

A

B

C

FIG. IIID-31. Photographs of carbon intervertebral fusion cages. (**A**) Brantigan cages. (**B**) Wedge cages in two profile views. (**C**) Steffee ramps (these cages manufactured by Acromed).

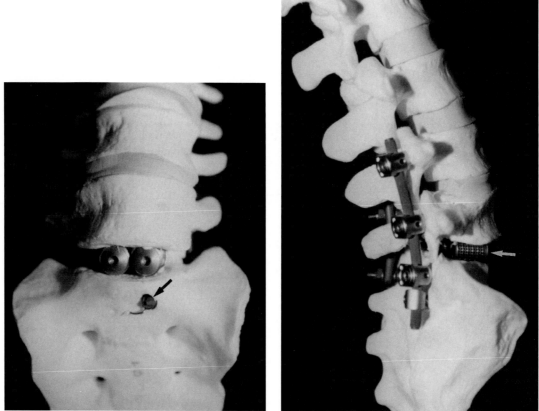

A

B

FIG. IIID-32. Synthetic spine model showing disk implants from the Sofamor Danek group. (**A**) A frontal view shows the disk cages at the L5–S1 level. Also noted is a left-sided pedicle screw (*arrow*) that perforates an anterosacral cortex at S1. (**B**) A lateral view shows the CCD 2 and Dyna-Lok for L4-5 fusion. Also shown are intervertebral fusion cages (*arrow*) at L5–S1.

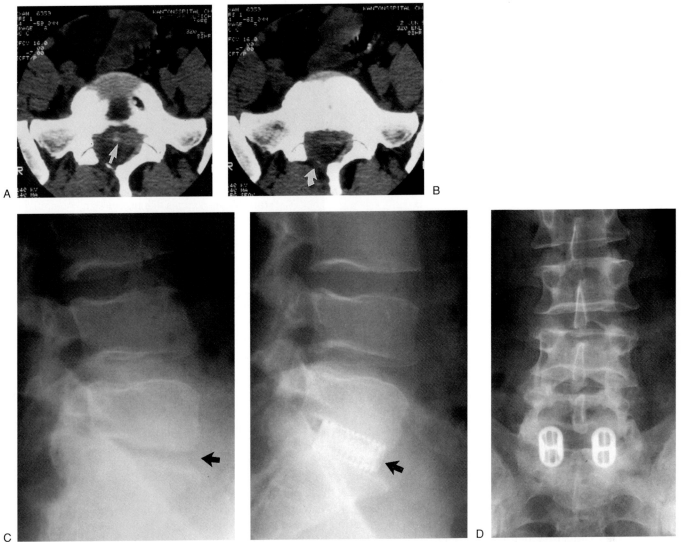

FIG. IIID-33. Recurrent disk herniation following prior diskectomy with treatment with Ray threaded fusion cages. (**A**) Axial CT demonstrates a recurrent left L5–S1 disk herniation (*straight arrow*). (**B**) Adjacent axial CT shows the right hemilaminectomy defect (*curved arrow*). (**C**) Lateral radiograph of the lumbosacral spine demonstrates a loss in height of the L5–S1 intervertebral disk height (*arrow*). (**D**) The postoperative lateral radiograph shows the Ray threaded fusion cages (*arrow*). There is an increase in disk height at L5–S1 because of the insertion of these fusion cages. A diskectomy was also carried out at the time of the cage positioning. (**E**) Anteroposterior radiograph postoperatively showing the two Ray threaded fusion cages at L5–S1.

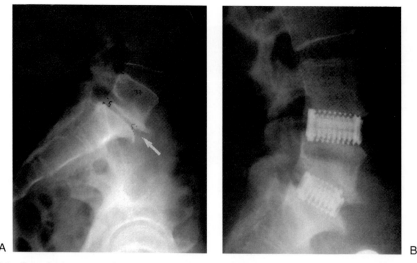

FIG. IIID-34. Ray fusion cage insertion for disk herniation and instability at L4-5 and L5–S1. (**A**) Preoperative lateral radiograph demonstrates the marked disk space narrowing at L5–S1 (*arrow*) and the mild anterolisthesis at this level. (**B**) Postoperative radiograph shows the Ray disc fusion cages in place at L4-5 and L5–S1. There has been a restoration of the disk height at L5–S1 and a preservation of the overall lumbar lordosis.

determined by flexion and extension radiographs showing no motion, AP films confirming the absence of a radiolucent halo around the implant, and CT demonstrating maintained or increased bone density within the implant. In his series of 149 patients, Leclercq (44) found a 94% fusion rate at 1 year, and Ray (43) found a solid fusion in 96% of 127 patients after 2 years without supplemental pedicle screw fixation. Other titanium cages have been developed by Bagby and Kuslich (''BAK'' cages) (45) and recently by the Sofamor-Danek group (Fig. IIID-32).

Some indications for fusion cage insertion are large median disk prolapse requiring a bilateral approach and recurrent disk herniation with mild to moderate instability (16). Since August 1994, we have operated on 30 patients and implanted 21 pairs of carbon cages or ramps and 10 pairs of titanium cages with promising results in previously unoperated spines and some recurrent disk herniation operations. However, in patients with multiple previous operations and degenerative problems at three or more levels, the results were less satisfactory.

The fusion cages restore a certain amount of disk-space height and stabilize the motion segment (Figs. IIID-33, IIID-34, and IIID-35). The intervertebral foramina are enlarged postoperatively, and theoretically, no further disk herniations should occur. Titanium cages have been successfully implanted in cases of grade 1 spondylolisthesis and after facetectomy, without additional posterior implants (42,43,45). For patients with spondylolisthesis of higher grades, or in cases of major instability after laminectomies and facetectomies, the combination of an-

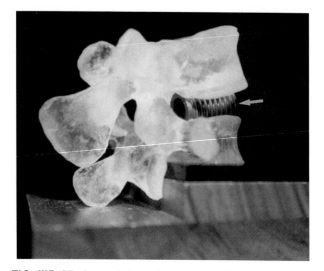

FIG. IIID-35. Lateral view of synthetic spine model demonstrating Ray's threaded fusion titanium cages (*arrow*).

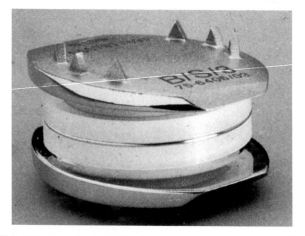

FIG. IIID-36. Photograph of Link disc prosthesis (33). (Picture provided by Waldemar Link GMBH and Co.)

terior column support by cages with posterior column reconstruction by means of VSP plates and screws gives one of the most stable and resistant constructs (22).

A very stiff arthrodesis means additional stresses from load transfer to the adjacent segments (21). These segments may decompensate later and become unstable or stenotic as a result of reactive hypertrophic degenerative changes. Occasionally, additional disk herniations may occur at adjacent spinal levels (12,15,16,20,21).

Preserving function is the goal of functional disk endoprostheses such as the Link SB Charité model (Fig. IIID-36) (46). A multicenter retrospective study including 93 patients with predominantly degenerative disk derangement reported pain relief in a significant number of patients. Unfortunately, there was no significant improvement in work status (43.5% unable to work before surgery; 42% unable to work after surgery). Device failure, migration, or dislocation occurred in 6.5% of cases. This rather extensive operation has not established itself as a routine procedure, and further studies are warranted (46).

CONCLUSIONS

Conventional radiographs are routinely used in the postoperative assessment of patients having undergone spinal instrumentation. They show the position of bone grafts and metallic hardware and the degree of achieved deformity correction and enable the measurement of angles and curvatures that can be compared with preoperative radiographs. The assessment of the solid bony fusion provided by the bone grafts, and also of bone resorption and instrumentation failure, is easily done with conventional radiographs.

In patients with a failed spondylodesis, a more demanding neuroradiologic work-up is needed. Conventional myelography, if possible with dynamic flexion and extension views, is still indicated in patients with ferromagnetic implants, which produce significant artifacts on CT and MR imaging. A postmyelographic CT may yield further useful information concerning the levels above and below the surgical appliance and even at instrumented segments if the amount of metal within the cross-sectioned area is relatively small. In patients with MR-compatible titanium or carbon cage implants, the best analysis is provided by MR imaging.

Instrumentation failure resulting in pseudarthrosis is frequently a consequence of insufficient compensation for a weak anterior column (i.e., insufficient or absent load sharing). A basic biomechanical understanding of spinal instrumentation will help to better analyze the preoperative images, to optimize the planned procedure, and to interpret the postoperative imaging studies in patients with the failed spondylodesis syndrome.

ACKNOWLEDGMENTS

The authors would like to thank Dr. Marcus Lütolf, Head of the Radiology Department, Kantonsspital Chur, for the x-rays, myelograms, CTs, and MRs; Mrs. S. Haas and S. Zarra for the photographic work; and S. Andreoli for typing the manuscript.

REFERENCES

1. Harrington PR: Surgical instrumentation for management of scoliosis. *J Bone Joint Surg* 1960;42A:1948.
2. Roy Camille R, Demeulenaere C: Ostéosynthèse du rachis dorsal, lombaire et lombo-sacré par plaques métalliques vissées dans les pédicules vertébraux et les apophyses articulaires. *Presse Med* 1970; 78:1947.
3. Benini A, Magerl F: *Die degenerative Instabilität der Lendenwirbelsäule.* Bern: Hans Huber, 1991.
4. Cotrel Y, Dubousset J, Guillaumat M: New universal instrumentation in spinal surgery. *Clin Orthop* 1988;227:10.
5. Dick W: *Innere Fixation von Brust- und Lendenwirbelfrakturen. Aktuelle Probleme in Chirurgie und Orthopädie, Bd. 28.* Bern: Hans Huber, 1987.
6. Grob D, Magerl F: Dorsale Spondylodese der Halswirbelsäule mit Hakenplatte. *Orthopäde* 1987;15:55–61.
7. Louis R: *Surgery of the Spine.* Berlin: Springer-Verlag, 1983.
8. Magerl F: Translaminäre Verschraubung der Intervertebralgelenke. In: Weber BG, Magerl F, eds. *Fixateur externe.* Berlin: Springer.
9. Steffee AD, Brantigan JW: The variable screw placement spinal fixation system. *Spine* 1993;18(9):1160–1172.
10. Van Heeswijk WCHJ, Stengs C, Slot GH, et al: Spinal fusion for low back pain using H-frame instrumentation. *Orthop Int Ed* 1993; 1:471–478.
11. Benini A: Lumbale Diskektomie ohne oder mit Spondylodese? Revival eines alten Dilemmas. *Orthopäde* 1989;127:276–285.
12. Benzel EC: Biomechanics of lumbar and lumbosacral spine fractures. In: REA GL, Miller CA, eds. *Spinal Trauma: Current Evaluation and Management.* American Association of Neurological Surgeons, 1993:165–195.
13. Hollowell JP, Larson SJ: Indications for lumbar fusion. *Neurosurg* 1995;5:125–140.
14. Jacobs RP, Mack CA, Fessler RG: Pedicle screws: Biomechanics, uses and current assessment of outcome. *Neurosurg Q* 1994;4:39–50.
15. Kaech DL: Lumbar disc herniation, spinal stenosis and segmental instability. Diagnostic and therapeutic strategies. *Ces Slov Neurol Neurochir* 1995;58/91(1):6–27.
16. Kaech DL: Lumbar disc herniation, spinal stenosis and segmental instability: Role of diagnostic imaging. *Riv Neuroradiol* 1995; 8(Suppl 1):99–109.
17. Kaech D, Kalvach P: Disc herniation, stenosis and instability of the cervical spine. *Riv Neuroradiol* 1995;8(Suppl 1):111–119.
18. Riley LH III: Review of spinal instrumentation. *Neurosurg Q* 1992; 2(4):243–258.
19. Wittenberg RH, Shea M, Swartz DE, et al: Importance of bone mineral density in instrumentated spinal fusions. *Spine* 1991;16: 647.
20. Follett KA, Dirks BA: Etiology and evaluation of the failed back surgery syndrome. *Neurosurg Q* 1993;3(1):40–59.
21. Lee CK: Acclerated degeneration of the segment adjacent to a lumbar fusion. *Spine* 1988;13(3):375–377.
22. Brantigan JW, Steffee AD: A carbon fiber implant to aid interbody lumbar fusion. Two year clinical results in the first 26 patients. *Spine* 1993;18:2106–2117.
23. Brantigan JW: Pseudarthrosis rate after allograft posterior lumbar interbody fusion with pedicle screw and plate fixation. *Spine* 1994; 19:1271–1280.
24. Morscher E, Jung H, Suter H: Die vordere Verplattung der Halswirbelsäule mit dem Hohlschrauben-Plattensystem. *Chirurg* 1986;57: 702.
25. Markwalder TM, Reulen HJ: Diagnostic approach in instability

and irritative state of a "lumbar motion segment" following disc surgery—failed back surgery syndrome. *Acta Neurochir [Wien]* 1989;99:51–57.

26. Markwalder TM, Battaglia M: Failed back surgery syndrome part I: Analysis of the clinical presentation and results of testing procedures for instability of the lumbar spine in 171 patients. *Acta Neurochir [Wien]* 1993;123:129–134.

27. Heller JG, Whitecloud TS III, Butler JC, et al: Complications of spinal surgery. In: Herkowitz HN, Garfin SR, Baldeston RA, et al, eds. *The Spine,* 3rd ed. Philadelphia: WB Saunders, 1992:1817–1898.

28. Meier C, Reulen HJ, Huber P, Mumenthaler M: Meningoradiculoneuritis mimicking vertebral disc herniation. A "neurosurgical" complication of Lyme-borreliosis. *Acta Neurochir* 1989;98:42–46.

29. Jeanmonod D, Magnin M, Morel A: Thalamus and neurogenic pain: Physiological, anatomical and clinical data. *Neuroreport* 1993;4:475–478.

30. Jinkins JR: The pathoanatomic basis of somatic, autonomic and neurogenic syndromes originating in the lumbosacral spine. *Riv Neuroradiol* 1995;8(Suppl 1):35–51.

31. Kotilainen E, Alanen A, Parkkola R, et al: Cross-sectional areas of lumbar muscles after surgical treatment of lumbar disc herniation. *Acta Neurochir [Wien]* 1995;133:7–12.

32. Louis R: Spinal stability as defined by the three column spine concept. *Anat Clin* 1985;7:33.

33. Denis F: The three column spine and its significance in the classification of acute thoracolumbar spinal injuries. *Spine* 1983;8:817–831.

34. Denis F: Spinal stability as defined by the three column spine concept in acute spinal trauma. *Clin Orthop* 1984;189:65–76.

35. Roy Camille R: *L'instabilité lombaire 10ème cours de chirurgie intervertébrale par voie percutanée avec discoscopie.* Zurich: Balgrist, 1991.

36. Holt BT, McCormack T, Gaines RW: Short segment fusion—anterior or posterior approach. The load-sharing classification of spine fractures. *Spine* 1993;7:189–197.

37. Weinstein JN, Spratt KF, Spengler D, et al: Spinal pedicle fixation: Reliability and validity of roentgenogram besed assessment and surgical factors on screw placement. *Spine* 1988;13:1012–1018.

38. White AA, Panjabi MM: *Clinical Biomechanics.* Philadelphia: JB Lippincott, 1978:35–42.

39. MacNab I: *Backache.* Baltimore: Williams & Wilkins, 1977.

40. Lebwohl NH, Starr JK: Surgical management of thoracolumbar fractures. In: Greenberg J, ed. *Handbook of Head and Spine.* New York: Marcel Dekker, 1993:593–646.

41. Plötz GMJ, Benini A: Surgical treatment of degenerative spondylolisthesis in the lumbar spine: No reposition without prior decompression. *Acta Neurochir [Wien]* 1995;137:188–191.

42. Ray CD: Posterior lumbar interbody fusion by implanted threaded titanium cages. In: White A, ed. *Spinal Medicine and Surgery.* St. Louis: Mosby-Yearbook, 1995.

43. Ray CD: Ray threaded fusion cage: Clinical study results—two years follow-up. *Spine Surg Clin Update* 1995;002.

44. Leclercq TA: Posterior lumbar interbody fusion using the Ray threaded fusion cage. *J Clin Neurosci* 1995;2(2):129–131.

45. Kuslich SD: Experimental and clinical results of the BAKT (Bagby and Kuslich) fusion cage. In: *4th International Spine Symposium München,* September 22–23, 1995.

46. Griffith SL, Shekolov AP, Büttner-Janz K, et al: A multicenter retrospective study of the clinical results of the LINK® SB Charité intervertebral prosthesis. *Spine* 1994;19:1842–1849.

47. Dickmann CA, Fessler RG, MacMillan M, Haid RW: Transpedicular screw-rod fixation of the lumbar spine: Operative technique and outcome in 104 cases. *J Neurosurg* 1992;77:860–870.

48. Bereiter H, Melcher GA, Gautier E, Huggler AH: Erfahrungen mit Bio-Oss, einem bovinen Apatit, bei verschiedenen klinischen Indikationsbereiche. *Hefte Unfallheilkd* 1991;216:117–126.

Subject Index

ISBN 0-397-58406-7

9 780397 584062